OXFORD MEDICAL PUBLICATIONS

Psychogeriatric Service Delivery: An International
Perspective

Psychogeriatric Service Delivery: An International Perspective

Edited by

Brian Draper

Conjoint Associate Professor, School of Psychiatry and
School of Public Health and Community Medicine,
University of New South Wales, Sydney,
and Senior Staff Specialist and Assistant Director,
Academic Department for Old Age Psychiatry,
Prince of Wales Hospital, Randwick,
New South Wales, Australia

Pamela Melding

Clinical Senior Lecturer,
Department of Psychological Medicine,
University of Auckland,
Mental Health Services for Older Adults,
North Shore Hospital, Waitemata District Health Board,
Auckland, New Zealand.

Henry Brodaty

Professor of Psychogeriatrics, School of Psychiatry,
University of New South Wales, Sydney,
and Director, Academic Department for Old Age Psychiatry,
Prince of Wales Hospital, Randwick,
New South Wales, Australia

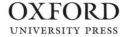

OXFORD
UNIVERSITY PRESS

OXFORD
UNIVERSITY PRESS

Great Clarendon Street, Oxford OX2 6DP

Oxford University Press is a department of the University of Oxford.
It furthers the University's objective of excellence in research, scholarship,
and education by publishing worldwide in

Oxford New York

Auckland Bangkok Buenos Aires Cape Town Chennai
Dar es Salaam Delhi Hong Kong Istanbul Karachi Kolkata
Kuala Lumpur Madrid Melbourne Mexico City Mumbai Nairobi
São Paulo Shanghai Taipei Tokyo Toronto

Oxford is a registered trade mark of Oxford University Press
in the UK and in certain other countries

Published in the United States
by Oxford University Press Inc., New York

A catalogue record for this title is available from the British Library

Library of Congress Cataloging in Publication Data
(Data available)

ISBN 0 19 852825 6 (Pbk)

10 9 8 7 6 5 4 3 2 1

Typeset by Cepha Imaging Pvt. Ltd., Bangalore, India
Printed in Great Britain
on acid-free paper by Ashford Colour Press Ltd.

Foreword

There are several terms to describe our specialty – psychogeriatrics, old age psychiatry, mental health of older people, psychiatry of old age or geriatric psychiatry. Each has their proponents and opponents determined by personal experience and the influence of others, whether they be medical colleagues or politicians. The old notion of psychogeriatric encompasses the concept of "psycho" and "geriatric" neither of which is a concept which attracts positive connotations, similar to someone being called "demented". Some people change their title on a whim and some let it stand either due to a dogged determination to retain the status quo or simply that they have so many other things to think about that it is just not a priority.

What is unique in the specialty, whatever its name, is the extraordinary energy, enthusiasm and dedication that the individual practitioners possess, coming from a relatively low base of public interest. A certain type of individual is attracted to the specialty with degrees of opportunism and altruism being core features, most people having a mixture of the two. As a relatively young discipline, it is easy to see how things have developed over the years and in some ways this reflects the way that society views the medical profession and its elderly citizens. It is absolutely fascinating to see how in different countries and cultures, the rise of the discipline serves to meet the needs of older patients with mental health problems. To have, in this one volume, an analysis of services is a superb achievement and provides a fascinating window on our specialty. One cannot imagine a book on orthopaedic service delivery or ophthalmology service delivery being devised to encompass such diversity. This reflects the wide array of approaches and developments which have taken place and will take place to manage what is, arguably, the most important of all specialties in psychiatry and probably in medicine.

The genius of Brian Draper, Pam Melding and Henry Brodaty in bringing together a collection of essays on the subject cannot be underestimated. The contributions are uniquely thoughtful and thought-provoking and attest to the complete lack of self-satisfaction which is so often present in medical specialties. It used to be said that practitioners of geriatric medicine, who were at the forefront of community based services, were "the barefoot doctors" but with the retreat of that specialty back into the breast of general medicine, old age psychiatrists, for a number of years, have had the right to claim that accolade. The number of older people around and their increasing political muscle makes the organisation of services a must and something which probably has been ignored for too long but cannot be forgotten for much longer. The sheer ingenuity of people who create services from next to no resources and capitalize on that enthusiasm and energy which rests within its practitioners from every discipline has to be admired and is ably demonstrated in this book. However, complacency is nowhere to be seen and the continuing questioning of the role that the doctor plays in the development of services is commonplace. Skills that have traditionally been the purview of the medical profession are now successfully and widely embraced by nurses, occupational therapists, social workers and physiotherapists and this has to be applauded.

Every contribution in this volume could stand alone as being an indicator of the vibrance and viability of this discipline. This book includes everything from the early beginnings of services, to tracking their progress in developing and developed countries through methods of evaluation, quality of care, involvement of consumers and looking to the future.

Every practitioner involved with or interested in older people with mental health problems could benefit from reading this compendium as could managers and administrators of services who could see just what could be achieved in a short time by people dedicated to a cause. I once got into trouble by failing to correct a proof reading error (not picked up by a computerized spellchecker) when I referred to a book as a milestone but it appeared as a millstone. This contribution really does deserve the accolade of milestone.

Alistair Burns
Professor of Old Age Psychiatry
University of Manchester
Past President, International Psychogeriatric Association

Preface

In an ageing world, the delivery of psychogeriatric services in an effective and efficient manner is an increasing concern for health service providers and administrators in both developed and developing countries. Each year life expectancy increases by approximately 6 weeks per annum. The effect will be to increase the population aged over 65 years, with the cohorts over the age of 80 years having the greatest increases in comparison to younger age groups. These are worldwide trends. Even today, health service delivery need is greatest in older populations who compose more than 50 per cent of hospital populations and health and disability service budgets. Ageing populations also portend an increase in the numbers of older people who will have mental health problems and dementia in particular. These demographic and epidemiological trends were envisaged over twenty years ago by Tom Arie and David Jolley (1983) in *The Rising Tide*. Despite awareness of these anticipated needs, mental health services for older people have been slow to develop in many places or in some countries not at all. As the 'baby boom' generations of the post Second World War II period reach retirement there is a pressing need to address future delivery of psychogeriatric services in an effective and efficient manner.

International consensus about the principles of psychogeriatric service delivery emphasizes community care and de-institutionalization, services configured to meet the full range of mental disorders seen in the elderly and multidisciplinary services, including collaboration with geriatric medicine services (Wertheimer, 1997). However, the practical implementation of these principles varies considerably both within and between countries. This book provides a guide on how to organize these services through scholarly reviews of available evidence and descriptions of services that exist around the world. The main aim of this volume will be to bring together the theory and practice of psychogeriatric service delivery from an international perspective. There is no single ideal way of delivering services but by having the opportunity to examine the different perspectives, ideas and evidence base for their effectiveness, readers will have a greater range of options to apply to their own unique needs.

The first section concentrates on the context and theory of psychogeriatric service delivery. In Chapter 1 John Snowdon and Tom Arie provide a historical context by addressing the reasons that psychogeriatric services were felt to be necessary when they first started to be developed around 50 years ago. It draws widely on experiences in the UK, Canada and the US as these have been best documented, but acknowledges that around the world services have developed with different emphases depending on local culture and traditions, patterns of health service funding, and the demography. The chapter reviews why and how these multifaceted services have developed.

Former President of the International Psychogeriatric Association and of the World Psychiatric Association (WPA) Section on Geriatric Psychiatry, Edmond Chiu, has outlined the principles of psychogeriatric service delivery in Chapter 2. His chapter is based upon the consensus statement in *The Organisation of Care in the Psychiatry of the Elderly* that was formulated by the WPA Section of Geriatric Psychiatry under the chairmanship of the late Jean Wertheimer: this is an official Technical Consensus Statement approved by both the World Health Organization (WHO) and WPA (WHO, 1997). The chapter provides a generic best practice model that identifies care needs relevant across developing and developed countries. It also describes the components of service delivery necessary for a comprehensive and effective psychogeriatric service.

How do psychogeriatric services fit into the matrix of other health service priorities around the world? Martin Prince and Peter Trebilco have examined this question from a public health perspective in Chapter 3 by considering the priorities of health care in developing countries in which the majority of the older people in the world reside. The chapter emphasizes the use of population health data and the significance of the social determinants of health as an important framework for health care. It draws on the practical experience obtained by Alzheimer's Disease International's 10/66 project that has been examining the impact of dementia in developing countries and provides us with some sensible suggestions about the style of service delivery that is appropriate and affordable.

The theoretical issues of needs analysis are integral to the planning of psychogeriatric services at both national and local levels. But, as Pamela Melding points out in Chapter 4, it is not always easy to establish who needs services. Her chapter covers the three major paradigms that have fundamentally influenced health care service planning and resource allocation. These are the ethics of allocating resources in health care, the social science of health economics, and 'evidence-based medicine' with its emphasis on clinical efficacy. These are discussed within the various contexts in which these issues have to be considered, for example, politics, culture, economics, and the care system.

Using an evidence-based medicine paradigm, Brian Draper and Lee-Fay Low have examined the quality of the available evidence for the effectiveness of psychogeriatric services within the context of the generic best practice model proposed in the WPA/WHO Technical Consensus Statement. Despite little formal evaluation of the overall model, they show that many components of the model now have high quality evidence that supports their effectiveness. The style of service delivery in community and outreach work that is best practice can now be reasonably established, though gaps in knowledge remain with acute and long term institutional care.

Although the principles of service delivery described by Edmond Chiu in Chapter 2 are relevant to all countries, their practical application varies considerably. Many factors contribute to this including economic development, culture, health system philosophy and funding and opportunities for training. This is accentuated by ageing demographics. For example, it is understandable that in developing African nations that have limited economic resources and with only around 5% of the population aged 60 years and over (United Nations Secretariat, 1998), that other health issues relating to younger people take precedence in health care planning and delivery. But of course, Africa, Asia and Latin America are ageing rapidly. This is reflected in Chapter 13 where Olusegun Baiyewu and Felix Potocnik describe the situation in Nigeria and South Africa. The circumstances in parts of Asia – as described by Helen Chiu in Chapter 9 – and Latin America – as described by Sergio Tamai in Chapter 11 – are similar. Clearly, the model of psychogeriatric service delivery that is feasible in poor developing countries is vastly different to that in rich developed countries. It is more likely to be reliant upon primary health care with a few tertiary referral specialist services to provide expert advice.

Cultural factors have an impact upon service delivery in all countries. In developed countries, migrant and indigenous populations need to be accommodated within mainstream services and this is often difficult to achieve, with reports of underservicing and culturally inappropriate services. In developing countries, cultural factors may inadvertently hinder service delivery to older people through a mix of religious beliefs, family attitudes and organization. For example, in Arabic countries such as Lebanon, the necessity of obedience to parents that is within the principles of the Islamic religion results in intense resistance from families about the use of institutions (Naboulsi, 1999). The rapid urbanization of many countries such as the Philippines is affecting the capacity of families to care for parents as women migrate to work and traditional family functions are altered (Eleazar, 1998).

But economic resources and an ageing population are not sufficient in themselves to guarantee the development of adequate psychogeriatric services. This can be seen in Europe where 20% of the population is aged 60 years and over. Using the Ageing Index (the number of people aged 65 and over per 100 youths under age 15) as an indicator of age structure, in 2000 17 out of the 20 countries with the highest age index scores were located in Europe (Kinsella, Velkov and the US Census Bureau, 2001). Yet few European countries have achieved the style of service organization described in the WPA consensus statement with old age mental health services that treat the full range of mental disorders in a variety of settings (Wertheimer, 1997). For example, a 1997 survey found that only the Netherlands, UK and Switzerland had a full range of long term, hospital-based and community-based old age mental health services in many parts of the country (Reifler and Cohen, 1998). The tendency in Europe is for the work to be split between adult psychiatry, neuropsychiatry, neurology and geriatric medicine, as can be seen in some of the countries described in Chapter 12, which comprises contributions from France (Karen Ritchie and Joanna Norton), Germany (Alexander Kurz and Julia Hartmann), Poland (Tadeusz Parnowski), Romania (Catalina Tudose) and Sweden (Sture Eriksson). The European Union of Medical Specialists (UEMS) Section for Psychiatry recently surveyed its membership and discovered that there was widespread disagreement about the possibility of setting up specific services for the old age mentally ill and extending the role of psychiatry in dementia care (Mann *et al.*, 2001).

'Lack of resources' was the main reason for negative responses, though this is not necessarily economic resources but also includes the way in which health resources are distributed within a country. In some countries, this may be a sign of a maldistribution of resources with an over-reliance on institutional care and an undersupply of community resources.

A recent survey of the WPA section on geriatric psychiatry identified postgraduate training in old age psychiatry as 'the most pressing need to provide more effective support for older people with mental disorders' (Camus *et al.*, 2003). This training includes subspecialty training of old age psychiatrists as well as the training of neurologists, geriatricians, primary care physicians and other health professionals. The presence of academic old age psychiatry in a country has been cited as an important prerequisite to improve training, but there are some well-developed countries that do not have any chairs in old age psychiatry and services in these countries are poorly developed (Camus *et al.*, 2003; Draper, 2003).

Health system philosophy and related funding issues are also important. The contrast between services in the US (as described by Soo Borson, Christopher Colenda and Mary Lessig), Canada (as described by Ken Shulman and Carole Cohen), the UK (as described by John Wattis) and Australia and New Zealand (the editors) in some areas is quite stark. It is not simply due to private versus public models of health care but also the way in which individual countries decide to organize services within those models. And this can vary significantly within a country, as witnessed by the major differences between states of Australia.

Of course not all countries could be covered in the space available, but we hope that those included provide an insight into the different approaches being taken and the various stages of development that exist around the world.

Section three concentrates on solutions to psychogeriatric service delivery. In Chapter 14, Ajit Shah and Shirish Bhatkal have comprehensively examined practical issues in core acute psychogeriatric service delivery in hospital and community settings. They cover topics from local planning to hands-on approaches to service delivery, which range from how to organize initial assessments to sensible suggestions about how to equip a service and ward design.

John Snowdon has considered the role of psychogeriatric services in long-term residential aged care in Chapter 15. He indicates that there is marked variability in the availability and utilization of long-term residential care in different cultures. The chapter gives examples of how psychogeriatric services have been provided and ways by which such services have responded to specific problems. It aims to provoke consideration of the development and funding of the provision of mental health services in this setting, and concludes by speculating about what might be an ideal aged care facility.

Some service delivery components are more specialized and may not be regarded as core business for all services. David Conn has addressed the pros and cons of running services such as day hospitals, memory clinics, consultation liaison services, services for younger people with dementia and respite care in Chapter 16. He also considers the particular requirements of an academic psychogeriatric service and covers issues such as research ethics, training and teaching.

How do you ensure continuity of care in a complex health service system? Psychogeriatric services lie at an intersection between adult mental health, geriatric medicine and in some countries, neurology, so service relationships and borders can create enormous difficulties for consumers and service providers alike. In Chapter 17 Pamela Melding has examined practical approaches to this important question by considering interfaces inside the service – for example, between hospital and community psychogeriatric care – and outside the service – for example, with general practitioners, geriatricians, nursing homes and welfare services.

The delivery of services to rural and regional areas is often a challenge, even in developed countries. In Chapter 18 Jane Neese presents a review of rural mental health, barriers and service delivery issues related to the older adult population. While focusing on the United States, many of the issues identified are relevant to rural areas in other countries. As noted in the chapter, there are certain advantages to service delivery in rural settings including less duplication and fragmentation of services. There is also evidence that due to limited resources, service providers may develop more effective partnerships with other community resources.

Henry Brodaty and Lee-Fay Low have examined the partnerships of carers and consumers with psychogeriatric services in Chapter 19. The many roles that carers have in assessment and treatment are discussed including ethical, quality of life and medico-legal concerns. There is also a timely reminder that carers have their own needs that are too often unmet by services. Consumer participation in the planning and implementation of health care is increasingly being recognized as critical to the development of health systems. This chapter reviews how consumer participation in psychogeriatric services can be facilitated and looks at the increasingly important impact of consumer organizations and support groups.

Ongoing evaluation of outcomes is a critical component of ensuring the quality of service delivery. In Chapter 20, Alastair Macdonald has examined the nature of service delivery evaluation, including the use of clinical audits and routine clinical outcome measurement (RCOM). His experience of using the HoNOS65+ in RCOM is discussed with many sensible suggestions about implementation of such a programme. This is very useful for health professionals working in places where RCOM is mandatory.

How do you decide upon which services to deliver when there are limited resources? Few services around the world would regard themselves as being adequately resourced. In the penultimate chapter, Tom Dening and K. S. Shaji consider this vexing question from the viewpoint of developed and developing countries, with particular reference to the United Kingdom and India. The ethical dilemmas posed by rationing of services at the coalface are discussed with some useful ideas about how to approach it.

In the final chapter, the editors have consulted astrologers, mystics, oracles, clairvoyants and even gazed into their own crystal balls to contemplate the future of psychogeriatric service delivery over the next 20 years. We reflect on the possible impact of an ageing population in developed countries (the baby boomer generation) and developing countries (improved health care in younger years) upon service delivery. The organization of services is likely to evolve with increased involvement of consumers and a better understanding of what constitutes best practice. Technological changes, including improvements in information technology with increased use of telemedicine and the Internet, better pharmacological treatments for depression and dementia and improved diagnostic tools such as neuroimaging will all change best practice. Ethical issues such as euthanasia and how to ration services will continue to require informed consideration.

In bringing this volume together, we have been acutely aware of the different terminology used to describe mental health service delivery for older people. We have used the term 'psychogeriatric services', though there are many alternatives that essentially mean the same thing. In North America, the preferred term is 'geriatric psychiatry services', in the UK the term is 'older people's mental health services', and other terms used elsewhere include 'aged care psychiatry services', 'old age psychiatry services' and 'old age mental health services'. Due to these regional variations, we have deliberately decided not to impose uniformity upon the chapters. Hence the reader should be aware that these differences of terminology between chapters do not necessarily mean that the authors are describing different types of services. However, in some countries it would seem that psychogeriatric services focus almost entirely on dementia care, while in others the broad range of mental disorders is encompassed. We have taken the view that psychogeriatric services should cover the full gamut of mental disorders.

An international perspective is always critical to any volume such as this. We have had great pleasure in working with our authors from five continents and would like to thank them for their excellent contributions. Of course it is not feasible to have authors from all countries but we are proud that there are contributors from 15 – Australia, Brazil, Canada, China, France, Germany, India, New Zealand, Nigeria, Poland, Romania, South Africa, Sweden, the UK and the USA.

We would also like to thank Oxford University Press and Martin Baum, Carol Maxwell, and Richard Marley for their helpful assistance throughout this project.

Brian Draper   *May 2004*
Pamela Melding
Henry Brodaty

References

Arie, T. and Jolley, D. (1983) The Rising Tide. *BMJ*, **286**, 325–6.

Camus, V., Katona, C., de Mendonca Lima, C.A., *et al.* (2003) Teaching and training in old age psychiatry: a general survey of the World Psychiatric Association member societies. *International Journal of Geriatric Psychiatry*, **18**, 694–9.

Draper, B. (2003) Training in old age psychiatry. *International Journal of Geriatric Psychiatry*, **18**, 683–5.

Eleazar, J.G. (1998) Psychogeriatrics and geriatrics are 'late bloomers' in the Philippines. *IPA Bulletin*, **15** (2), 8–9.

Kinsella, K., Velkoff, V., and U.S. Census Bureau (2001) *An Aging World: 2001*. Washington, DC: US Government Printing Office.

Mann, A., Furedi, J., Hagemo, E., *et al.* (2001) *Report of the European Union of Medical Specialists Section of Psychiatry – Old Age Psychiatry*. http://www.uemspsychiatry.org/section/reports/oldAge.pdf Accessed 12 December 2003

Naboulsi, M. (1999) Old age institutions in Arabic countries: the status of Lebanon. *IPA Bulletin*, **16** (4), 18.

Reifler, B.V. and Cohen, W. (1998) Practice of geriatric psychiatry and mental health services for the elderly: results of an international survey. *International Psychogeriatrics*, **10**, 351–7.

United Nations Secretariat, The Population Division, Department of Economic and Social Affairs, United Nations Secretariat (1998) *World Population Prospects, The 1998 Revision, Volume II: Sex and Age*. http://www.un.org/esa/socdev/ageing/agewpop1.htm accessed 16 January, 2004.

Wertheimer, J. (1997) Psychiatry of the elderly: a consensus statement. *International Journal of Geriatric Psychiatry*, **12**, 432–5.

World Health Organization (1997) *Organization of Care in Psychiatry of the Elderly – a technical consensus statement*. WHO/MSA/MNH/MND/97.3. Genvea: World Health Organization. The Consensus documents are available on the WPA Website: www.wpanet.org

Contents

Section 3

Contributors

Tom Arie
Kenninghall
Norwich, UK

Olusegun Baiyewu
Department of Psychiatry
University College Hospital
Ibadan, Nigeria

Shirish Bhatkal
John Connolly Unit
West London Mental Health NHS Trust
Southall, UK

Soo Borson
Department of Psychiatry & Behavioural
Sciences
University of Washington Medical Center
Seattle WA
USA

Henry Brodaty
Academic Department for Old Age
Psychiatry
School of Psychiatry
University of New South Wales
Sydney, New South Wales
Australia

Edmond Chiu
Academic Unit for Psychiatry of
Old Age
University of Melbourne
Kew, Victoria
Australia

Helen Chiu
Department of Psychiatry
Chinese University of Hong Kong
Shatin NT
Hong Kong

Carole A. Cohen
Department of Psychiatry
Faculty of Medicine
University of Toronto
Toronto ON
Canada

Christopher Colenda
College of Medicine
The Texas A & M University System
College Station TX
USA

David K Conn
Baycrest Centre for Geriatric Care
University of Toronto
Toronto ON
Canada

Tom Dening
Fulbourn Hospital
Cambridge, UK

Brian Draper
Academic Department for Old Age
Psychiatry
School of Psychiatry and
School of Public Health and
Community Medicine
University of New South Wales
Sydney, New South Wales
Australia

Sture Eriksson
Umea University
Umea, Sweden

Julia Hartmann
Department of Psychiatry &
Psychotherapy
Munich Technical University
Munich, Germany

Alexander Kurz
Department of Psychiatry &
Psychotherapy
Munich Technical University
Munich, Germany

Mary C. Lessig
Department of Psychiatry & Behavioural
Sciences University of Washington
Medical Center
Seattle WA
USA

Lee-Fay Low
Academic Department for Old Age
Psychiatry
Prince of Wales Hospital
Randwick, New South Wales
Australia

Alastair Macdonald
Academic Department
Ladywell House
Lewisham
London, UK

Pamela Melding
Mental Health Services for
Older Adults
Waitemata District Health Board
Auckland, New Zealand

Jane Neese
College of Health and Human Services
University of North Carolina
Charlotte NC
USA

Joanna Norton
INSERM
Hôpital de la Colombiere
Montpellier, France

Tadeusz Parnowski
Institute of Psychiatry and Neurology
Psychogeriatric Department
Warsaw, Poland

Felix Potocnik
University of Stellenbosch
Western Cape, South Africa

Martin Prince
Section of Epidemiology
Institute of Psychiatry
London, UK

Karen Ritchie
INSERM
Hôpital de la Colombiere
Montpellier, France

Ajit Shah
John Connolly Unit
West London Mental Health NHS Trust
Southall, UK

K.S. Shaji
Medical College
Thrissur
Kerala, India

Kenneth I. Shulman
Department of Psychiatry
Sunnybrook & Women's
Toronto ON
Canada

John Snowdon
Rozelle Hospital
Rozelle, New South Wales
Australia

Sergio Tamai
Sao Paulo
Brazil

Peter Trebilco
School of Public Health & Community
Medicine
University of New South Wales
Sydney, New South Wales
Australia

Catalina Tudose
Department of Psychiatry
Medical University "Carol Davila"
Bucharest
Romania

John Wattis
Ageing and Mental Health
Research Group Huddersfield University
Huddersfield, UK

Section 1

Chapter 1

A history of psychogeriatric services

John Snowdon and Tom Arie

Fifty years ago there were no local comprehensive old age psychiatry services anywhere in the world – at least, none that we know of. In mental hospitals there were, however, wards in which all or most of the inpatients were elderly. The number of psychiatric hospital beds in the United Kingdom (UK) occupied by elderly patients reached a peak in the mid-1950s (Cooper, 1991). In 1955, in the United States (US), 1.4 per cent of those aged 75 years or more were accommodated in state or county mental hospitals (Eisdorfer, 1977). Most older psychiatric inpatients were in long-stay wards and had little contact with psychiatrists. Elderly mentally ill people tended to be accorded low priority within psychiatry. There had been little research devoted specifically to the epidemiology and treatment of mental disorders in old age, and management tended to be custodial rather than assertive. Development of mental disorders in old age was commonly attributed to 'senility' and chances of recovery were usually predicted as poor.

Now, in 2004, there are comprehensive old age psychiatry services in many parts of the world: an International Psychogeriatric Association thrives, as does the Geriatric Psychiatry section of the World Psychiatric Association. Meetings and journals devoted to the mental disorders of old age abound.

There is great variation in the way these services are organized and funded; local culture and traditions, patterns of health service funding, and the demography – all these are important. The aims of this chapter will be to review why and how these multifaceted services have developed. It will not be possible to consider developments in all countries; we shall concentrate on those that have been documented and which we know best.

Post-war pioneers in aged care in Britain

In 1948, the British National Health Service (NHS) was established. Everyone was to be registered with a general practitioner (GP) who would provide a 24-hour service, at no cost to the patient. At the same time, responsibility for the sick and infirm aged poor in the UK was transferred from local authorities to the Hospital Boards, local authorities retaining responsibility for residential services.

The pioneer of 'geriatrics' in Britain was Dr Marjory Warren (Millard and Higgs, 1989), who worked in what had been a large old infirmary in London, and who with a handful of colleagues founded the Medical Society for the Care of the Aged, which subsequently became the British Geriatrics Society. The way in which that specialty developed both inspired and informed development, twenty years later, of the first old age psychiatry services, and the new 'psychogeriatricians' were warmly welcomed by their geriatrician colleagues.

During the early years of the NHS, it was common for geriatricians to be expected to deal with cases of severe dementia. As discussed by Godber (1978), physical illnesses are frequently the reason for admission to acute hospitals of people with severe cognitive or psychiatric problems. Lack of domiciliary supervision may necessitate admission, but after relieving the acute condition, geriatricians were commonly faced with social factors that made a return home impossible. Generally there was little support from psychiatric services.

> The specialty as a whole found old people an encumbrance, particularly if they suffered from dementia. Functional illness was undertreated and the standard response to a presentation of dementia was avoidance, or consideration solely of the option of institutional care.
>
> Godber and Rosenvinge, 1998

Researchers reported low rates of recognition by GPs of dementia and depression among their patients (Williamson *et al.*, 1964), but even when problems were identified, patients were rarely referred by GPs for specialist advice and treatment (Shepherd *et al.*, 1966).

Because of non-involvement by psychiatrists, some geriatricians developed physician-run dementia services. Where geriatricians ran hospital-based services that catered for all disorders among elderly people, concerns about 'misplacement' (being admitted to the 'wrong' unit, psychiatric or geriatric) did not arise. Prinsley (1973), a geriatric physician, described a 'psychogeriatric' unit which catered for a range of psychiatric illnesses presenting in old age, where there was minimal cross-consultation with psychiatrists. Evidently the unit filled a gap in local services, but considerable concern should surely have been expressed about a geriatrician having to extend responsibilities beyond the field of his own expertise and training. The eventual development of old age psychiatry services largely removed the need for geriatricians to act as substitutes for unavailable psychiatrists.

Developing positive ideas and attitudes

In the 1950s, prognostic studies by Roth (1955) gave impetus to reviewing attitudes to treatment of mentally ill elderly people. They differentiated clinical entities amongst older inpatients at a large mental hospital, and then reported the outcomes for five groups at 6 months and 2 years. Their research revealed that inpatients with affective disorders have a much better prognosis than those with dementia. After 2 years, 20 per cent of the depressive subgroup had died, but another 65 per cent had been discharged from hospital; 80 per cent in the dementia subgroups had died. At that time, 80 per cent of inpatients with paranoid psychosis were still alive after 2 years, but most were still in hospital.

Roth later became professor of psychological medicine in Newcastle (UK), where he and collaborators such as the psychiatrists Kay, Kiloh, Blessed and Bergmann, and the pathologist Tomlinson, studied the epidemiology and clinical aspects of the main forms of psychiatric illness in old age and their relationship to changes which could be observed in the post-mortem brain. In London, Corsellis (1962) published a monograph on *Mental Illness and the Ageing Brain*, and Post (1965) described clinical presentations in late life in one of the first textbooks in this field. Reports of a series of scandals in long-stay care prompted consideration of how management of the psychiatric problems of older people could be improved (Arie, 2002). Meticulous studies such as those of Roth laid the basis for better understanding and encouraged positive attitudes by showing that many old age mental disorders were very responsive to treatment.

In the US in 1955, research on human ageing was commenced at the National Institute of Mental Health (Butler, 1975a). Researchers examined the contributions of personality and environmental factors to adaptation in late life. During an 11-year follow-up of initially healthy individuals it was concluded that 'senility is not an inevitable outcome of aging', and that decline of intellectual abilities is a consequence of specific diseases rather than being attributable to the 'process of aging'. In 1959, the World Health Organization (WHO) convened the first meeting of its Expert Committee on Mental Health Problems of Ageing and Aged. In 1965, a conference of the World Psychiatric Association devoted to 'Mental Disorders in the Aged' provided impetus for new developments.

Availability of the phenothiazines and antidepressants, and the demonstrable benefits of electroconvulsive therapy (Post, 1978), provided new optimism. The 'social psychiatry' movement, and community mental health services such as those in 'the Worthing experiment' (Grad and Sainsbury, 1963) may have provided ideas on what could be done. Colwell and Post (1959) declared that the scope for community action in the case of elderly psychiatric patients was frighteningly large, and called for scientifically conducted assessments of the value of community care for such people. Lecturing to a Canadian audience, Macmillan (1960), the superintendent of a mental hospital in Nottingham, espoused the opportunities for prevention of old age mental disorders provided by a community mental health service. For example, he discussed benefits derived from attendance at day centres or day hospitals by solitary old people and those whose relatives have to go to work. 'If adequate and timely help is given, rejection can be halted' (and by 'rejection' he meant 'the relative's determination to be free from what has become an intolerable burden'). Macmillan argued that it would surely be logical to provide more and more community services (including joint medical assessments and domiciliary visits) rather than more and more residential accommodation. Bower (1964) delivered an enthusiastic address in Melbourne in 1963, describing a visit to England, and noting that 'domiciliary visiting, carried out by a social worker and senior psychiatrist, proved to be vastly superior to outpatient treatment'. He said that British GPs had at first been opposed to this service, but now considered it most valuable. A few years later, Macmillan and Shaw (1966) showed the advantages of community interventions in cases of squalor.

Early developments in old age psychiatry were documented by Arie and Isaacs (1977), who referred to descriptions by a handful of younger workers of the local services that they were establishing. Epidemiological studies, such as those of Kay *et al.* (1964), were important in defining the scale of the problem of old age mental disorders.

Barker (1998) referred to the development of geriatrics and Busse (2002) described the growth of old age psychiatry, in the US. Shulman (1994) referred to pockets of interest and activity in the US and Canada, naming Busse and Pfeiffer (1973), Goldfarb, Stern and Kral. In the 1970s, a study team from the American Psychiatric Association described ten 'creative' mental health services for the elderly (Glasscote *et al.*, 1977), of which four were in England, four in the US, and one each in Stockholm and Copenhagen. Shulman (1981) described his local university-based service in Toronto, largely modelled on the British pattern, but with innovations of its own. Shulman (1994) commented that the UK's higher proportion of elderly people led to the development of specialized geriatric services much earlier than in North America. In Europe, the percentage of persons aged over 65 years reached 10 to 15 per cent much earlier than in other continents, but the demographic factor was not the only determinant of the timing of developments in health services for older people. The type and extent of development of services differed between countries, even when they had similar proportions of older people in their populations.

Developments in the US

Butler (1975a) defined ageism as 'the process of systematically stereotyping and discriminating against people because they are old', and he added, 'psychiatry has shown a sense of futility and therapeutic nihilism about old age'. He argued that many of the conditions labelled 'senility' are actually manifestations of socio-economic or medical problems that could be resolved with prompt, appropriate treatment. He referred to public mental hospitals that 'in general do not have active treatment programmes that recognize the capacity of older people to change'. This was at a time when disproportionately few older persons in the US were attending mental health specialists, community services or even primary care practitioners for assessment and treatment of mental health problems. Services for the aged represented only 2 per cent of the work of outpatient psychiatric clinics and 4 per cent of community mental health services (Cohen, 1976).

Social and community psychiatry movements developed slowly, as society changed following the Second World War. It is relevant to compare trends in community provision for the aged in the US and Britain. Shenfield (1962) noted that American projects (e.g. 'creative leisure' programmes) appeared to be based on a middle-class concept of ageing, whereas in Britain and parts of Europe, interest had spread more broadly, and included domiciliary services provided by local authorities and voluntary societies.

A 1961 report in the US called for the creation of a network of Community Mental Health Centers (CMHCs) and an end to the traditional dependence on massive state mental hospitals (Butler, 1975a). Financial incentive to discharge patients from state hospitals was provided by the Medicare and Medicaid amendments to the Social Security Act of 1965. Until then, public-sector care of mentally ill people was the responsibility of state governments. Medicaid covered convalescent and nursing home care, but state hospitals remained a state responsibility. Between 1969 and 1973 the number of aged patients in state mental hospitals decreased by 40 per cent. Transfer was to 'the community', which included nursing homes, foster care facilities and welfare hotels, where psychiatric services were virtually non-existent (Butler, 1975a).

In the mid-1970s, new legislation required CMHCs to develop programmes for the aged. Cohen (1976) drew attention to the financial and practical difficulties inherent in providing a complete range of services to people who commonly needed medical evaluation and home visits.

Butler (1975a) referred to the 'dumping syndrome'. He said that in New York State, patients in nursing homes under Medicaid

> do not receive psychiatric care: in fact, they often receive only minimal physical care. This money . . . could better be spent in giving an older person and his/her family a choice of various facilities and services in the community.

He referred to a US Senate report concerning numerous examples of cruelty and negligence in nursing homes, and of 'kickbacks to nursing home operators from suppliers'. (In England there had been comparable reports of abuses in public institutions for the aged.) The US Senate commented on the very high cost of aged care services that appeared to be poorly distributed, and drew attention to inappropriate care of debatable quality (Maddox and Glass, 1989).

It is said (Millard and Higgs, 1989) that 'Why Survive? Being Old in America' (Butler, 1975b), which won a Pulitzer prize, led to the establishment of the National Institute on Aging. Protest can make governments act!

A government initiative in the 1980s established through the Veterans Administration a network of GRECCs (Geriatric Research, Education and Clinical Centres), which contributed greatly to development of old age services, and especially perhaps to the education of specialists (Barker, 1998).

Developing comprehensive psychogeriatric services

Mental health services for older people have evolved in different ways and with varying pace in Britain and the US over the last fifty years, but the need for evolution has been propelled by similar factors in these two countries. Ageing of the population together with the negative attitudes held by many about old age and elderly people, understanding of pathology, increasing effectiveness of treatments, and a considerable growth in expectations have all been contributing factors.

Because the proportion of elderly people increased, health professionals needed to spend more time on their care and treatment, but 'ageists' resented the diversion of time to treat people whom they regarded as untreatable. Proportionally little time was given to their care, and many older patients were moved to back wards or (to deal with overcrowding) residential facilities. There were some who advocated for the needs and rights of infirm people, and who highlighted examples of negligence or abuse of elderly people in institutions. There was an impetus towards provision of domiciliary and community services, but differences in funding and organization of services meant that Britain was in a more favourable position to respond to the impetus than was the US.

In both Britain and North America in the late 1960s, health care for older people was commonly conducted in shabby settings. Innovators in Britain considered it would be an intriguing challenge to test whether work with older people, if done well and with adequate resources in good accommodation, would be viewed as attractive and give as much professional satisfaction as other branches of health care. These enthusiasts had increasing contact with staff in the Department of Health and Social Security (DHSS), who were already grappling with a growing literature on misplacement of older people in inappropriate hospital settings. In 1970 the Department proposed that 'Psychogeriatric Assessment Units' (PGUs) should be set up in general hospitals, to be run jointly by geriatricians and psychiatrists. It was proposed that at least one psychiatrist in each district should take responsibility for liaising with the geriatric and social services, and that their collaboration should centre on the PGU. Initially the focus was to be on dementia. In due course, the government issued guidelines on levels of provision of service for mental illness related to old age (DHSS, 1972), including recommendations for the number of beds and day-places to be allocated for older people with functional mental illness, ambulant patients with dementia, and 'graduates' (those who had become old while in psychiatric hospitals). The guidelines defined the respective responsibilities of psychiatrists and geriatricians, and of social services, for the care of dementia, and a document agreed by the Royal College of Psychiatrists and the British Geriatrics Society fleshed out the detailed basis for this collaboration in Guidelines that have been widely used, and which were later updated (Royal College of Psychiatrists, 1992). In simple terms, non-ambulant physically disabled people with dementia were to be the responsibility of geriatric medical services, behaviourally disturbed ambulant people would be the responsibility of psychiatrists, and the social services would be responsible for ambulant people who were not severely disturbed. Each service was to give ready support to the others.

These proposals were congenial to those psychiatrists in Britain who, from the late 1960s onwards, organized part of their local psychiatric services to meet the special needs of old people. They began to meet as a group to discuss their experiences and for mutual support. A cluster of pioneers (e.g. Whitehead, 1969; Arie, 1970; Pitt, 1974) described the establishment of local services. In Jolley's (1995) retrospective look at the importance of one of these developments he stated that:

> The lead was from the front: all patients were seen by a senior doctor, at home or wherever, quickly and effectively. Concern for staff morale, interest in collaboration with Geriatric Medicine and Social Services, awareness of differences in referral rates from differing parts of the patch, were key points identified during the first year.

By 1981, government policy was firmly endorsing the establishment of such specialized local psychiatric services for old people (DHSS, 1981).

Arie and Jolley (1982) described the principles underlying the provision of comprehensive old age psychiatry services in Britain – flexibility, responsiveness, availability, unhierarchical use of staff, domiciliary assessment, and willingness to collaborate with other services and agencies.

By 1980, some 120 consultant psychiatrists in the UK had psychiatry of old age as their main activity (Wattis *et al.*, 1981). By 1992 there were more than 300, and at the time of writing there are some 500. A few services limited their clientele to those suffering from organic mental disorders, but most took on all types of mental disorder presenting among elderly people from a defined catchment area, and domiciliary consultation was usually a lynchpin of their procedure. Dening (1992) noted marked differences in emphasis between seven community-orientated old age psychiatry services in England that he visited in 1991. A controversial issue was whether all patients should initially be seen by a psychiatrist (practised in a majority of services) or whether assessments by non-medical professionals were acceptable. Some services accepted referrals only from GPs and geriatricians, while others accepted them from families and other sources. All services emphasized the importance of liaising with GPs. Dening suggested that recent changes to the NHS and community care legislation in Britain would have a considerable impact on the way services were to be provided.

A joint working party of the Royal Colleges of Physicians and of Psychiatrists (1989) endorsed the comprehensive model of psychogeriatric services and made recommendations concerning the number of nurses and other health professionals to be employed in the community arm of each such service, per 20,000 elderly. Co-location of psychogeriatric and geriatric services (or at least their acute services) was recommended, where possible. In Nottingham (UK) a Department of Health Care of the Elderly combined geriatrics and psychogeriatrics into a single University department, headed by a psychiatrist, but with differentiated services. These arrangements brought together teaching, research and services, and ensured optimal liaison and co-responsibility for patients when possible, and prevented patients from 'falling between two stools' (Arie, 2002). That old age psychiatry was separate from the remaining psychiatric services had its disadvantages, but they were minimized by close collaboration and cross-membership of committees, and sharing in duty rotas, and of course in the psychiatric training scheme. Indeed, a psychogeriatrician took his turn as chairman of the psychiatric staff committee. As Pitt put it (cited by Shulman, 1994), geriatric psychiatry is part of the family of psychiatry, but is married to geriatrics.

Reifler *et al.* (1982) discussed the work of a psychogeriatric outreach team in the US. The most common reasons for referral were inability to care for self (35 per cent), being forgetful or confused (34 per cent), bizarre behaviour (28 per cent) and bizarre thought (22 per cent). Dementia was diagnosed more often than depression. Levy (1985) commented that home visits by private practitioners in the US had become a rarity, and psychiatric home evaluations were relatively unknown. Unfavourable reimbursement patterns and reliance on sophisticated medical centres were cited as possible reasons. He described 176 patients he saw at home in Brooklyn in 1983, most referred by a community agency or the patient's family, and he referred to 'the striking failure of local family practitioners to make use of psychiatric services for the elderly'. Discussing the small referral rate for black and Hispanic patients he suggested that unawareness of medical services, cultural resistance to psychiatric intervention, and ability to care for such problems within the community without assistance, might be explanations.

At the same time, Lipowski (1983) was drawing attention to the needs of elderly medical-surgical inpatients with psychiatric problems in general hospitals. He said that nursing staff resisted their transfer to psychiatric wards, and he called for debate and decisions on a national scale. His solution was for liaison psychiatrists to take over the role of geropsychiatric consultants in general hospitals.

As illustrated above, reports from the 1980s reveal that community provision of psychogeriatric services was feasible in the US, but it seems that the system of funding restricted its availability. Shulman (1981) contrasted the US, where financial restrictions on the amount of billing allowed in a given period of time could influence the treatment available for elderly patients, with Canada (with a modified form of universal health care) and Britain, where treatment was equally available to all. An 'epidemiological' approach to service planning – that is to say, planning for defined populations – was most readily feasible in Britain.

Developments in Canada

Shulman (1994) drew attention to Martin Rodenburg's single-handed pioneering effort to develop a comprehensive psychogeriatric service in Kingston, Ontario. Teitelbaum *et al.* (1996) provided details of the Kingston service that evolved. Shulman (1981) described how his service in Toronto developed from a general hospital base, and wrote that a unique problem in North America was the lack of a defined catchment area for most general hospitals. He emphasized the importance of collaboration with geriatric medicine but noted very few examples of an effective and collegial partnership. In the Toronto service, patients referred because of organic brain disorders were seen in their homes, whereas functionally ill or depressed patients were seen in health care settings. He emphasized too the importance of a multidisciplinary follow-up clinic for those discharged from hospital.

Shulman (1981) referred to the traditionally poor service given by psychiatrists to people with dementia, and stated that patients suffering from dementia have been dealt with largely by social services in nursing home settings. In this regard, Canada and Australia in the early 1980s differed from Britain, where long-term care for people with dementia was provided more in hospitals than in nursing homes. Only from the Thatcher years did the nursing home industry mushroom in Britain; long-stay care was the first major 'privatization' of health services in Britain.

Harris *et al.* (1990) showed that a multidisciplinary outpatient psychogeriatric programme can provide an effective service. They compared statistics concerning the psychiatric diagnoses of patients seen by various other North American psychogeriatric services in the 1980s, with medians of about 47 per cent organic mental disorder and 32 per cent mood disorder.

Stolee *et al.* (1994) noted considerable variation in the way Canadian geriatric psychiatry outreach services had developed. They operated from varying bases (hospitals, long-term care facilities, community centres), there was wide variation in the disciplines represented on the teams, their goals and target populations varied, and so did the method of mental health consultation. Ginsburg *et al.* (1998) questioned 38 outreach teams in Ontario and noted wide variations in practice. Nine had no psychiatrists directly affiliated with them.

It is apparent from the above that Canada's old age psychiatry services evolved community-oriented services comparable to those in Britain, during the 1970s and 1980s, and to a greater extent than in the US. The health care systems of some provinces facilitated such developments more than did those of others.

Development of old age psychiatry services around the world

Psychiatric services for elderly people have evolved in many parts of the world, as described in issues of the *Bulletin of the International Psychogeriatric Association*. Specialized mental health services for the elderly in the Netherlands (where over 12 per cent of the population is aged more than 65 years) began to develop in the 1970s (Heeren, 1998). In the early 1980s the newly established Regional Institutes for Outpatient Mental Health Care all included separate departments for the elderly, and by 1990 most general psychiatric hospitals also had separate facilities for elderly people.

Bramesfeld (2003) noted that nearly countrywide community-oriented gerontopsychiatric services are available in the UK and Switzerland, but that services in Denmark, Sweden and France are mainly focused on dementia. There are few mobile gerontopsychiatric teams in Germany and none in France. The six specialized old age psychiatry services in France have day-clinic, inpatient and outpatient departments, but in that country 'gerontologists seem to be particularly important for treating psychiatric diseased persons'. Reasons why countries with similar proportions of elderly people have such different provision of services for mentally ill older persons have yet to be clarified in the literature.

The first special unit in Denmark for psychogeriatric patients was developed in 1976 (Abelskov, 1998), and now most counties are reported to have psychogeriatric services. Norway (16 per cent aged over 65 years) developed its first department of old age psychiatry in 1971, and special units and departments of old age psychiatry had been established in 15 out of 19 counties by 1999 (Engedal, 1999).

In contrast, in countries such as Belarus, with 13 per cent aged over 65 years, old age psychiatry hardly exists (Solodkaya, 1999). Health care is limited and specialist education is lacking, especially in relation to aged health, because of the poor economic situation.

Only 7.4 per cent of the population of Thailand was aged over 60 years in 1990, and until recently there were no specialized psychogeriatric services. Ten of the 350 psychiatrists in the country were working part-time in old age psychiatry (Nivataphand, 1999). In Korea (8.3 per cent aged over 65 years in 2003) most psychiatric hospitals have not yet established separate geriatric wards (Oh and Cheon, 2001) but over 10 per cent of the country's 1850 psychiatrists are members of the Korean Association for Geriatric Psychiatry, and a multidisciplinary community-oriented approach has been widely adopted (Suh, 2003). Systematic development of psychogeriatric services in Hong Kong (10 per cent aged over 65 years) began in 1994 (Chiu et al., 1998), with a multidisciplinary community-oriented approach based on the Nottingham (UK) model.

Japan's population aged over 65 years rose rapidly, from 8 per cent in 1975 to over 15 per cent in 2000, and the Japan Psychogeriatric Society was formed in 1983 (IPA, 2000). Hasegawa made notable contributions to the specialty both at home and internationally.

Psychogeriatrics as a separate service within psychiatry began in New Zealand in the late 1970s, in some measure shaped by experience of the service developed by Arie. In Australia although establishment of community services was recommended by Bower (1964), they were not widely developed until the 1980s. Even then, some eminent Australian psychiatrists argued that psychiatric resources need not be allocated for elderly persons with behavioural or psychiatric disorders because (they said) geriatricians were just as capable of doing the work (Andrews, 1990). In spite of this, services did develop, and by 1992, a majority of elderly people in Australia lived in the catchment areas of variably comprehensive old age psychiatry services, with ratios of 0.37 psychiatrist, 0.42 social or welfare worker, 0.46 occupational therapist and 0.59 community nurse to 10,000 elderly (Snowdon et al., 1995).

Reifler and Cohen (1998) sent questionnaires to members of the IPA, and used the data to rate the stage of development of old age psychiatry services and of the specialty of geriatric psychiatry in the various countries of which they were citizens. Not all countries returned enough questionnaires to allow meaningful ratings to be made, but it was interesting to see how far the services in some countries had evolved.

A survey in 2001 of World Psychiatric Association (WPA) member-societies (Camus et al., 2003) revealed that 40 of the 48 responding countries provided some specific psychiatric services for older people, and that 13 of the 48 recognized old age psychiatry as a subspecialty. Non-responders to the survey included the US, Canada and Spain. Conclusions about progress in development of old age psychiatry around the world are limited by having reports from only a quarter of the world's countries. Nevertheless, there was evidence that the establishment of specific curricula and guidelines for training in old age psychiatry facilitate official recognition of the subspecialty.

The picture obtained from the surveys and from other published details is sketchy. It would be good to look at how services in India, for example, have evolved, and compare them with developments in South American countries. However, this account is not meant to be comprehensive and certainly is not meant to imply that slower or different evolution is being criticized. This chapter is about history, and one of the points to be made is that different economic situations and different cultures lead to different ways of dealing with old age mental health problems. One observation to be made is that in some circumscribed regions, where extended families take interest in all people in their communities, whatever their age, people with dementia are well able to continue to live in their villages or centres, even if behavioural or cognitive problems are severe. They provide their own, non-medical, non-health-care service and do not 'require' specialist services. Cultures cope differently with mental disorders.

Reifler and Cohen (1998) deemed the Netherlands, UK and Switzerland to have the best-developed services in early 1998, though 15 other countries were regarded as well on their way in development. The UK, US and Finland were rated as the leaders (remembering that the questionnaires were answered by citizens of the countries whose services they were rating) in development of geriatric psychiatry as a profession, with training and a certification process for geriatric psychiatrists and acceptance of the specialty by the profession. Since 1998, it is probable that several other countries have fulfilled criteria to reach the level of these leaders.

Returning to consideration of the US and UK, but adding Ireland, Reifler (1997) commented that the US was the most entrepreneurial, and Britain's greatest strength was its uniformity and comprehensiveness. In Ireland, the first old age psychiatrist was appointed in 1989, and services were in place in only a few areas when Reifler wrote his report. A nationwide system of services was being developed. Reifler commented that geriatric psychiatry as a specialty was more advanced in the UK and Ireland than in the US. There is no doubt, however, that research and interest in the specialty in the US have developed considerably in the six years since that investigation.

Towards maturity

The Czech Psychogeriatric Association dates back to 1968, and the European Association for Geriatric Psychiatry first met in Germany in 1971. The American Association for Geriatric Psychiatry was founded in 1978, which was the year when the

Royal College of Psychiatrists officially formed its Section of Psychiatry of Old Age, though a less formal 'Group' had been in existence in the College since 1973. A comparable Canadian Section (of its Psychiatric Association) was formed at about that time. The Dutch equivalent was founded in 1981, and the Japan Psychogeriatric Society soon after. The Australian and New Zealand College's Section was formed in 1987 and is now a Faculty (as is the British equivalent). Korea, Hong Kong, Romania, Spain and other countries have formed comparable Associations, which indicates acceptance by the members and by their countries' psychiatrists that old age psychiatry is distinct and identifiable as a specialty. Old age psychiatry was recognized as a specialty in Britain, with specific higher training requirements, in 1989. The Canadian Academy of Geriatric Psychiatry was established in 1993. The American Board of Psychiatry and Neurology (ABPN) has administered examinations in geriatric psychiatry since 1991, and in twelve years over 2500 psychiatrists obtained this further qualification. Since 1997, the ABPN's exam has been called 'certification in the subspecialty of geriatric psychiatry' (Bragg and Warshaw, 2003).

These various Associations have been active in support and education of those working in psychogeriatric services. The Geriatric Section of the WPA has collaborated in organizing consensus conferences. One such meeting resulted in a Curriculum document, aimed at training leaders in the provision of comprehensive specialist mental health services for older people as recommended in various WHO/WPA consensus statements (Gustafson et al., 2003). The organization which has taken the most active role in promoting development of old age psychiatry services around the world has been the International Psychogeriatric Association (IPA), the origins and development of which have been recorded by Finkel (2001a,b,c) in three issues of the IPA Bulletin. The proposal for its inception came from members of the 1980 British Council course in Nottingham. These courses provided education and impetus to psychiatrists who have gone on to be leaders in the field all over the world. Professors Chiu and Ames from Australia have recently been running similar courses for geriatric psychiatrists in Asia. The Romanian Geriatric Psychiatry Association has organized continuing education meetings in Eastern Europe (N. Tătaru, personal communication).

Another sign of its development is the fact that over 20 countries can now claim to have one or more academic chairs of old age psychiatry (Camus et al., 2003).

The hugely successful and rapidly proliferating Alzheimer's Associations and Societies and other non-government bodies have been important as effective lobbyists and in a prime role as 'supporters of the supporters'.

The present and future

'Early developments were shaped by the self-evidently unmet need of gross morbidity in older people. In most of the world, this is still the case' (Arie and Jolley, 1999). Many countries are making progress in developing services for older people with mental health problems, though others have met barriers. A major obstacle in so-called developed countries has been 'rationing'. The situation in Britain, the pioneer country in development of psychogeriatric services, is illustrative.

Jolley (1999) reviewed progress in implementation of the recommendations published by the Royal College of Physicians and Royal College of Psychiatrists (1989). One recommendation was that resources, workload, manpower and training facilities should be identified and the data used by the DHSS to ensure that policies were being effectively implemented 'in what has long been recognised as a priority area'. Jolley noted, however, that

> Policy and priorities have become harder to identify as a consequence of the successive changes in the NHS. 'Planning' has been superseded by 'purchasing' and, more recently, by 'commissioning'. National guidelines have been eschewed and local bargaining championed as the means of determining priorities. Within this poorly defined framework health authorities and other purchasers have not always given priority to the needs of older people with mental illness. Many health authorities have failed to make an appropriate contribution to long-term care of the severely mentally ill and incapacitated. Rather, they have chosen to spend their revenue on other groups of patients. Those older people who would previously have received care in hospital have been thrown into the means-tested and inadequately regulated environment of social provision.

He went on to note the 40 per cent decrease in long-stay beds in both geriatric and psychiatric units and hospitals, with a consequent increase in the role of teams that provide support and education to those in residential facilities.

Britain maintained its long-term care provision in hospitals long after the US, Canada and Australia had moved patients out to nursing homes. In the 1980s, aspects of care that were formerly provided in publicly funded facilities were handed over to the commercial sector. The government maintained a divide between social services and health, and gave social workers the purchasing role in arranging accommodation. Funding was given to local authorities for community care. In fact, domiciliary services have improved, and a higher proportion of people are able to stay at home longer than was the case twenty years ago, but care for those too disturbed to live at home, but who can no longer be admitted to facilities that are run by old age psychiatry services, must surely be a cause for concern. Neither the funding, nor, in many places, the division of responsibilities, has worked out satisfactorily. There have been examples in other countries of more appropriate arrangements for those who formerly would have been in long-stay hospital beds. In the Australian state of Victoria, psychogeriatric nursing homes have taken over this role. Psychiatric expertise is available, and psychogeriatricians are involved in decisions about who no longer needs to be in such a specialist facility.

Blazer (1998) has discussed potential problems faced by geriatric psychiatry once it has matured. He noted that in the UK in recent years, more responsibility has been placed on the GP to allocate resources for the care of patients. He declared, 'at the very time that geriatric psychiatry has "come of age", we must demonstrate once again the specific expertise that can be marshalled to care for older adults experiencing psychiatric disorders'.

Jeste *et al.* (1999) considered that the current health care system in the US serves mentally ill older adults poorly and is unprepared to meet an upcoming crisis in geriatric mental health. They recommended formulation of a 15- to 25-year plan for research, including health services research. They stated that

> The recently developed models of managed mental health care do not assure quality medical health care, clarify the role of cognitive and psychosocial rehabilitation, or identify the optimal mix of services necessary to maintain the older patient with severe persistent mental disorders in the community as long as possible.

Bartels *et al.* (1999) argued that current mental health services for elderly people are largely fragmented and underutilized due to the battle between the federal and state governments over the costs of Medicaid and limitations in Medicare coverage, and commented that deinstitutionalization has left many older persons with decreased access to mental health care in both community and long-term settings. Mental health specialty services for older persons tend to be a low priority in managed health care organizations compared with medical and surgical specialty services. Bartels *et al.* (1999) made recommendations for innovative models of care, and urged quests for data describing the costs and outcomes of such models.

All is not total gloom in relation to current and future provision of old age psychiatric services in the US. Colenda and van Dooren (1993) discussed the benefits of ensuring that CMHCs develop specialized old age services that work well. They stated that a network of neighbourhood 'gatekeepers' is critical to the success of outreach programmes. Their final comment is worth repetition: in discussing the future of the health care system, they said 'one measure of the system's success is how well the public and private mental health sectors provide compassionate mental health care for individuals who are disenfranchised and at risk of not receiving the care they deserve'.

This chapter is on history rather than on prediction of the future. Nevertheless, our proposals for the future should be based partly on what we have observed to work well in the past. We have discussed advances and setbacks, and considered how things that start well can go wrong, and why. Countries that have funds and are early in their development of old age services can learn from the mistakes of others. Advocates need to ensure that their governments are concerned with the quality of life of people in all age-groups rather than just with their country's total wealth and status. Mental health is an important determinant of that quality.

The changing context of services

The relevance of and need for old age psychiatry is recognized now in both developed and developing countries; in the latter, although the proportion of old people is lower than in developed countries, the rate of increase is usually even more rapid. Services will evolve differently, and innovation and variety are already evident. Arie (2000) has considered factors that will influence developments in the near future. In medicine there is the amazing promise of the neurosciences, of molecular biology and of genetics in understanding mental disorders; the availability of new methods of investigation, mostly non-invasive; and the development of new treatments, physical and psychological. Electronics provides almost unimaginable possibilities ranging from brain-implanted stimulation, via information systems, to prosthetic home environments.

All this is against a background of demographic change and changes in the status of old people, patterns of work and retirement, and pension policies. Along with this, in rich countries, is a huge growth of expectations in a much better informed and less passively accepting public. The role and status of doctors, and their relationship and interchangeability with other professions, is already in flux. Perhaps we shall also be exploring the possibilities of a new occupational category, an 'age care practitioner', filling, at different levels of training, a wide range of tasks in the care of the aged.

Ethical questions, including those concerned with mental capacity and with the end of life, often hitherto ignored or denied, are becoming the subject of open and often very spirited debate, and of legislation.

One can safely make two conclusions about the future. First, the bulk of the world's mental morbidity in old age, like the great bulk of the suffering due to all illness, will still for the foreseeable future be untreated, despite the existence of effective treatments. Second, in spite of the technical advances which will become available, there will everywhere continue to be a place for the trained and informed practitioner.

References

Abelskov, K. (1998) Psychogeriatrics in Denmark: growing, but not yet a recognized specialty. *IPA Bulletin*, **15** (1), 11.

Andrews, G. (1990) Health services research and the future of Australian psychiatry. *Australian and New Zealand Journal of Psychiatry*, **24**, 435–6.

Arie, T. (1970) The first year of the Goodmayes psychiatric service for old people. *Lancet*, **ii**, 1179–82.

Arie, T. (2000) What's coming next in services? *Hong Kong Journal of Psychiatry*, **10** (2), 8–10.

Arie, T. (2002) The development in Britain. In J. R. M. Copeland, M. T. Abou-Saleh and D. G. Blazer (eds.) *Principles and Practice of Geriatric Psychiatry*, 2nd edn, pp. 9–11. Wiley, London.

Arie, T. and Isaacs, A.D. (1977) The development of psychiatric services for the elderly in Britain. In F. Post and A. D. Isaacs (eds.) *Studies in Geriatric Psychiatry*, pp. 241–6. John Wiley, Chichester.

Arie, T. and Jolley, D. (1982) Making services work: organisation and style of psychogeriatric services. In R. Levy and F. Post (eds.) *The Psychiatry of Late Life*, pp. 222–51. Blackwell, Oxford.

Arie, T. and Jolley, D. (1999) Psychogeriatrics. In H. Freeman (ed.) *A Century of Psychiatry*, pp. 260–4. Mosby-Wolfe, London.

Barker, W.H. (1998) Geriatrics in North America. In Tallis *et al.* (eds.) *Brocklehurst's Textbook of Geriatric Medicine and Gerontology*, 5th edn, pp. 1499–511. Churchill Livingstone, Edinburgh.

Bartels, S.J., Levine, K.J., and Shea, D. (1999) Community-based long-term care for older persons with severe and persistent mental illness in an era of managed care. *Psychiatric Services*, **50**, 1189–97.

Blazer, D.G. (1998) Geriatric psychiatry matures: advantages and problems as the psychiatry of old age grows older. *Current Opinion in Psychiatry*, **11**, 401–3.

Bower, H.M. (1964) Old age in Western society. Lecture II: psychiatric aspects. *Medical Journal of Australia,* **2,** 325–31.

Bragg, E.J. and Warshaw, G.A. (2003) Evolution of geriatric medicine fellowship training in the United States. *American Journal of Geriatric Psychiatry,* **11,** 280–90.

Bramesfeld, A. (2003) Service provision for elderly depressed persons and political and professional awareness for this subject: a comparison of six European countries. *International Journal of Geriatric Psychiatry,* **18,** 392–401.

Busse, E.W. (2002) Scope and development in the twentieth century. In J. R. M. Copeland, M. T. Abou-Saleh and D. G. Blazer (eds.) *Principles and Practice of Geriatric Psychiatry,* 2nd edn, pp. 7–8. Wiley, London.

Busse, E. and Pfeiffer, E. (1973) *Mental Illness in Later Life.* American Psychiatric Press, Washington, DC.

Butler, R.N. (1975a) Psychiatry and the elderly: an overview. *American Journal of Psychiatry,* **132,** 893–900.

Butler, R.N. (1975b) *Why Survive? Being Old in America.* Harper and Row, New York.

Camus, V., Katona, C., de Mendonça Lima, C. A., *et al.* (2003) Teaching and training in old age psychiatry: a general survey of the World Psychiatric Association member-societies. *International Journal of Geriatric Psychiatry,* **18,** 694–9.

Chiu, H.F.K., Pan, P.C., Li, S.W., and Tsang, M.H.L. (1998) Psychogeriatrics in Hong Kong: building the framework. *IPA Bulletin,* **15,** 10–13.

Cohen, G.D. (1976) Mental health services and the elderly: needs and options. *American Journal of Psychiatry,* **133,** 65–8.

Colenda, C.C. and van Dooren, H. (1993) Opportunities for improving community mental health services for elderly persons. *Hospital and Community Psychiatry,* **44,** 531–3.

Colwell, C. and Post, F. (1959) Community needs of elderly psychiatric patients. *British Medical Journal,* **2,** 214. Reprinted in H. Freeman and J. Farndale (eds.) *Trends in the Mental Health Services,* pp. 251–60. Pergamon, Oxford.

Cooper, B. (1991) Principles of service provision in old age psychiatry. In R. Jacoby and C. Oppenheimer (eds.) *Psychiatry in the Elderly,* pp. 274–300. Oxford University Press, Oxford.

Corsellis, J.A.N. (1962) *Mental Illness and the Ageing Brain,* Maudsley monograph no.9. Oxford University Press, London.

Dening,T. (1992) Community psychiatry of old age: a UK perspective. *International Journal of Geriatric Psychiatry,* **7,** 757–66.

Department of Health and Social Security (1972) *Services for Mental Illness Related to Old Age.* Circular HM (72) **71,** London: HMSO

Department of Health and Social Security (1981) *Growing Older.* London: HMSO.

Eisdorfer, C. (1977) Evaluation of the quality of psychiatric care for the aged. *American Journal of Psychiatry,* **134,** 315–17.

Engedal, K. (1999) Old age psychiatry in Norway: providing specialist services to the mentally ill. *IPA Bulletin,* **16,** 10.

Finkel, S. (2001a) History of IPA, part 1. *IPA Bulletin,* **16,** (2) 6–9.

Finkel, S. (2001b) History of IPA, part 2. *IPA Bulletin,* **16,** (3) 6–7.

Finkel, S. (2001c) History of IPA, part 3. *IPA Bulletin,* **16,** (4) 8–11.

Ginsburg, L., Hamilton, P., Madora, P., Robichaud, L., and White, J. (1998) Geriatric psychiatry outreach practices in the province of Ontario: the role of the psychiatrist. *Canadian Journal of Psychiatry,* **43,** 386–90.

Glasscote, R.M., Gudeman, J.E., and Miles, D.G. (1977) *Creative Mental Health Services for the Elderly*. American Psychiatric Association, Washington.

Godber, C. (1978) Conflict and collaboration between geriatric medicine and psychiatry. In B. Isaacs (ed.) *Recent Advances in Geriatric Medicine*, pp. 131–42. Churchill Livingstone, London.

Godber, C. and Rosenvinge, H. (1998) Services. In R. Butler and B. Pitt (eds.) *Seminars in Old Age Psychiatry*, pp. 193–208. Gaskell, London.

Grad, J. and Sainsbury, P. (1963) Evaluating a community care service. In H. Freeman and J. Farndale (eds.) *Trends in the Mental Health Services*, pp. 303–17. Pergamon, London.

Gustafson, L., Burns, A., Katona, C., *et al.* (2003) Skill-based objectives for specialist training in old age psychiatry. *International Journal of Geriatric Psychiatry*, **18**, 686–93.

Harris, A.G., Marriott, J.A.S., and Robertson, J. (1990) Issues in the evaluation of a community psychogeriatric service. *Canadian Journal of Psychiatry*, **35**, 215–22.

Heeren, T. (1998) Mental health care for the elderly in the Netherlands. *IPA Bulletin*, **15** (4), 16.

IPA (2000) Japan Psychogeriatric Society. *IPA Bulletin*, **17**, 21.

Jeste, D.V., Alexopoulos, G.S., Bartels, S.J. *et al.* (1999) Consensus statement on the upcoming crisis in geriatric mental health. Research agenda for the next two decades. *Archives of General Psychiatry*, **56**, 848–53.

Jolley, D. (1995) The first year of the Goodmayes psychiatric service for old people. Thomas Arie. Commentary. *International Journal of Geriatric Psychiatry*, **10**, 930–2.

Jolley, D.J. (1999) Care of older people with mental illness. Progress in the implementation of recommendations 1989–1998. *Psychiatric Bulletin*, **23**, 117–20.

Kay, D.W.K., Beamish, P., and Roth, M. (1964) Old age mental disorders in Newcastle-upon-Tyne. Part 1: a study of prevalence. *British Journal of Psychiatry*, **110**, 146–58.

Levy, M.T. (1985) Psychiatric assessment of elderly patients in the home. A survey of 176 cases. *Journal of the American Geriatrics Society*, **33**, 9–12.

Lipowski, Z.J. (1983) The need to integrate liaison psychiatry and geropsychiatry. *American Journal of Psychiatry*, **140**, 1003–5.

Macmillan, D. (1960) Preventive geriatrics. Opportunities of a community mental health service. *Lancet*, **ii**, 1439–41.

Macmillan, D. and Shaw, P. (1966) Senile breakdown in standards of personal and environmental cleanliness. *British Medical Journal*, **2**, 1032–7.

Maddox, G.L. and Glass, T.A. (1989) The continuum of care: movement toward the community. In E. W. Busse and D. G. Blazer (eds.) *Geriatric Psychiatry*, pp. 635–7. American Psychiatric Press, Washington.

Millard, P.H. and Higgs, P. (1989) Geriatric medicine beyond the hospital. *Age and Ageing*, **18**, 1–3.

Nivataphand, R. (1999) Psychogeriatrics in Thailand. *IPA Bulletin*, **16** (1), 17.

Oh, B.H. and Cheon, J.S. (2001) Mental health and the elderly in Korea. *IPA Bulletin*, **18** (3), 17.

Pitt, B. (1974) *Psychogeriatrics*. Churchill Livingstone, Edinburgh.

Post, F. (1965) *The Clinical Psychiatry of Late Life*. Pergamon, Oxford.

Post, F. (1978) Then and now. *British Journal of Psychiatry*, **133**, 83–6.

Prinsley, D.M. (1973) Psychogeriatric ward for mentally disturbed elderly patients. *BMJ* **iv**, 169–70.

Reifler, B.V. (1997) The practice of geriatric psychiatry in three countries: observations of an American in the British Isles. *International Journal of Geriatric Psychiatry*, **12**, 795–807.

Reifler, B.V., Kethley, A., O'Neill, P., Hanley, R., Lewis, S., and Stenchever, D. (1982) Five-year experience of a community outreach program for the elderly. *American Journal of Psychiatry*, **139**, 220–3.

Reifler, B. V. and Cohen, W. (1998) Practice of geriatric psychiatry and mental health services for the elderly: results of an international survey. *International Psychogeriatrics*, **10**, 351–7.

Roth, M. (1955) The natural history of mental disorder in old age. *Journal of Mental Science*, **101**, 281–301.

Royal College of Physicians and the Royal College of Psychiatrists (1989) *Care of Elderly People with Mental Illness. Specialist services and medical training.* Royal College of Physicians of London and Royal College of Psychiatrists, London.

Royal College of Psychiatrists (1992) Revised guidelines for collaboration between physicians in geriatric medicine and psychiatrist of old age. *Psychiatric Bulletin*, **16**, 583–4.

Shenfield, B.E. (1962) American experience in ageing as viewed by a European. In J. Kaplan and G. J. Aldridge (eds.) *Social Welfare of the Ageing.* Columbia University Press, New York. (Cited by Slater E and Roth M, 1969. *Clinical psychiatry. Third edition*, p. 562. Bailliere, Tindall and Cassell, London.)

Shepherd, B., Cooper, B., Brown, A.C., and Kalton, G.W. (1966) *Psychiatric Illness in General Practice.* Oxford University Press, London.

Shulman, K. (1981) Service innovations in geriatric psychiatry. In T. Arie (eds.) *Essays in Old Age Medicine, Psychiatry and Services*, pp. 214–23. Croom Helm, London.

Shulman, K.I. (1994) The future of geriatric psychiatry. *Canadian Journal of Psychiatry*, **39** (suppl. 1), 54–8.

Snowdon, J., Ames, D., Chiu, E., and Wattis, J. (1995) A survey of psychiatric services for elderly people in Australia. *Australian and New Zealand Journal of Psychiatry*, **29**, 207–14.

Solodkaya, T. (1999) Current state of old age psychiatry in Belarus. *IPA Bulletin*, **16** (1), 15–16.

Stolee, P., LeClair, J.K., and Kessler, L. (1994) Geriatric psychiatry consultation in the community. *Canadian Journal of Psychiatry*, **39** (Suppl. 1), 527–32.

Suh, G.-H. (2003) Psychogeriatrics in Korea. *IPA Bulletin*, **20** (1), 7–9.

Teitelbaum, L., Cotton, D., Ginsburg, M.L., and Nashed, Y.H. (1996) Psychogeriatric consultation services: effect and effectiveness. *Canadian Journal of Psychiatry*, **41**, 638–44.

Wattis, J., Wattis, L., and Arie, T. (1981) Psychogeriatrics: a national survey of a new branch of psychiatry. *BMJ* **282**, 1529–33.

Whitehead, T. (1969) *In the Service of Old Age. The welfare of psychogeriatric patients.* Penguin, London.

Williamson, J., Stokoe, I.H., Gray, S., *et al.* (1964) Old people at home. Their unreported needs. *Lancet* (May 23), 1117–20.

Chapter 2

Principles and best practice model of psychogeriatric service delivery

Edmond Chiu

The early principles of psychogeriatric service delivery were established in the United Kingdom in the 1960s (see Chapter 1) by pioneers such as Tom Arie, Brice Pitt, David Jolly and Felix Post. Pitt in his *Psychogeriatrics: – an introduction to the psychiatry of old age* (1982) said:

> The principal aim of a psychogeriatric service must be to meet the needs of old people in its community. Usually the service operates from the psychiatric hospital or unit of the area, but it is concerned not nearly or even mostly with old people already in hospital, but with the development of *comprehensive assessment, treatment and care for the elderly mentally ill at large.*
>
> (My emphasis)

Tom Arie, since the 1970s, has consistently affirmed and taught 'services have concerned themselves not only with the best interest of those who are patients, but also with the population of potential patients within a local community' (Jolly and Arie, 1992).

The concept of a psychogeriatric team has been the central pillar of the development in the United Kingdom. A consultant psychiatrist, committed to psychogeriatrics, leads a team. In those countries where this has reached a speciality status (e.g. UK, USA, Canada and Australasia) the psychogeriatrician is the recognized specialist psychiatrist to head such a multidisciplinary team of nurses, social workers, psychologists (clinical and/or neuropsychologists), occupational therapists, physiotherapists and other allied health professionals such as speech pathologists, podiatrists, and music therapists.

The managed care system (Reifler, 1997) in the US differs significantly from that of the British and Irish systems, which are well coordinated. The central activities of Domiciliary Visits (DVs) and community teams are also elements missing from the US model. A national framework with remarkable consistency both in structure and individual components was the major distinguishing feature between UK and the US. By implication, Reifler commented that the 'one-payer' system permits the model in UK whereas the managed care system in the US prevents the development of such a structure of service delivery.

To determine a country's development of service models Reifler proposed a 'simple skeletal outline' of four stages in both the development of the profession and the development of services for the mentally ill elderly (Table 2.1).

Table 2.1 Four stages in the development of the profession and services of treatment of the mentally ill (Reifler, 1997)

	Development of geriatric psychiatry	Development of services for mentally ill elderly
Stage 1	No criteria for designation of geriatric psychiatrist; practitioners are self-designated	Only very basic services are available, usually in general psychiatric facilities only
Stage 2	Certification process for geriatric psychiatrists exists and is well accepted by the professional community	Separate and/or specialized programmes beginning to be established, including long-term care and community-based programmes
Stage 3	National need for geriatric psychiatrists established and mechanisms in place to accomplish this	Full range of long-term, hospital-based and community-based programmes exist in many parts of the nation
Stage 4	Nation has a full complement of credentialed geriatric psychiatrists, sufficient to meet the needs of the entire country	Entire spectrum of service for mentally ill elderly exists throughout the country with access for all in need

While the differing models exist between UK, US, Australia, Canada and other more developed nations (see Chapters 7–14), the Asian varieties are worth a brief description.

Hong Kong has been strongly influenced by the Arie model and has developed a model very similar to the UK, Australia and New Zealand. It has area-based services, led by a consultant psychiatrist. Community teams, inpatient and outpatient services, memory clinics and day centres are integrated and coordinated to provide care to a defined population. Long-term mental hospitals, although still in existence, play a less central role.

By contrast, economically successful Singapore has as its centrepiece of mental health care delivery for the elderly a large mental hospital at Woodbridge Hospital, (opened in 1993) with only embryonic attempts at community teams. That the psychogeriatric ward at Woodbridge Hospital was the first ward to be 'open' in 2002 reflects the dramatically different model of service delivery, which has an implied policy supporting institutionalization.

China, having awoken from its 'cultural revolution' and now opening up to the rest of the world, is trying very hard to catch up in its mental health service development. It has funded two demonstration projects (one in Beijing, the other in Shanghai) to test out what is the appropriate model for this large populous country within the next few years. China will soon show the world her own evolved model of mental health service delivery to the mentally ill elderly.

Another emerging model, which is of interest, is that of Indonesia, a country with a population of 200,000,000 of whom 7.6 per cent are elderly. It now has a defined Government policy, a recognized subspecialty (since 1996) of old age psychiatrists and 23 psychiatrists working in this speciality, though none exclusively with older people. While there are no community-based teams and shortages of acute care, home care, nurses and allied health professionals, it has moved rapidly to develop a professional infrastructure to take the country forward from its minimalist status.

An international consensus model on the organization of care

Recognizing that in different countries there are different developments with different socio-economic and political contexts, varying levels of fiscal and professional commitment, the late Jean Wertheimer, as Chairman of the World Psychiatric Association Section of Geriatric Psychiatry, led the development of a Consensus Statement in the Organisation of Care in the Psychiatry of the Elderly, an official Technical Consensus Statement approved by both WHO and WPA (WHO/MSA/MNH/97.3) and posted on the WPA website to be freely available in the public domain (WHO, 1997).

This statement was the product of a Consensus Conference held in Lausanne in April 14–16 1997 hosted by the Lausanne University Psychogeriatric Service, which was headed by Jean Wertheimer. With great vision and perspicacity, he brought together a comprehensive group of professionals from relevant professional organizations and NGOs (see the Appendix at the end of this chapter) to work towards an agreed best model for the development of psychogeriatric services worldwide. The experience of developed countries (UK, Australia, Switzerland, France) influenced the initial discussions. This was modified and adapted for international (including less developed countries) suitability by the contributions from international organizations and NGOs such as International Psychogeriatric Association, World Health Organization, World Federation of Mental Health, Alzheimer's Disease International, International Federation of Social Workers, International Council of Nurses and International Union of Psychological Science as well as by individuals from Zimbabwe and India.

This document provides a generic best practice model, establishing both general and specific principles, identifying care needs, described components of service necessary for a comprehensive and effective psychogeriatric team and service system. The remainder of the chapter will draw heavily from this document.

General principles

Psychiatry of the Elderly is a complex discipline, confronted with intricate problems pertaining not only to mental health and behaviour but also the physical health and relational, environmental, spiritual and social matters. The situations, which this discipline is facing, are thus closely linked to the family nucleus, the local customs and culture, the general organization of Public Health and social assistance. The organization of care in Old Age Psychiatry must be worked out along the perspectives of the Primary Health Care Strategy of the WHO (Declaration of Alma Ata, 1978), focus on the patients and their families, and yet be integrated into the medical and social network designed for the population in general and the elderly in particular. However, this integration must not be synonymous with dilution and loss of specificity. On the contrary, since collaboration is necessary, it is therefore indispensable that competencies, specific care and structures adapted to Old Age Psychiatry, be solidly developed. Care of the elderly requires a strong contribution from Old Age Psychiatry.

> Jean Wertheimer in the Introduction to the Consensus Statement

From this foundation we can move forward to the enumeration of the essential general principles of this document, which stated:

> Good health and life of good quality are fundamental human rights. This applies equally to people of all age groups and to people with mental disorders.
>
> All people have the right of access to a range of services that can respond to their health and social needs. These needs should be met appropriately for the cultural setting and in accordance with scientific knowledge and ethical requirements.
>
> Governments have a responsibility to improve and maintain the general and mental health of older people and to support their families and carers by the provision of health and social measures adapted to the specific needs of the local community.
>
> Older people with mental health problems and their families and carers have the right to participate individually and collectively in the planning and implementation of their health care.
>
> Services should be designed for the promotion of mental health in old age as well as for the assessment, diagnosis and management of the full range of mental disorders and disabilities encountered by older people.
>
> Governments need to recognize the crucial role of non-governmental agencies and work in partnership with them.
>
> Preparing for increasing life expectancy and ensuing health risks calls for significant social innovations at the individual and societal level, which must be founded on a knowledge base drawn from contributions by, and collaboration among, the medical, behavioural, psychological, biological and social sciences.
>
> In developing countries it may be difficult to provide resources for the provision of care. This, however, does not invalidate the aims of helping the elderly by the application of the principles listed above and the specific principles that follow.

> Consensus Statement pp. 2–3

Specific principles

It is in this section that the essential governing specific principles of best practice are declared. These can be referred to as the C.A.R.I.T.A.S. principles. The word C.A.R.I.T.A.S. is an acronym borrowed from the Latin motto of the Sisters of Charity Health Service in St Vincent's Hospital, Melbourne: – Caritas Christi urget nos (the love of Christ urges us). This acronym was proposed by the author to the Consensus Group, which accepted it in the form of agreed specific principles, specified in pages 3–4 of the Consensus Document.

Good quality care for older people with mental health problems is:

Comprehensive

Accessible

Responsive

Individualized

Transdisciplinary

Accountable

Systemic

A **comprehensive service** should take into account all aspects of the patient's physical, psychological and social needs and wishes and be patient-centred.

An **accessible** service is user-friendly and readily available, minimizing the geographical, cultural, financial, political and linguistic obstacles to obtaining care.

A **responsive** service is one that listens to and understands the problems brought to its attention and acts promptly and appropriately.

An **individualized** service focuses on each person with a mental health problem in his or her family and community context. The planning of care must be tailored for and acceptable to the individual and family, and should aim wherever possible to maintain and support the person within their home environment.

A **transdisciplinary** approach goes beyond traditional professional boundaries to optimize the contributions of people with a range of personal and professional skills. Such an approach also facilitates collaboration with voluntary and other agencies to provide a comprehensive range of community orientated services.

An **accountable** service is one that accepts responsibility for assuring the quality of the service it delivers and monitors this in partnership with patients and their families. Such a service must be ethically and culturally sensitive.

A **systemic** approach flexibly integrates all available services to ensure continuity of care and coordinates all levels of service providers including local, provincial and national governments and community organizations.

The transdisciplinary principle needs further explanation. In less developed countries, with few professional disciplines beyond doctor and nurse, the concepts of multidisciplinary and interdisciplinary can be difficult to apply. Our Zimbabwean colleague, Dr Juliet Dube-Ndebele suggested, and the Consensus Group agreed, that the concept principle of transdisciplinary – which has the core value of transcending disciplinary boundaries to be inclusive of all available skills from professional, lay and voluntary groups – should be promoted instead of the traditional multidisciplinary or interdisciplinary principles.

Care needs

These needs include the following comprehensive list:

Prevention

There are several specific circumstances within the psychiatry of old age where preventative strategies may be useful. Vascular dementia may be prevented by appropriate measures that reduce risk of cerebrovascular accident. These include identification of those at high risk of CVA (screening for, followed by treatment of, hypertension and atrial fibrillation, early identification and good control of diabetes), low-dose aspirin and encouragement towards healthy lifestyle (diet, exercise, non-smoking). Similarly depression may be prevented by facilitating meaningful social contact and recognizing circumstances that increase individual risk (bereavement, social isolation, institution-alization, poverty). Encouraging continued social and intellectual activity in old age might protect against both depression and dementia. Recognition of impending carer burnout and provision of appropriate support can prevent crises of care.

Early identification

Early identification of mental disorders of old age (such as depression, dementia, delirium, delusional disorders, anxiety disorders, alcohol and substance abuse and dependence) may facilitate access to services and effective management and reduce stress both for the individual and the carer(s). Greater vigilance is required with certain populations who have an increased risk of depression such as those with neurological conditions, those in residential care and those who are carers, as well as those who are more likely to suicide such as those with depression, chronic pain or substance abuse. Abrupt change in behaviour or personality should alert the clinical team to the possibility of treatable mental disorder. Carers and families are in the best position to recognize such change. Screening (e.g. Mini Mental State Examination for dementia, Geriatric Depression Scale for depression) may have a role but requires training in true case recognition as well as in administration of screening instruments.

Comprehensive medical and social assessment (including diagnosis)

Wherever possible, initial assessment should be in the individual's home environment. All care professionals should be trained in comprehensive initial assessment and good record keeping. The purposes of such assessment are to identify problems (including practical difficulties), resources and needs (from the points of view of the individual and the care network), to make a working diagnosis and to generate an initial manage-ment plan (which may include further assessment or specialist referral). A diagnostic formulation is important both to allow rational care planning and to inform patients and carers as to the current situation, management options and outlook. Timely referral as appropriate (to hospital specialists, social services, voluntary organizations etc.) is integral both to the initial assessment and to subsequent management (see below).

Management (more than just treatment)

Management is more than treatment in the medical sense. A coherent and comprehen-sive care plan should critically review diagnoses and address the individual's physical, psychological, social, spiritual and material needs as well as specific psychiatric diagnoses. The needs of the carer network and of the local community must also be addressed. Progress must be monitored in follow-up and risk of relapse considered. Prophylactic treatment may play an important role. The primary goal of management is, as far as possible, to maintain or improve the quality of life of patients and their carers while respecting their autonomy. Quality management also includes special care for dying persons and their families.

Continuing care, support and review of the individual and carer(s)

Patients with severe mental illness, particularly those with dementia, may need considerable support in maintaining self-care and activities of daily living. In some cases continuous supervision may be necessary. The ability of informal carers to meet these needs, and the resultant burdens on carers, need to be monitored closely and emerging problems addressed promptly. Practical and regular help with household and personal care may considerably enhance quality of life. Counselling and emotional support for carers may play a crucial role. A proactive approach is more efficient as well as more humane than one that is crisis-driven. Emerging physical problems may require active medical treatment.

Information, advice and counselling

Patients and carers need easy access to readily understandable and accurate information concerning diagnosis, management options and implications and available support resources. Educating patients and carers and promoting discussion are important components in care planning, which may facilitate compliance, particularly in the context of long-term prophylaxis. A systematic multidisciplinary approach to record keeping and information sharing (within the confines of confidentiality) is highly desirable.

Regular breaks (respite)

The provision of breaks from caring may be crucial in enabling informal carers to continue in their caring role. Such respite may take many forms and should be as flexible and responsive as possible to individual needs and circumstances. Respite may be required at different times of day or night and may be offered both in the patient's home and in appropriate alternative settings such as day centres, day hospitals and residential facilities. Using scarce residential facilities for respite rather than exclusively for continuing care may increase their effectiveness considerably.

Advocacy

The legal rights and financial and other personal interests of such patients must be protected. Some older people with mental disorders (particularly those with dementia) may not be able to represent their interests effectively, manage their affairs or agree to what is proposed for them. This is particularly problematic for patients who are alone and where there is a conflict between individual and family interests. Patient advocates (who have neither a carer nor a service provider role for the patient concerned) may be important, as may reference to advance directives.

Residential care

Though care should be provided in patients' homes as long as possible, it must be recognized that care in an alternative residential setting may be the only way of meeting patients' needs effectively or avoiding intolerable carer burden. Such care will always be necessary, particularly for people who have no relatives available or willing to look after them.

Spiritual and leisure needs

Older people with mental health problems need the opportunity to express and discuss spiritual needs and observe their religious practices. Meaningful and appropriate recreational and leisure activities may contribute substantially to quality of life. Appropriate provision and support in these areas should be considered in both community and residential settings.

Descriptors of components of service

In this section of the document, the service components and organizational details are described.

The relationship between our patients, their families/carers and the component of the service is eloquently represented by the 'Surround with Care' idea and well illustrated by the following figure:

The minimal list of components is: (as represented by the alphabet in Figure 2.1)

- Community mental health teams for older people
- Inpatient service
- Day hospitals
- Outpatient services
- Hospital respite care
- Continuing hospital care
- Liaison services
- Primary care collaboration
- Community and social support services
- Preventative programmes

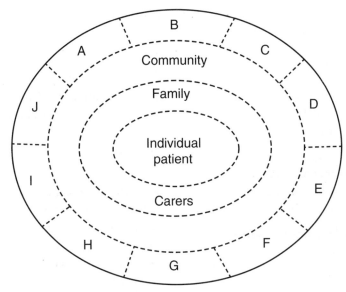

Figure 2.1 Surround with care.

Best practice

This Consensus Statement not only provides the basic framework for organization of psychogeriatric services, it can also provide the basis for the development of best practice measures and monitoring of the quality of organizational structure in the delivery of psychogeriatric services.

The listed domains can be readily converted to items for quality evaluation. For any psychogeriatric service in place or being developed, this document forms the foundation for the evaluation of quality service delivery and practice. Every health authority should benchmark and measure its performance against the principles and the domains of this document.

Conclusion

The final two paragraphs of this document (page 13) are worth reproduction here:

> The attainment of the best possible quality of life of elderly people with mental disorders and their carers is paramount and is the ultimate guiding principle in organization of care.

> Good services should always be under-pinned by good research.

Appendix

Consensus Meeting on Organization of Care in Old Age Psychiatry
    Organized by the World Psychiatric Association, Section of Geriatric Psychiatry
    Co-sponsored by the World Health Organization

Hosted by the Lausanne University Psychogeriatrics Service
Lausanne April 14–16 1997

List of participants

Alzheimer's Disease International
Dr Nori Graham, President
(Co-Rapporteur)
London, England

Swiss Alzheimer Association
Mr Oskar Diener, General Secretary
Yverdon-les-Bains, Switzerland

International Council of Nurses
Ms Anne-Francoise Dufey
Lausanne, Switzerland

International Federation of Social Workers
Ms Anne O'Loughlin
President, Irish Association of Social Workers
Dublin, Ireland

International Psychogeriatric Association
Prof. Raymond Levy, President (Chair)
London, England

International Union of Psychological Science
Prof. Kurt Pawlik, Past President
Hamburg, Germany

Lausanne University Psychogeriatric Service
Dr Vincent Camus
Lausanne, Switzerland
Dr Carlos de Mendonca Lima
Lausanne Switzerland

Medicus Mundi Internationalis
Dr Kojo Koranteng
Basel, Switzerland

World Federation for Mental Health
Ms Beverly Benson Long, President
Atlanta, USA
Prof. John R. M. Copeland
Liverpool, England

World Health Organization
Dr Jose Manoel Bertolote
Mental Disorders Control
Division of Mental Health and
Prevention of Substance Abuse
Geneva, Switzerland
Dr Juliet Dube-Ndebele
Consultant, Regional Office for Africa
Harare, Zimbabwe
Dr Helmut Sell
Regional Advisor, Health and Behaviour
Regional Office for South-East Asia
New Delhi, India

World Psychiatric Association
Prof. Norman Sartorius, President
Geneva, Switzerland
Prof. Jean Wertheimer, Chairperson
Geriatric Psychiatry Section (GPS)
Lausanne, Switzerland
Prof. Oluwafermi Agbayewa
Member, GPS
Vancouver, Canada
Professor Edmond Chiu
Member, GPS
Melbourne, Australia
Prof. Cornelius Katona
(Co-Rapporteur)
Member, GPS
London, England

Prof. Jean-Marie Leger
Member, GPS
Limoges, France

Secretariat
Mrs Suzanne Scheuner
Mrs Tina Anderson

References

Jolly, D. and Arie, T. (1992) Developments in psychogeriatric services. In T. Arie (ed.) *Recent Advances in Psychogeriatrics*, pp. 117–35. Churchill Livingstone, Edinburgh.

Pitt, B. (1982) A psychogeriatric service. In *Psychogeriatrics – an Introduction to the Psychiatry of Old Age*, 2nd edn, pp. 130–41. Churchill Livingstone: Edinburgh.

Reifler, B.V. (1997) The practice of geriatric psychiatry in three countries: observations of an American in the British Isles. *International Journal of Geriatric Psychiatry*, **12**, 795–807.

World Health Organization. (1997) *Organization of Care in Psychiatry of the Elderly – A Technical Consensus Statement*. WHO/MSA/MNH/MND/97.3. World Health Organization, Geneva. The Consensus documents are available on the WPA Website: www.wpanet.org

Chapter 3

Mental health services for older people: a developing countries perspective

Martin Prince and Peter Trebilco

Ageing in the developing world

By 1990, a clear majority (58 per cent) of the world's population aged 60 years and over was already to be found living in developing countries. By 2020 this proportion will have risen to 67 per cent. Over this period of 30 years this oldest sector of the population will have increased in number by 200 per cent in developing countries as compared to 68 per cent in the developed world (Murray and Lopez, 1996). This demographic transition will be accompanied by unprecedented economic growth and industrialization, and by profound changes in social organization and in the pattern of family life.

For older people, mental health conditions are an important cause of morbidity and premature mortality. Among the neuropsychiatric conditions, dementia and major depression were the two leading contributors accounting respectively for one quarter and one sixth of all Disease Adjusted Life Years (DALYs) in this group (Murray and Lopez, 1996). If the age-specific prevalence of dementia in developing countries matches that observed in developed countries, then by 2025 nearly three-quarters of all cases would be living in the developing world, a total of 24 million people out of the estimated 32 millions living with dementia worldwide (Prince, 1997).

Public health

In the developing world, a public health model that considers the use of population health data and the significance of the social determinants of health is an important framework for health care. 'New public health' factors emerged from the Ottawa Charter (WHO, 1986) and were described by Professor Fran Baum:

> The new public health is the *totality of the activities organised by society collectively (primarily lead by government) to protect people from disease and to promote health.* These activities occur in all sectors and will include *the adoption of policies which support health.* They will also ensure that *social, physical, economic and natural environments promote health.* The new public health is based on a belief that the *participation of communities in activities to promote health* is as essential

to the success of those activities as is the participation of experts. The new public health works to ensure that *practices of the government and private sector (including the health sector) do not detract from health and wherever possible promote health.*

Baum 1998, p. 29, emphasis added

If public health theories are to be put into policy, and health promotion activities undertaken, or if preventive operations are to be attempted, then the government, at whatever level the interventions are being planned, must have the political will to reorient supplies and services.

Services

It is easy to forget that therapeutic advances have made available to mental health practitioners several of the more efficacious interventions in biomedicine (Eisenberg, 1999). This is certainly true of old age psychiatry. For late-life depression we have antidepressants and stepped care, multidisciplinary interventions (Banerjee *et al.*, 1996; Blanchard *et al.*, 1995; Unutzer *et al.*, 2002). For dementia, psychosocial interventions for caregivers (Brodaty *et al.*, 2003b), behavioural management strategies (Brodaty *et al.*, 2003a) and the new anticholinesterase drugs (Farlow, 2002) have all been shown to be at least moderately effective. Our limitation is more in delivering effective interventions to all those who might benefit. This is most marked in developing countries, where there are very few psychiatrists or other mental health professionals. The World Health Organization (WHO) surveyed the mental health resources available for 2000 (the Year of Mental Health) and found fewer than one psychiatrist per 100,000 population across India, China and much of the rest of South and South East Asia, and fewer than one psychiatrist per million population in most of sub-Saharan Africa (WHO Atlas Project, 2002). The WHO has called the mismatch between the need for interventions and the limited resources to implement them the 'Mental Health Gap'. Arguably, the dearth of specialist services in the developing world is such that they will not, for the foreseeable future, be able to provide any kind of accessible national specialist service. The WHO's recommendation is that mental health services be organized at the level of primary care, but this has been little implemented. Centralized hospital-based services provide limited care to small numbers of patients with serious mental illness; for the rest the burden of care falls upon the family, the community, and traditional healers. Awareness and understanding of common mental disorders is low at all levels of society. People with mental illness are often stigmatized, and neither recognized nor treated appropriately by health services.

Economic challenges

Table 3.1 lists the population, per capita GDP, adjusted life expectancy and literacy from selected countries. The overall picture is challenging. The low annual income of individuals from countries such as Bangladesh, Ethiopia, and India means that the standard of living of the great majority of the persons in these populous parts of the

Table 3.1 Population size, income, life expectancy and literacy levels in twelve selected countries

Country	Population millions[a] ($US)[a]	GDP per capita	Adjusted life expectancy[b]	Literacy per cent[a]
Bangladesh	138.4	1700	49.9	43
Brazil	182.0	7600	59.1	86
China	1287.0	4400	62.3	86
Ethiopia	66.6	750	33.5	43
India	1049.7	2540	53.2	60
Indonesia	234.9	3100	59.7	89
Japan	127.2	28000	74.5	99
Mexico	104.9	9000	65.0	92
Nicaragua	5.1	2500	58.1	68
Russian Federation	144.5	9300	61.3	99
Taiwan	22.6	18000	74.0[a]	86
USA	290.3	37600	70.0	97

[a]Data are from 2003 CIA World Fact Book accessed on http://www.theodora.com/wfb2003/

[b]Data are from World Health Organization (2000) Disability adjusted healthy lifestyle expectancy at birth table (www.photius.com/rankings/healthy_life-table2.html)

world will have poor diet, infectious diseases and often dangerous working and living environments. Table 3.1 also shows estimates of life expectancy in the same countries. If so few will reach the ages when diseases of old age could be expected to manifest themselves, the target populations for psychogeriatric services will be comparatively small and there will be less demand on clinical, welfare and other social resources. Just because there is a small percentage of a population does not excuse governments from responsibility, but requirements for the considerable costs of efficacious services will be smaller than for those countries with a larger elderly population.

Service development

An unconsidered imposition of western models of care on developing countries would be highly inappropriate, and unlikely to succeed. New service development needs to recognize the sociocultural and regional factors that modulate health perceptions, illness presentations, and interactions between the potential consumers and providers of health care services (Patel, 2003). A 'health systems approach' involves first a careful analysis of these factors; local socio-demography, patterns of disease, culturally determined beliefs and practices, existing resources, prevailing government policy and macro and microeconomics. This analysis should then inform the prioritization, design and delivery of new services. In most developing countries, there is, as a rule, little if any formal health or social welfare provision, coupled with a heavy reliance on informal care from families. However, within this broad generalization there are important regional and cultural variations.

A health systems approach

What then are the contextual factors, knowledge of which should shape the development of responsive mental health services for older people in developing countries?

Attitudes towards older people

In many developing countries older persons are accorded great respect, both within the extended families that they head, and in society as a whole. In Ghana for example, the aged enjoy high status as mediators and experts on social problems, folklore and tradition. 'The elderly were regarded as a symbol of deity, an affront to an older person was an affront to the gods requiring costly expiation' (Apt, 1996).

This system of beliefs is widely held across the African continent. In south-eastern Asia the Confucian moral principle of supporting, loving and respecting the elderly is traditionally rooted in the family and practised throughout society, not only in China and Chinese-dominated societies but also, for example, in Japan and Thailand (Phillips, 2000). The related concept of 'filial piety' demands respect, honour and duty of care from the son towards the parents. In India also, older persons are venerated, a typical formulation being that 'parents are next to God. The family must respect and treat them well' (Patel and Prince, 2001). Others though have identified an inherent fatalism in traditional Indian attitudes towards ageing. The Hindi phrase *sathiyana*, customarily translated as senility, more literally means 'sixtyish' (Cohen, 1995). Dravidian languages have similar constructs, simultaneously conveying the concept of advanced chronological age and inevitable decline (Shaji *et al.*, 2002b). The final stages in the classical cycle of life, Vanaprastha and Sanyasa, encourage a 'disengagement' of older persons allowing both preparation for death and a seamless intergenerational transfer of goods, property and power. Proper observance of Vanaprastha was said to require two things (Dandekar, 1996): a) while handing over the household responsibility, one should go and live like a rishi, and b) leaving the son in charge, one should go to the forest to pray. Such disengagement is rare in practice. However, for older Indians the sociological and psychological influence of these principles is acknowledged still to be profound and pervasive (Rao, 1986). Indeed, viewed through this prism, western sensibilities can seem mystifying to Indian commentators:

> People (in rural India) are not scared of death. They take it as inevitable. Lacking medication for illness in old age, there is relatively less medicated survival compared to the situation in the industrially advanced world. The nursing homes of the West sometimes give the impression that they are waiting rooms for the dead before they are buried. Lying in their beds with a variety of tubes in their bodies they make a tragic picture of the attempts of modern medication to ward off death …. Another limitation of medication is that it raises hopes that death

can be sidestepped. This has such a pitiable effect on people's attitudes that in certain societies even the terminally ill elderly have to be trained to face inevitable death.

Dandekar, 1996

Of course, attitudes towards ageing are not a constant. In focus group discussions carried out in South India many older participants felt that respect for them was on the wane (Patel and Prince, 2001): 'the values that were taught by our elders about oneself and towards others are now being purposely forgotten resulting in more hardships in later life and less respect towards older people'.

The younger generation were reported not to enjoy the company of the older generation in social gatherings and tended to avoid them. Some older people remarked that nowadays their married children 'told them what to do'. In Japan also it has been suggested that 'respect for the elderly may be more symbolic than substantial'. Recent research suggests a preponderance of negative over positive stereotypes (Phillips, 2000).

Living arrangements

The living arrangements of older people vary dramatically across the globe. These cannot, however, be stereotyped in terms of straightforward regional or developed/developing country differences. Instead cultural influences seem to predominate. In most developing countries older people, whether or not widowed, typically live with their families in multi-generational households. The concept of living alone is alien and dreaded. For example 96 per cent of older Chinese and 88 per cent of Ghanaians live with younger relatives. However, in Japan, a highly industrialized and economically developed country, until recently, 87 per cent of older people also lived with younger relatives. Conversely, in the UK, only 25 per cent of older persons live with younger family members, and most live alone (35 per cent) or with their spouse (40 per cent). Most of those who live alone do so because they are widowed. While such countries are generally economically developed, it seems that their nuclear family structures predated the industrial revolution. In the UK historical evidence suggests that extended multi-generational family units have always been the exception, children always having tended to leave home and set up their own household when they marry. For young and old alike, the independence that comes from having one's own household is greatly valued.

In many developing countries traditional family and kinship structures are widely perceived as under threat from the social and economic changes that accompany economic development and globalization (Tout, 1989).

1. Changing attitudes towards older people, as described above, are certainly one factor.

2. The education of women and their increasing participation in the workforce (generally seen as key positive development indicators) are another; tending to reduce both their availability for caregiving and their willingness to take on this additional role.

3. Migration is another issue; populations are increasingly mobile as education, cheap travel and flexible labour markets induce children to migrate to cities and abroad to seek work. In India, Venkoba Rao has coined an acronym to describe this growing social phenomenon – PICA, Parents in India, Children Abroad. 'Push factors' are also important – in the economic catastrophe of the 1980s 2 million Ghanaians left the country in search of economic betterment. Sixty-three per cent of older persons have lost the support of one or more of their children who have migrated to distant places in Ghana or abroad.

4. Declining fertility in the course of the final demographic transition has also had an impact. Its effects are perhaps most evident in China where the one-child family law leaves increasing numbers of older people, particularly those with a daughter, bereft of family support.

5. In sub-Saharan Africa changing patterns of morbidity and mortality are more relevant; the ravages of the HIV/AIDS epidemic has 'orphaned' parents as well as children, as bereaved older persons are robbed of the expectation of economic and practical support into later life.

Family support

All over the world the family remains the cornerstone of care for older people who have lost the capacity for independent living, whether as a result of dementia or other mental disorder. However, stereotypes abound and have the potential to mislead. Thus, in developed countries with their comprehensive health and social care systems the vital caring role of families, and their need for support, is often overlooked. This is true for example in the UK, where despite nuclear family structures and contrary to supposition, there is a strong tradition which persists today for local children to provide support for their infirm parents. Conversely, in developing countries the reliability and universality of the family care system is often overestimated. Older people are among the most vulnerable groups in the developing world, in part because of the continuing myths that surround their place in society (Tout, 1989). It is often assumed that their welfare is assured by the existence of the extended family. Arguably, the greatest obstacle to providing effective support and care for older persons with mental illness and their families in developing countries is the lack of awareness of the problem amongst policy makers, health care providers and the community. Mythologizing the caring role of the family evidently carries the risk of perpetuating complacency.

The 10/66 Dementia Research Group's multicentre pilot study is the first systematic, comprehensive assessment of care arrangements for people with dementia in the developing world, and of the impacts upon their family caregivers (The 10/66 Dementia Research Group, 2004). As in the EUROCARE study with data from 14 European countries (Schneider et al., 1999), most caregivers in developing countries were older women caring for their husbands or younger women caring for a parent.

Caring was associated with substantial psychological strain as evidenced by high rates of psychiatric morbidity and high levels of caregiver strain. These parameters were again very similar to those reported in the EUROCARE study. However, some aspects were radically different. People with dementia in developing countries typically live in large households, with extended families. Larger families were associated with lower caregiver strain; however, this effect was small, applied only where the principal caregiver was co-resident and indeed seemed to operate in the opposite direction where the caregiver is non-resident, perhaps because of the increased potential for family conflict.

Government policy – the role of state vs. the role of family

There is a tendency for governments that have less developed centralized welfare and benefit systems to bolster traditional family care arrangements through coercive legislation or fiscal or social incentives. Thus, in the People's Republic of China, the Communist Party has enshrined the Confucian principle in the 1980 Marriage Law giving parents who have lost the ability to earn the right to claim support from their children. Breaches are theoretically punishable by up to five years imprisonment. In Japan, the legal sanction compelling children to care for parents has only recently been repealed. Social incentives have also been popular in South-East Asia. In Japan, the government still exhorts families to care for older persons 'who have created our prosperity' and provides incentives including tax breaks for family caregivers of those over 70 and loans for home modifications. In countries with social housing programmes such as Singapore and Hong Kong SAR, family caregivers of older persons find themselves prioritized on the housing waiting list. Even within the European Union, government policy varies widely from states that assume a statutory responsibility to provide comprehensive care on demand (e.g. some Scandinavian countries) to those that provide negligible services and place a legal responsibility on families to provide financial and practical support (e.g. some southern European countries).

Sources of income for older people

It is unlikely that governments in developing regions will be able in the near future to raise general standards of income to levels that ensure universal good nutrition, adequate housing, employment and social stability for the whole population. Population growth – Calhoun (1997) estimates the world average as 15.7 per cent – outstrips economic growth (ranging between 1.0 per cent and 13.3 per cent in 1997). Furthermore, the least developed regions that have the greatest population growth tend to have relatively stagnating economies. Therefore poverty will remain, and income differentials between the least and most developed regions are forecast to grow. Redistributive efforts, through international aid, the International Monetary Fund and the World Bank will have minimal impact.

Many, but by no means all, economically developed countries have made provision for universal pension schemes, disability living allowances, and caregiver benefits. These can make a crucial contribution to easing the plight of people with dementia, and those who care for them. In low-income countries a small minority of older persons has even a basic subsistence pension, and more comprehensive schemes are unlikely to be feasible in the near future under even the most optimistic predictions. This is unfortunate, for an older person's pension, however nugatory, can make an important guaranteed contribution to the family budget.

For these reasons, older people in developing countries often work for as long as their health permits. In 1990, the UN estimated that in developing regions of the world 45 per cent of those aged 60–64 years and 28 per cent of those aged 65 years or over were engaged in remunerated work. This figure, if anything underestimates the true extent of their economic productivity; many are involved in part-time or informal employment, which is often under-reported. Additionally they contribute to an important but unquantified extent to their family's broader welfare. They may supervise grandchildren while parents work, they care for adult children with congenital disabilities, they engage in voluntary work and in informal education of younger generations. With the onset of disability, older people are instead dependent on their children for housing, food, and money, as well as personal care. One of the key findings from the 10/66 Dementia Research group's caregiver pilot study (The 10/66 Dementia Research Group, 2004), is that caregiving in the developing world is associated with substantial economic disadvantage. A high proportion of caregivers have had to cut back on their paid work to care. Many caregivers need and obtain additional support, and while this is often informal unpaid care from friends and other family members, paid caregivers are also relatively common. People with dementia in developing countries are heavy users of health services, and associated direct costs are high. Compensatory financial support is negligible; few older people in developing countries receive government or occupational pensions, and virtually none of the people with dementia in this study received disability pensions. Caregivers are commonly in paid employment, and almost none received any form of caregiver allowance. The combination of reduced family incomes and increased family expenditure on care is obviously particularly stressful in lower income countries where so many households exist at or near to subsistence level. This may be literally beyond the limited resources of some families. In the absence of a safety net, lack of family support arising from whatever cause can be catastrophic. Indigence is a clear and documented problem among older persons in many developing countries (Tout, 1989). The extent to which people with dementia suffer this fate is as yet unknown.

Knowledge, attitudes and beliefs

Alzheimer's Disease International and its member national societies have identified raising awareness of dementia among the general community and among health workers as a global priority (Graham and Brodaty, 1997). There has been relatively little formal study of the extent of awareness in developing countries. One index is that of media coverage. In one of its earliest ventures, the 10/66 Dementia Research Group reported a search of Indian broadsheet newspapers (*The Times of India* and the *Hindu*), which failed to unearth a single article about the disease (The 10/66 Dementia Research Group, 2000). While much remains to be done the growth of awareness in some developed countries has been striking: in the UK, a similar search of the columns of just one national newspaper revealed 57 articles over an 18 month period, covering dementia from many different perspectives. Knowledge, attitudes and beliefs can also be accessed through qualitative research studies. Three recent studies from India tend to agree regarding the extent of awareness in the different communities studied (with a mixture of focus group discussion and open-ended interviews) (Patel and Prince, 2001; Cohen, 1995; Shaji *et al.*, 2002b). First, the typical features of dementia are widely recognized, and indeed named 'Chinnan' (literally childishness) in Malyalam language in Kerala (Shaji *et al.*, 2002b), 'nerva frakese' (tired brain) in Konkani language in Goa (Patel and Prince, 2001), and 'weak brain' in Hindi in Banares (Cohen, 1995). However, in none of these settings was there any awareness of dementia as an organic brain syndrome, or indeed as any kind of medical condition. Rather it was perceived as a normal, anticipated part of ageing. In Goa the likely causes were cited as 'neglect by family members, abuse, tension and lack of love' (Patel and Prince, 2001). In Kerala it was reported that most caregivers tended to misinterpret symptoms of the disease and to designate these as deliberate misbehaviour by the person with dementia (Shaji *et al.*, 2002b).

This general lack of awareness has important consequences. First, there is no structured training on the recognition and management of dementia at any level of the health service. Second, in the absence of understanding regarding its origins dementia is stigmatized, for example sufferers are specifically excluded from residential care, and often denied admission to hospital facilities. Third, there is no constituency to place pressure on the government or policy-makers to start to provide more responsive dementia care services (Shaji *et al.*, 2002b). Fourth, while families are the main caregivers, they must do so with little or no support or understanding from other individuals or agencies. Cohen (1995), on the evidence of his research in Banares, speaks of the 'outsider narrative' for dementia, that is the explanation of a neighbour, relative or passer by as

> that the old person receives inadequate respect or support from a particular child. Family members will be far more likely to speak of weak brain, when they speak of it at all as a natural phenomenon, as but old age. Certain kinds of behaviors of old persons, particularly yelling and wandering, are difficult to contain within household space and, when associated with accusations of mistreatment, ultimately require alternative explanations from family insiders against the outside narrative of the Bad Family.

This construction is a counterpoint to the suggestion from Goa that dementia is associated with, indeed caused by, family neglect. Behavioural symptoms of dementia;

wandering, calling out, making accusations; may be taken by outsiders as prima facie evidence of neglect or abuse. Caregivers then face a double jeopardy, the strain of care heightened by the stigma and blame that attaches to them because of the disturbed behaviour of their relative. This notion is supported by the open-ended responses of some caregivers to the question 'What do you find most difficult about looking after your relative?'

> Family members think we are the cause for his illness – they think we deserve all that is happening to us. Other than family, we don't really care.
>
> Caregiver, Bangalore, India

> She keeps wanting to go home. She feels cheated and deceived. She behaves like a child and greets me instead of me greeting her. She behaves embarrassingly. We continue locking the door every time. We feel ashamed; it is a useless life.
>
> Caregiver, Anambra, Nigeria

Such evidence argues powerfully for the benefits of broad dissemination of appropriately structured information about dementia (The 10/66 Dementia Research Group, in press).

Community services

Until recently there has been surprisingly little information regarding the nature of services available for people with dementia in developing countries, the extent of help-seeking and the effectiveness of care. Even now with the rising interest in epidemiological research, generalizable quantitative data are not available. Nevertheless, it seems clear that dementia in the developing world tends to be a hidden problem. Perceived to be part of normal ageing and not a health condition, affected families rarely present to health services who are ignorant of most cases in their community. However, lack of help-seeking should not be presumed to reflect a lack of need; K. S. Shaji, working with the 10/66 Dementia Research Group in Kerala, Southern India, commented of the caregivers of the 17 older persons with dementia:

> Many caregivers expressed a wish to know more about the disease and its management. Most said that they would be interested to attend meetings of support groups or training programs for caregivers. However, none of the people with dementia was in regular contact with any health care facility. Visits to outpatient care facilities were perceived as neither feasible nor useful. None of the caregivers ever received any advice from anybody regarding management of their relatives at home. They said that they were learning from their own experience and were unhappy not to be receiving any help from health professionals. They had not come into contact with any non-governmental or governmental agency that offered special services for people suffering from dementia.
>
> Shaji et al., 2002a

In Goa too, unsurprisingly perhaps, given the fatalistic view of 'brain weakness', primary health care doctors said that they were not consulted, and had little or no direct experience of the problem in their community (Patel and Prince, 2001).

This experience contrasted with that of the local multi-purpose health workers, who both recognized the dementia vignette and identified many of their active community caseload as sufferers. Thus, both in Goa and Kerala, there was little evidence of active help-seeking by families in need. While normalization of the experience of dementia may provide part of the explanation, it is also the case that developing country health services are generally ill-equipped to meet the needs of older persons. Health care, even at the primary care level is clinic-based; the older person must attend the clinic, often involving a long journey and waiting time in the clinic, to receive care. Even if they can get to the clinic the assessment and treatment that they receive is orientated towards acute rather than chronic conditions. The perception is that the former may be treatable, the latter intractable and not within the realm of responsibility of health services. Indeed in the experience of the author, the diagnosis of dementia is often made specifically to exclude older persons from receiving care. Thus, for example, in a Soweto township, nurses in a community clinic were trained to discriminate between dementia and delirium. Cases of delirium were referred to hospital for treatment of the underlying acute disorder whereas cases of dementia were returned home for family care. In Goa, psychiatry interns were advised not to admit older people with dementia for fear that their families might be reluctant to take them back.

The 10/66 Dementia Research Group's caregiver pilot study (2004) indicated that people with dementia were using primary and secondary care health services. Only 33 per cent of people with dementia in India, 11 per cent in China and SE Asia and 18 per cent in Latin America had used no health services at all in the previous three months. In all centres, particularly in India and Latin America, there was heavy use of private medical services. The economic strain arising from use of health services was unevenly distributed. Thus, while health care services are cheaper in low income countries, in relative terms families from the poorer countries spent a greater proportion of their income on health care for the person with dementia. They also tended selectively to use the more expensive services of private doctors. One may speculate that this reflects the caregivers' perception of the relative unresponsiveness of the cheaper government medical services.

Residential care

Residential care homes are widespread in many developed countries, where as many as one half of all those with dementia may be cared for in these settings. As yet they are rare in developing countries; governments, as part of their policy to bolster traditional family care arrangements, have either not encouraged or officially discouraged their development. However, in the most rapidly developing regions, their numbers are rising fast. In the initial stages of their development homes are run by government or by charities to cater for those few older persons who have no family to care for them. In India (Patel and Prince, 2001) older persons entered such homes when they are relatively well, usually because they lacked a family to care for them in the event of deteriorating health, or because they feared becoming a burden on their relatives, feared inadequate support, and therefore wished to maintain their independence from the family. This constellation has been reported in two previous Indian ethnographic studies (Cohen, 1995; Vatuk, 1990): it has been referred to as 'dependency anxiety' (Vatuk, 1990) and differentiated from what Vatuk terms 'Western feelings of guilt and low self-worth associated with the shame of dependence upon one's children'. In Goa, residents of old age homes described their reasons for moving into residential care (Patel and Prince, 2001).

> In a few cases chronic deteriorating health or acute episodes of illness were mentioned as reasons for admission. However in many cases the older persons were in good health, and 'approaching age' or worries about ability to look after oneself in the future underpinned the move. Many of the residents had no family to look after them. One lady for example, had two daughters who died when they were young; she fell ill, and having no one too look after her, her neighbours admitted her to the home. However, many had family who were either unwilling or unable to support them. This theme was reflected in the many residents who complained that their family never visited them after their admission to the home. Several reasons were cited for the withdrawal of family support. In some cases children had migrated abroad. In several cases the resident had quarreled with family members. Others reported that families did not want to care for older persons because of the 'financial burden' of doing so. 'Nobody wishes to care for old folk if they have no money.' Residents had experienced being 'shuffled from family to family'; at least in the old age home they had security. Many residents expressed bewilderment that their families seemed to have forgotten them after their admission.

Goan old age homes, as a rule, did not admit those with permanent disabilities and specifically excluded those with dementia. Thus, there was no local continuing care provision for those with dementia, or for those who lacked both family support and financial means (Patel and Prince, 2001). The homes themselves were adequate in some respects but concerns were expressed about the isolation of residents from their families and from their local community, and at the lack of structured activities. These homes undoubtedly represent a transitional phase in what is likely to become an extended network of public and private sector facilities.

The way ahead
Awareness

Many of the most important priorities with respect to improving mental health care for older persons impinge only indirectly upon service development and improvement. They have more to do with creating the climate that fosters such advances. Alzheimer's Disease International, the international non-governmental organization that supports people with dementia and their caregivers worldwide, has contributed enormously over the last decade. Its role has been to build and strengthen Alzheimer associations throughout the world, so they are better able to meet the needs of people with dementia and their families. It now has 64 national members, an increase of 50 per cent in less than a decade, with most new members being developing country associations. National associations create a framework for positive engagement between clinicians, researchers, caregivers and people with dementia. They raise funds, disseminate information, and act as powerful advocates with government, policymakers and media. World Alzheimer's Day, on 21 September each year is a cornerstone of the campaign to 'name the condition', improving awareness of dementia as a health condition. Better awareness is a necessary precondition for appropriate help-seeking, and lack of awareness is a public health problem for which population level interventions of this kind are most appropriate.

A role for research

The 10/66 Dementia Research Group is a network of researchers from developing countries that draws attention through its title to the relative paucity of population-based research into dementia in the developing world. Only 10 per cent of research effort is targeted at those developing regions where currently two-thirds of those with the disorder are thought to live (The 10/66 Dementia Research Group, 2000). More good quality epidemiological and health services research, appropriately disseminated, can help to generate awareness, shape health and social policy, and encourage the development of better services for those with mental disorders and their caregivers (Jenkins, 1998). In a consensus statement, the 10/66 Group highlighted two processes in particular by which well conducted research might inform policy (The 10/66 Dementia Research Group, 2000):

1. By estimating the magnitude of the problem through local epidemiological studies. These would inevitably have greater impact on regional policy-makers, garner more publicity and create more awareness than would projections based upon prevalence data from elsewhere applied to local population distributions.

2. By emphasizing the impact on family and other informal carers. A widely accepted notion within society of the family as endlessly supportive caregivers allows governments to continue to accord a low priority to the needs of older people with dementia and other disabling conditions. Assumptions of this kind may be challenged, usefully, by descriptive studies of care arrangements for older people. Even where care is exemplary, it is essential that the impact of providing care on the family, and on the wider community be quantified. Impact should be considered in practical, psychological and in economic terms. Data of this kind provide an evidence base for the coming debate on the relative role of state and family, formal and informal care. Strong and effective arguments can be mounted for community support services for people with dementia and their caregivers. Again, it is desirable that any new services that are developed as demonstration projects be assessed for effectiveness and cost-effectiveness.

Specialist services

Biomedical practitioners in developing countries are understandably drawn to the rapidly evolving clinical discipline of dementia care. Many also develop research interests and are keen to contribute to the growing literature. Centres of excellence have been and will continue to be established in prestigious national and regional institutions. Such initiatives, possibly including memory clinics, neuroimaging and other technical diagnostics, and multidisciplinary expertise are generally to be welcomed. They have an important role in raising awareness often out of all proportion to the cover of the service that they are able to deliver. Quite apart from their visibility to policy-makers they can play a key role in exposing generations of doctors and paramedical staff to training and experience in this field. The problem arises if this model is seen as the end rather than the beginning of service development. The model is simply not generalizable; the severe resource limitations with respect to specialist doctors, indeed with respect to doctors of any kind, will mean that the needs of only a tiny proportion of the population of people with dementia will be met in this way. The limited resource of specialist doctors must also be used to lead the development of feasible frameworks for national service delivery, focusing upon existing community health resources.

Primary care and community services

Many developing countries have in place some comprehensive community-based primary care systems staffed by doctors, nurses and generic multi-purpose health workers. There is certainly a need here for more training in the basic curriculum to move beyond the current preoccupation with prevention and simple curative interventions. The resource implications of chronic disease management may be enormous; however, every developed country has seen increasing proportions of its health budgets consumed in this way. Developing countries such as India and China, witnessing previously unprecedented rates of demographic ageing, are certain to be profoundly affected, the only question being the extent to which they are able to manage the change.

Four community-based initiatives in Southern India suggest some sustainable models.

Dementia case-finding in Kerala

Minimally trained locally based community multi-purpose health workers (MPHWs) are a core component of many developing country health services. The role of the MPHW is principally preventative, the focus being upon child and maternal health, infectious diseases, nutrition and reproductive health. Previous research had indicated that MPHWs were aware of the problems of the elderly but 'were not adequately trained or officially expected to deliver any services in these fields' (Nair *et al.*, 2001). However, this is at least an outreach service; they visit many if not most homes in their catchment area district on a regular basis, and politeness demands that they enquire after the health of older family members. In Goa, it was the MPHWs, rather than the clinic-based primary care doctors who were aware of cases of dementia in the community (Patel and Prince, 2001). They are thus potentially well-placed to act as key informants in the identification of older persons with dementia. In Kerala, Southern India, MPHWs (known in India as Anganwadi workers) after a half day training session covering typical dementia presentations, were able to draw up a list of possibly affected older persons. Two-thirds were subsequently found to be suffering from DSM IV dementia, while others had other chronic mental health conditions with associated unmet need (Shaji *et al.*, 2002a). In the pilot study it was possible to secure the cooperation of MPHWs with only a small financial incentive. Since the Integrated Child Development Scheme operates across India, this dementia case identification strategy could be generalized nationwide. Identification of cases creates the potential for intervention after assessment of unmet need.

The 10/66 Dementia Research Group Indian network's caregiver intervention

The 10/66 DRG in India has developed a brief caregiver education and training intervention to be administered by Anganwadi and other MPHWs after further training. The fully manualized intervention is delivered in five half-hour sessions. It is designed to provide family caregivers with information about the dementia syndrome, and training in strategies to better manage common behavioural problems at home. After an initial assessment with the main caregiver, all extended family members are encouraged to attend so that the family shares knowledge and understanding of the process, and so that the supportive function of the family network can be maximized. The intervention is supported by cartoon drawings summarizing some of the basic educational messages, to be used as drop off material particularly for families with low levels of literacy. The effectiveness of the intervention is to be tested in randomized controlled trials in Chennai and Vellore in Southern India, and in adapted versions in the Dominican Republic, Moscow and Beijing.

A flexible homecare intervention in Goa

Goa is one of India's most economically developed and demographically aged states with 8 per cent of the population aged 65 or over. There are an estimated three thousand persons with dementia. For affected families home care is already a relatively popular option. Traditionally these services are provided by young female nurses from another southern Indian state. There are limitations, however. Only full time employment is possible. The nurse comes to live with the family and only nursing care is provided: support with cooking, cleaning, washing and other domiciliary support must be provided by a female member of the family. Indeed a female member of the family must be available at all times to chaperone the young nurse. Perhaps most importantly the young nurses have no training in or experience of dementia care. The Sangath Child and Family NGO, working with the Goa Chapter of ARDSI, India's national Alzheimer's Association, has developed a flexible homecare programme in which a cohort of local dementia nurses and homecare workers will be specially trained. These may then be employed by local families to provide care inputs according to need (for example twilight care for those with mobility impairment, daytime respite for working caregivers). The service is supported by a 36-bed dementia care home for respite care and assessment. The cost-effectiveness of the new intervention is to be assessed in a randomized controlled trial.

Comprehensive community care models

There are as yet very few examples of integrated community oriented programmes seeking to provide comprehensive dementia care for whole populations. It is no accident that two should come from Kerala, the southern Indian state where the focus upon education and funding of public medical services has resulted in a life expectancy of 70 for men and 74 in women, even though the per capita GDP is only around the norm for India. ARDSI is based in Cochin, Kerala. Under the leadership of Dr Jacob Roy it has pioneered the development of memory clinics (diagnosis), day care centres (respite care), Geriatric nurse training centres (homecare), guidance and counselling (caregiver education) and caregiver support groups. Professor K. S. Shaji, the convenor of the Indian Psychiatric Society's Geriatric Psychiatry Interest Group has detected that decentralized planning, under the new panchaythi raj system of governance in Kerala, has enabled the development and implementation of programmes at the local level. This has given opportunities to develop and test models for dementia care. One such initiative is in progress at the Talikulam Rural Development Block in the Thrissur District of Kerala. A monthly dementia care clinic is established in the Primary Health centre where a neurologist and a psychiatrist liaise with primary care staff. The catchment area population is about one hundred thousand of whom ten thousand are aged sixty years or more.

Residential care

Good quality, well-regulated residential care has a role to play in all societies, for those with no family supports, and for those where family support capacity is exhausted, both as temporary respite and for provision of longer-term care. Absence of regulation, staff training and quality assurance is a serious concern in developed and developing countries alike. Important priorities would include a system of registration and inspection of homes, training of careworkers, and provision of medical services for residents.

Equity

The gross disparities in resources within and between developed and developing countries are leading to serious concerns regarding the flouting of the central ethical principle of distributive justice. The globalization of biomedicine has in part accounted for the emergence of both awareness of the problem and tensions between the previously relatively isolated health systems. Aged care programmes in the west are increasingly dependent upon migrant careworkers and trained nursing staff recruited directly from developing countries to fill low pay jobs. Conversely the costs of therapeutic interventions, particularly new drugs, are often simply beyond the means of health care systems in the developing world. These are rising fast as the pharmaceutical companies seek to recoup the huge research and development costs associated with bringing new 'smart drugs' to the market. The geopolitical and economic significance of the ensuing disputes is signified by the controversy over the treatment of HIV/AIDS in South Africa. When President Mandela declared a public health emergency to permit use of much cheaper generic alternatives to the standard and effective triple therapy, US Vice President Al Gore sided with the pharmaceutical companies in their attempt to enforce their patent rights. New drug treatments in psychiatry are also very expensive. Anticholinesterase therapies for Alzheimer's disease are beyond the reach of all but the richest families in most developing countries. The same would be true for most SSRI antidepressants and 'atypical' antipsychotic drugs, each of which are generally favoured in the West for use in older patients over the older and cheaper tricyclic antidepressants and 'typical' antipsychotic drugs because of their better safety and side-effect profiles. The advent of a disease-modifying, as opposed to symptomatic treatment for Alzheimer's disease, would introduce similar ethical concerns regarding accessibility to those that have arisen in relation to the management of HIV/AIDS in low income countries.

Equity is also an important issue *within* developing countries. Access to care is often entirely dependent upon means to pay. Quite apart from economic constraints, health care resources are grossly unevenly distributed between rural and urban districts. Most specialists, indeed most doctors, work in cities. Provision of even basic services to far-flung rural communities is an enormous challenge. We have seen earlier in this chapter the potential power of demonstration projects and centres of excellence as pathfinder services. A counter-argument would be that such new developments entrench existing inequities and draw resources away from cheaper public health initiatives whose benefits could be distributed more generally. Some low income countries with particularly striking achievements in health service development (Cuba is one example) have made it a principle that no service development be introduced in one area, or for one sector of the population that could not be introduced for all. Finally, it is clear that for a variety of reasons, in many parts of the world, older people do not have the same access to health care as do younger people. Intriguingly, the WHO's Global Burden of Disease report is itself intrinsically ageist (Murray and Lopez, 1996). A year of life lived in older age is accorded only approximately half the value of that of one lived in 'one's prime'. The net result is that the impact of diseases of ageing, particularly dementia, is greatly underestimated.

Ways to resolve limited funds and growing demands

The new public health is the totality of the activities organized by society collectively (primarily led by government) to protect people from disease and to promote health. Practices of the government and private sector (including the health sector) do not detract from health and wherever possible promote health.

Baum, 1998, p. 510

Society and government have essential roles to play in cohesive and comprehensive policy development and service delivery. Such policies need to strike an appropriate balance between those which seek to promote health and prevent disease (or in the case of dementia, delay its onset) and those which seek to cure or alleviate suffering through treatment or provision of support services. Social medicine is defined as: 'an approach to the prevention and treatment of disease that is based on the study of human heredity, environment, social structures, and cultural values' (Glanz, 1990, p. 304). Prevention, where it can be achieved, is clearly the best option, with enormous potential benefits for the quality of life of the individual, for family and carers, and for society as a whole. Primary preventive interventions can be highly cost-effective. 'The management of neurodegenerative disease is a major challenge for health care systems around the globe. Costs in the United States are estimated at between A\$40,000 and A\$50,000 per person per annum – US \$100bn in total each year. North American and European studies point to the concentration of huge costs in residential care services as well as upon informal family carers, and the potentially enormous cost-savings of postponing the severity of the disease' (Access Economics, 2003, p. 31). The primary prevention of dementia is therefore a relatively neglected area. Evidence from the developed world suggests that risk factors for vascular disease, including hypertension, smoking, type II diabetes, and hypercholesterolaemia may all be risk factors for Alzheimer's Disease as well as vascular dementia. The epidemic of smoking in developing countries, and the high and rising prevalence of type II diabetes in south and South-East Asia should therefore be particular causes of concern.

The Indian examples cited above demonstrate that development of mental health services for older people needs to be tailored to suit the health systems context. 'Health systems' here can be taken to include macroeconomic factors, social structures, cultural values and norms, and existing health and welfare policy and provision. For many low-income countries the most cost-effective way to manage chronic conditions in older people will be through supporting, educating and advising family caregivers. This may be supplemented by home nursing or paid homecare workers; however, to date most of the growth in this area has been that of untrained paid carers operating in the private sector. The direct and indirect costs of care in this model therefore tend to fall upon the family. Some governmental input whether in terms of allowances for people with dementia and/or caregivers, or subsidized care would be desirable and equitable. The next level of care to be prioritized would be respite care, both in day centres and (for longer periods) in residential or nursing homes. Such facilities (as for example is envisaged in Goa, above) could act also as training resource centres for caregivers. Day care and residential respite care are more expensive than home care, but nevertheless basic to a community's needs, particularly for people with more advanced dementia.

Residential care for older people is unlikely to be a priority for government investment, when the housing conditions of the general population remain poor, with homelessness, overcrowding and poor sanitation. Nevertheless, even in some of the poorest developing countries (e.g. China and India), nursing and residential care homes are opening up in the private sector to meet the demand from the growing affluent middle class. Similarly, low income countries lack the economic and human capital to contemplate widespread introduction of more sophisticated services; specialist multidisciplinary staff and community services backed up with memory clinics, outpatient, inpatient and day care facilities. Nevertheless, services comprising some of these elements are being established as demonstration projects (see the example of Kerala, above). The ethics of health care do require that governments take initial planning steps, now. The one certainty is that 'in the absence of clear strategies and policies, the old will absorb increasing proportions of the resources devoted to health care in developing countries' (Kalache, 1991). This shift in resource expenditure is of course likely to occur regardless. At least, if policies are well formulated, its consequences can be predicted and mitigated.

References

Access Economics Pty Ltd (2003) *The Dementia Epidemic: Economic Impact and Positive Solutions for Australia.* Prepared for Alzheimer's Australia, Canberra, Access Economics Pty Ltd.

Apt, N.A. (1996) *Coping with Old Age in a Changing Africa.* Aveburey, Aldershot.

Banerjee, S., Shamash, K., Macdonald, A.J.D., and Mann, A.H. (1996) Randomised controlled trial of effect of intervention by psychogeriatric team on depression in frail elderly people at home. *BMJ* **313**, 1058–61.

Baum, F. (1998) *The New Public Health: an Australian Perspective.* Oxford University Press, South Melbourne.

Blanchard, M.R., Waterreus, A., and Mann, A.H. (1995) The effect of primary care nurse intervention upon older people screened as depressed. *International Journal of Geriatric Psychiatry*, **10**, 289–98.

Brodaty, H., Draper, B.M., and Low, L.F. (2003a) Behavioural and psychological symptoms of dementia: a seven-tiered model of service delivery. *Medical Journal of Australia*, **178** (5), 231–4.

Brodaty, H., Green, A., and Koschera, A. (2003b) Meta-analysis of psychosocial interventions for caregivers of people with dementia. *Journal of the American Geriatrics Society*, **51** (5), 657–64.

Calhoun, D.R. (ed.) (1997) *1997 Britannica Book of the Year.* Encyclopedia Britannica, Inc, Chicago.

CIA World Fact Book (2003) GDP per capita http://www.photius.com/wfb1999/rankings/gdp_per_capita_0.html accessed 19 April 2004.

Cohen, L. (1995) Toward an anthropology of senility: anger, weakness, and Alzheimer's in Banaras, India. *Med Anthropol Q*, **9** (3), 314–34.

Dandekar, K. (1996) *The Elderly in India.* Sage, New Delhi.

Eisenberg, L. (1999) Psychiatry and neuroscience at the end of the century. *Current Opinion in Psychiatry*, **12** (6), 629–32.

Farlow, M.A. (2002) Clinical overview of cholinesterase inhibitors in Alzheimer's Disease. *International Psychogeriatrics*, **14** (Suppl. 1), 93–126.

Glanz, W.D. (ed.) (1990) *Mosby's Medical, Nursing, and Allied Health Dictionary*, vol. 6, 3rd edn, The C. V. Mosby Company, St Louis.

Graham, N. and Brodaty, H. (1997) Alzheimer's Disease International. *International Journal of Geriatric Psychiatry*, **12** (7), 691–2.

Jenkins, R. (1998) Linking epidemiology and disability measurement with mental health service policy and planning. *Epidemiologia e Psichiatria Sociale*, 120–6.

Kalache, A. (1991) Ageing is a Third World problem too. *International Journal of Geriatric Psychiatry* **6**, 617–618.

Murray, C.J.L. and Lopez, A.D. (1996) *The Global Burden of Disease. A comprehensive assessment of mortality and disability from diseases, injuries and risk factors in 1990 and projected to 2020.* Global Burden of Disease and Injury Series, vol. 1. Boston, The Harvard School of Public Health, Harvard University Press.

Nair, V., Thankappan, K., Sarma, P., and Vasan, R. (2001) Changing roles of grass-root level health workers in Kerala, India. *Health Policy Plan*, **16** (2), 171–9.

Patel, V. (2003) Health systems research: a pragmatic method of meeting mental health needs in low income countries. In G. Andrews and S. Henderson (eds.) *Unmet Need in Psychiatry*. Cambridge University Press, Cambridge, pp. 353–77.

Patel, V. and Prince, M. (2001) Ageing and mental health in a developing country: Who cares? Qualitative studies from Goa, India. *Psychological Medicine*, **31** (1), 29–38.

Phillips, D.R. (2000) *Ageing in the Asia Pacific Region.* Roultedge, London.

Prince, M.J. (1997) The need for research on dementia in developing countries. *Tropical Medicine and Health*, **2**, 993–1000.

Rao, V. A. (1986) Social psychiatry of old age in India. *Indian Journal of Social Psychiatry*, **2**, 3–14.

Schneider, J., Murray, J., Banerjee, S., and Mann, A. (1999) EUROCARE: a cross-national study of co-resident spouse carers for people with Alzheimer's Disease: I. Factors associated with carer burden. *International Journal of Geriatric Psychiatry*, **14** (8), 651–61.

Shaji, K.S., Arun Kishore, N.R., Lal, K.P., and Prince, M. (2002a) Revealing a hidden problem. An evaluation of a community dementia case-finding program from the Indian 10/66 Dementia Research Network. *International Journal of Geriatric Psychiatry*, **17** (3), 222–5.

Shaji, K.S., Smitha, K., Praveen Lal, K., and Prince, M. (2002b) Caregivers of patients with Alzheimer's Disease: a qualitative study from The Indian 10/66 Dementia Research Network. *International Journal of Geriatric Psychiatry*, **18**, 1–6.

The 10/66 Dementia Research Group (2000) Dementia in developing countries. A preliminary consensus statement from the 10/66 Dementia Research Group. *International Journal of Geriatric Psychiatry*, **15**, 14–20.

The 10/66 Dementia Research Group (2004) Care arrangements for people with dementia in developing countries. *International Journal of Geriatric Psychiatry*, **19**, 170–7.

The 10/66 Dementia Research Group (in press). Behavioural and Psychological Symptoms of Dementia in Developing Countries. *International Psychogeriatrics.*

Tout, K. (1989) *Ageing in Developing Countries.* Oxford University Press, Oxford.

Unutzer, J., Katon, W., Callahan, C.M., Williams, J.W. Jr., Hunkeler, E., Harpole, L., Hoffing, M., Della Penna, R.D., Noel, P.H., Lin, E.H., Arean, P.A., Hegel, M.T., Tang, L., Belin, T.R., Oishi, S., and Langston, C. (2002) Collaborative care management of late-life depression in the primary care setting: a randomized controlled trial. *JAMA*, **288** (22), 2836–45.

Vatuk, S. (1990) 'To be a burden on others': dependency anxiety among the elderly in India. In O. M. Lynch *Divine passions: The Social Construction of Emotion in India*. University of California Press, Berkeley, pp. 64–8.

World Health Organization (1986) *Ottawa Charter for Health Promotion, 1986.*
http://www.euro.who.int/AboutWHO/Policy/20010827_2 accessed 19 April 2004.

World Health Organization (2000) *Disability Adjusted Healthy Lifestyle Expectancy at Birth Table.*
www.photius.com/rankings/healthy_life-table2.html accessed 19 April 2004.

The World Health Organization Atlas Project (2002) *Mapping Mental Health Resources in the World*
http://www.cvdinfobase.ca/mh-atlas/ accessed 19 April 2004.

Chapter 4

Principles of planning health services

Pamela S. Melding

'Cheshire puss ... would you tell me, please, which way I ought to go from here?'

'That depends a good deal on where you want to get to,' said the Cat.

'I don't much care where –' said Alice.

'Then it doesn't matter which way you go' said the Cat.

'– so long as I get somewhere'. Alice added as an explanation.

'Oh you're sure to do that,' said the Cat, 'if only you walk long enough'.
Lewis Carroll, Alice in Wonderland, 1865

There are so many directions to follow in planning health services for a population that Alice's exchange with the Cheshire Cat in Lewis Carroll's classic story may seem like an exemplar. Planning health services on a national, statewide, or regional basis has multiple considerations to be taken into account and can be an overwhelming task. There are many key stakeholders including politicians, policy-makers, planners, purchasers, providers, practitioners, patients, potential patients, and premium or taxpayers (James, 1995). Some of these key stakeholders have multiple investments; all have points of view, and values that they want to have considered, and too often these are diametrically opposed. Demand for health care services continues to rise and it is apparent that health services are like a sponge that mops up resources without ever being saturated. Medical technology has advanced health care well beyond the ability to pay for all that is possible. Whilst the population is supportive of health care provision, there is a limit to how much they are prepared to pay in taxes, insurance or on fee for service. The dilemma of the twenty-first century is that we have a healthier but older population that expects the advanced health care they hear about in the media will be available *for them*. What the consumer expects, what the provider and practitioners are capable of or want to provide and what the funder or premium payer is prepared to pay for are often poles apart.

Geriatric psychiatry service development cannot be seen in isolation from other older people's health services or indeed the health care system in general. They are just one piece, albeit an important piece, in a complex jigsaw of services, all of which are important, and all paid for from a tax or insurance base that is usually much less than is optimal. Difficult decisions have to be made if not everything can be provided.

Services provided for one group may be at the expense of another – the 'opportunity cost'. The core of health policy and planning is about resource allocation – who gets what, where, and when.

Establishing who need services is not as obvious at it would first seem. Good information is vital but until very recently, health planners have had to work with poor information systems (such as population census data, manual hospital coding of discharge diagnoses, registration of deaths or other output statistics) that were often wrong. Even in this current computer age, accurate or meaningful health information systems are in their infancy in many places.

Many different health services have developed on a basis of poor information, ad hoc, to enhance professional interests, or because someone thought it was a 'good idea' rather than because there was real unmet need. Some technological services developed because they appealed to the public's sense of wonderment and need for 'miracles'. Some services have developed because of emotive media manipulation of public opinion (so called 'shroud-waving') influencing politicians. Services develop in urban areas that attract doctors or are close to universities and tertiary institutions needing training facilities. Some services develop because technology allows efficiencies. Sometimes, these efficiencies create more demand than anticipated so that limits have to be set or other opportunities forgone (Maynard, 2001). The result is often inequitable so that ability to access services may depend on locality rather than need.

Geriatric psychiatry services illustrate some of the deficiencies in past health service planning very well. They are not technology based and do not produce many 'miracles', so they lack the glamour and popular appeal of a heart or kidney transplant service. Potential recipients do not go out and lobby for services nor do advocates of geriatric psychiatry go out and manipulate media opinion by 'shroud-waving' threats. Therefore, in many countries, provision of geriatric psychiatry is less than ideal (see Section 2 of this book). If developed at all, they often earn the epithet of a 'Cinderella service'. However, the worldwide ageing phenomenon, the rapid increase in life expectancy, the rise of consumer lobby groups plus the increasing numbers of specialists in psychological medicine of the aged have begun to make health departments all over the world realize that attention needs to be directed towards elder care services.

Population ageing will have a major impact on health services. Older people are heavy users of all health services. They see their GP more often and take more pharmaceuticals than do younger adults (New Zealand Ministry of Health, 2002a). Medical and surgical discharge figures and hospital bed-day figures also reflect a disproportionately higher use of secondary services (Draper, 2001). Older people also need more costly home services and residential placements. The neurodegenerative diseases can take years to take their toll, but the person needs care throughout the illness and the cost (both monetary and non-monetary) of formal and informal care is enormous. As the population ages the already limited resources will need to be stretched further. It is also becoming evident that neglecting the effect of population ageing on utilization of health care services could increase costs further (Jacobzone *et al.*, 1998). It becomes a matter of urgency to develop services when the cost of not doing so starts to outstrip supply costs. Neglect and lack of provision of health incentives lead to more expensive health care ultimately because of delayed diagnoses, chronicity, and institutionalization. In addition, patients have poorer quality of life and carers have a greater burden. Inadequate service can lead to inappropriate diagnoses, poor assessment, more complications, higher rates of institutionalization, carer burnout and lowered morale.

Planners have to look at proposals to develop geriatric psychiatry services from a 'helicopter' perspective, rather like Alice's Cheshire Cat. How does geriatric psychiatry fit, not only into the total picture of a health service in general, but also into the schemata of services for older people such as geriatric medicine services, community support, and accommodation needs? Where does geriatric psychiatry fit in the mental health scheme of services? If geriatric psychiatry is developed, what is the opportunity cost? Even when geriatric psychiatry services are scheduled for development, numerous other questions arise. Why should the mentally ill older person have specialist services? Is there a real need? What would be the demand for such services? Could they be developed within existing services? Would the development of geriatric services be fair to others in the population needing health services? What would be the resource implications of geriatric psychiatry services? What evidence is that they are effective? What are the costs of the benefits and harms such services may have? Are they cost-effective? Are they cost-effective when compared to other services that need investment? Which principles will underpin the planning of such services?

In the last thirty years, some major paradigms have fundamentally influenced health care service planning. They are the three E's of resource allocation. The first is the *ethics* of allocating resources in health care, the second is the social science of health *economics* and its tools for assisting with resource decisions, and the third is '*evidence-based medicine*' with its emphasis on clinical *efficacy*. These three complimentary concepts provide powerful objective arguments against ad hoc development, the 'good idea' or 'shroud-waving' politically motivated service delivery. Today, health service planning, be it at a national, regional, area or local level needs to consider these paradigms.

Ethics

Arbitration between competing needs

Who, of the key stakeholders in the provision of health care should arbitrate between competing needs? In effect, this really means rationing, who gets access to health care and who does not. Maynard (1996) considers that 'in no country is there a clear and publicly accepted set of principles that can determine who gets what health care and when'. No one likes making decisions that might have an adverse effect on some people and attempts to do so usually invite harsh criticism. Health services have experimented with different key players for making these decisions (James, 1995; Robinson, 2001). Politicians, whose fortunes and ideologies change almost as frequently as their manifestos, have found that initiatives that increase costs, through expansions of benefits or access, win votes, but initiatives to control health care costs loses votes. Unsurprisingly, politicians would prefer others to make potentially politically damaging decisions. Health care organizations are accountable for their expenditure, and they are likely to arbitrate from this point of view rather than population need. When they ration or cut services, the public bombards them with condemnation. Health administrators also make easy scapegoats for public anger (James, 1995). Physicians prefer to be on the side of their patients, advocating for more resources and better quality, rather than taking on the social responsibility for managing costs (Robinson, 2001). Consumers are becoming more prominent as key decision-makers. The movement towards to consumerism is driven by a widespread skepticism of governments, health organization and professional control of service delivery, plus reduced social tolerance for interference with individual autonomy. In addition, the Internet technology revolution has given consumers the information they need to question traditional arbitrators of service delivery intelligently and assertively (Robinson, 2001).

Consumers vary enormously in their abilities to input into philosophical health care debates. Consumers who are younger, richer, more assertive, educated and less likely to be sick themselves are more likely to be appointed to Trustee Boards of Health Care organizations, advisory panels or make submissions on which services should be provided. The older, physically frail, and mentally ill consumers or actual service users are less likely to be invited to join panels that arbitrate, or even be consulted. However, various consumer organizations such as Age Concern, MIND, Grey Power, and Alzheimer Associations are increasing worldwide and these can act as proxies for consumers in health care debates. Similarly some ethnic groups have traditional leaders or elders who can advocate for their disadvantaged members.

Although the consumer is becoming more influential in the provision of health care services, there have been some problems with public opinion being the arbitrator of which services to provide. This was glaringly demonstrated by the Oregon experience in trying to define 'core health priorities' (Brannigan, 1993). The volunteer public panel were not initially grounded in ethical principles (Richmond et al., 1995) and their final list was heavily criticized as counterintuitive and discriminatory against the disabled (Donaldson et al., 1988). Other approaches utilizing public opinion have also proved contradictory (Bowling 1996). While there is criticism, usually from health professionals, that consumers are not yet sophisticated enough to take on the arbitrating role, this is a rather patronizing reaction. There is valid criticism that the role of consumers in key decisions of health care provision is still tokenistic (Richards, 1999). Nevertheless, there is an increasing trend towards consumers playing a greater role in arbitrating between competing needs, by default if not by design (Robinson, 2001; Smith, 1996). When it comes to planning services, consumers should certainly be involved, preferably at national level and definitely at local level to ensure that services will meet their expectations.

Ethics of distribution of health care

How should health care resources be distributed in a society? There is neither an easy answer to this question nor any common or right answer. The basic question is, what is 'fair' or equitable to a population? The problem with notions of fairness or justice is that many different interpretations and societal values can define it, and what might be considered fair or just in Australia or the UK is not necessarily viewed the same way in the USA or Asia. A society determines what is fair and equitable by its own values and judgement. According to Beauchamp and Walters (1989) there are six different principles upon which a theory of distributive justice or 'fairness' to the *individual* might be based. These are:

1. To each an equal share.
2. To each according to individual need.
3. To each according to acquisition in a free market.
4. To each according to individual effort.
5. To each according to their societal contribution.
6. To each according to merit.

The problem with 'health' per se is that its distribution amongst individuals is neither fair nor equitable. Theories of distributive justice for health care that rely on principles such as desert due to individual effort, the free market, merit or social worth are distinctly unfair to those people who, because of illness, are unable to make such contributions in the normally accepted social sense. In this category are the old, needy, frail and the mentally ill (Campbell *et al.*, 1992, p. 100). Egalitarianism or the principle of equal and impartial distribution, which superficially seems to have great appeal, can be a problem in health care distribution when resources are limited as scarcity of resources can have greater detrimental effects on some disadvantaged groups than on others (Campbell *et al.*, 1992, p. 100).

The utilitarian (or social welfare) theory of distributive justice considers what is fair to society as a whole rather than what is fair to the individual. According to this theory, resources should be distributed to benefit the greatest number of people. Consequently, the individual can be discriminated against for the greater good (Richmond *et al.*, 1995). Thus, with this theory, minorities such as the old, the terminal and mentally ill would be treated unfairly, as indeed they are in many jurisdictions. Utilitarian theory of distributive justice is the principle behind rationing decisions based on economic parameters such as quality adjusted life years (QALY) (see below).

The American philosopher, John Rawls (1921–2002), provided a philosophical framework of distributive justice known as the 'Difference' or 'Maximin' principle (1971) which considers both society and the individual. His theory states that if people considered what is justice under 'a veil of ignorance', i.e. no knowledge of our own personal social situation now or in the future, they would support two principles of justice. The first would require that each person be accorded the maximum amount of equal personal liberty compatible with the same amount for all other persons. The second principle recognizes that there *is* inequality in society and that it is just to permit such differences if the resultant inequalities enhance the position of the most disadvantaged in society. Rawls did not specifically apply his theory of justice to the distribution of health care. However, Amy Gutmann and Dennis Thompson (2002), drawing on Rawls, asserted that equality of opportunity, equal relief from pain and equal respect are the three central values at the foundation of a principle of equal access to health care. The 'Difference principle' has great appeal but is particularly criticized for two things. Ensuring that the position of the most disadvantaged is enhanced requires a lot of governance and government involvement, which does not sit well with libertarian societies or thinkers. The second is that equality of opportunity for access implies a health system concentrated on illness and disability rather than on health promotion.

When these ethical principles are applied to the provision of health care for a society in general, there can be no doubt that the Rawls' model would be most beneficial to older psychiatric patients, as they are amongst the most disadvantaged people in a society. Rawlsian 'justice' demands that their position in the distribution of health care be enhanced. However, the last ten to twenty years has seen the ascendancy of more utilitarian values influencing purchasing decisions, leaving the uneconomic old, disabled, and mentally ill patients marginalized in service provision.

Equity

Like distributive justice, equity also can have many meanings. Campbell *et al.* (1992) define equity as ensuring that people are treated in a fair and just manner by ignoring irrelevant differences between them but taking into account the relevant differences. However, there are other definitions of equity such as equal expenditure, equal access

Table 4.1 Ethical theories and geriatric psychiatry service delivery

Theory	Implication for geriatric psychiatry
Egalitarian	Health is not egalitarian; probably disadvantageous
Utilitarian	Disadvantages minorities and older people
Free market	Disadvantageous to older people
Social worth	Disadvantageous. Who decides social worth?
Individual effort	Disadvantageous to old and sick
Merit	Disadvantageous. Who decides what is meritorious?
Rawls 'difference principle'	Advantageous to geriatric and psychiatry populations

for equal need, and equal utilization of health care, equal health (Mooney, 1983). In 'Rawlsian' health service planning, equity means equality of opportunity of access for equal need or equality of outcome.

Health has many social determinants, and the size of the population is just one factor in determining population need. Others that have bearing on the need for health care services include socioeconomic status, overcrowding, education, housing quality, industry type, air pollution and of course, age strata. There are often inequities between urban and rural areas (See Neese, Chapter 18 this volume). Ethnic minorities or immigrant groups often have inequitable access to health care, because of lack of knowledge about the system, cultural or language barriers (Jones and Gill, 1998). When resources are seriously maldistributed, it may be impossible to take away from those oversupplied, to give to those areas in need, without having other social impacts such as redundancies, loss of teaching opportunities, increasing waitlists etc. For example, a university city with a small population but a long established medical and nursing school might have an oversupply of beds and facilities if compared to the rest of the population. Reducing the resources to be equitable with the rest of the population may result in the medical school no longer having sufficient facilities to ensure its viability.

Economics

The social science discipline of health economics started to emerge in the late1960s and early 1970s, as it was fast becoming obvious in countries with state run health services that demand would not plateau as the population got healthier (as predicted by their protagonists) but would continue to outstrip supply. This crisis coincided with a number of critical reviews on the effectiveness of health care interventions (Maynard and Sheldon, 1997, p. 149). A major tenet of health economics is the concept of '*opportunity costs*', which is the benefit obtainable by next best use of those resources (Donaldson, 2002). Health economics professes to provide objective analyses of the costs of health care that can assist in decisions regarding the allocation of scarce resources, so that the maximal benefits for the resources can be accrued to a society *as a whole*. Thus, health economists lean more to utilitarian principles of distributive justice than Rawlsian, which often puts them at odds with health care professionals. Nevertheless, the discipline of health economics has been very influential in bringing a societal perspective to planning and developing services.

Need versus demand and the health economics view

Whilst clinicians talk about need, health economists talk about demand. They are not the same thing. People normally go to the doctor when their symptoms are severe, chronic, or disabling or when they think the doctor can help (Hulka *et al.*, 1972). The individual will demand health care based on a recognized *felt* need. However, the technical expert, the doctor, may also detect *unperceived* need in an individual, creating demands for health care beyond that requested by the patient. The definition of the level of need represents the technical relationship between health status and health care. Once the technical expert has defined the level of need at the medical consultation, the subsequent demand for investigations, treatments, services, and involvement with other health professional staff is the core of resource consumption.

Economics is concerned with the supply and consumption of health care resources and the factors that influence them (Maynard and Sheldon, 1997, p. 161). Amongst these are need, barriers to accessing health care, and the drivers of provider behaviour such as the economists' 'bête noir', the 'agency relationship' and 'supplier-induced demand'. This arises when the clinician is both the agent who assesses the health need for the patient and the supplier who provides the solution. The doctor, in their position as supplier of health care solutions for the consumer, is able to bring about a level of consumption that might be different to that of a fully informed consumer able to choose autonomously – 'supplier-induced demand' (McGuire et al., 1988, p. 160).

Whilst it is obvious that supplier-induced demand may certainly occur when doctors need to maximize their income i.e. in fee for service situations, it less obviously can occur in publicly funded systems where the motivations may be very different, for example, career enhancement, teaching opportunities, or professional development. Supplier-induced demand also occurs when the consumer demands less than is technically desirable and is persuaded to consume more, or when new technologies appear where there were none before, such as the acetylcholinesterase inhibitor drugs for dementia (Maynard, 2001). Psychiatry and geriatric psychiatry are not immune from supplier-induced demand, as the consumer usually wants less than is desirable. The natural brake on exploitative supplier-induced demand is medical ethics influencing doctor behaviour and the fundamental medical principle of non-maleficence, 'primum non nocere': 'first, do no harm'.

Whilst the identification of need by the agency relationship is difficult for a lay person to evaluate objectively, the resulting demands (its outputs) are analysable. Health economists have vigorously challenged the traditional monopoly of the medical profession in influencing demand for health care. As a result, there has been polarization of views across the two camps, the economists arguing for controls on doctors' ability to induce consumption and physicians objecting on grounds of clinical freedom, together with scepticism on both sides as to the others' motivations. Thus, in some jurisdictions, expert clinicians have been excluded from health care decision-making on grounds of 'vested interests' (Hornblow, 1997) and from public consultation groups on grounds of 'provider capture'. The cash-strapped economically minded administrator may consider that the correct level of service should be the uninduced demand of felt need and attempt to limit any induced demand by limiting opportunities for case finding. Such a poor level of service would be a problem for mental health services as there is often a wide gap between the degree of felt and unfelt need in psychiatric patients

(Andrews *et al.*, 2001a). Population studies of mental health in Australia, UK, and USA showed that less than half people with significant comorbidities demanded health care to treat them (Andrews *et al.*, 2001b). The clinician will want to have services that have the ability to detect unperceived need and will use ethical arguments based on altruism and compassion.

Predicting demand/need

Information systems

Health planners have access to multiple sources of information of varying quality and usefulness. Demand information is easiest to collect such as hospital admission and throughput statistics, discharge data, mortality data, general practice consultations, and medical insurance claims or payments made. Many of these sources are imprecise and subject to human error or neglect in reporting. Computerized systems are still in their infancy and they are by no means universal. It can be particularly problematic to capture data about elderly people with complex comorbidities on these systems. Nevertheless, successful data from patient self-assessment (Wasson *et al.*, 1999) or comprehensive geriatric assessment (Department of Health, 2002) that do capture some of the complexity can be valuable in planning future services (see Chapter 17 of this volume on Integrating services).

Demography

The characteristics of the population are important in health service planning and especially age stratification, gender, and ethnic mix. So is any predicted change in demography in the near future. Services need to be developed to anticipate future increases in the elderly population and any ethnic or gender imbalances.

Epidemiology

Epidemiology measures health status in a population or health events and such information is invaluable to planners to determine the size of the health problems, their distribution, demography and impact on a community. Often epidemiological data is not available for a particular problem in a population and the results from well-designed overseas studies needs to be extrapolated to the particular situation. This approach, whilst useful, is fraught with problems and easily criticized as inappropriate on grounds of diverse environmental factors or differences in social determinants of health in the comparator countries. Other problems with interpretation of epidemiological studies include diverse methods of selection, different epidemiological instruments, screening versus diagnostic tools, severity criteria and varying periods used for prevalence (Cooper and Singh, 2000). Both prevalence and incident data are important to know for setting levels of access to services. In geriatric psychiatry many of the conditions are chronic so have high prevalence and low incidence e.g. in Alzheimer's disease the prevalence of the disorder for a population of 100,000 elderly may be 5 per cent or 5000 people per annum but the incidence of new cases will be much lower at 0.5 per cent or 500 new cases per annum. Despite the problems, planning has to start somewhere and epidemiology may be a much more useful path to take than that of demand data.

Efficiency and the concept of the health 'market'

While most people applaud efficiency gains, the concept of market forces in health systems is an anathema to most health professionals. Simply, the theory behind the health care 'market' goes something like this. *Health* is a fundamental concern of all people of all ages. It only has value to the individual and has no value in exchange. Markets in health, per se, cannot exist. Health has many inputs. Some such as genetics, lifestyle, occupational hazards and chance factors are difficult to assess but do influence health status and the demand for care. Social determinants of health such as housing, sanitation, education are also important factors impinging on health status. '*Health care*' is just one input into health. Whilst the exact relationship between health care and health status is difficult to assess, *health care* consumes measurable resources and *health care* does have value in exchange. Therefore, *health care* is a consumer commodity and markets in health care can exist. As health is unpredictable there also is '*risk*'. The individual takes up the management of risk, as user pays, or insurance, provided by insurance companies or the state through taxation. Even in countries where the costs of most health care are covered by insurance, the state may also be a major provider of insurance for a large portion of the population, usually the poor and needy. Thus, markets also exist in health care insurance. But why have markets and competition? The theory of managed markets in health care is that the quality, efficiency, and economy of health care delivery will improve if independent provider groups compete for consumers (Kronick *et al.*, 1993) as with any other consumer commodity. However, because the provision of health care exists in an imperfect market it has to be 'managed' to provide the incentives of the market under regulation to protect against market failure (Ham and Maynard, 1994). Money prices, time prices, waiting lists, and non-price rationing are devices used to manage the market equilibrium. Supply costs are controlled by competition in costs of production, alternative production techniques, input substitution (manpower, equipment, drugs), remuneration methods and incentives (Maynard and Sheldon, 1997, p. 161). Both the UK and New Zealand introduced the concepts of the managed market, business principles and competition into their health services in the early 1990s. However, New Zealand is currently walking away from its quasi-market place in the public sector, which did not provide the expected benefits despite huge restructuring costs (Hornblow, 1997).

Services for mentally ill older people have not been obvious targets to introduce the incentives of the health care market. In many parts of the world, even in those with managed health care markets, there is a shortfall of services and personnel working in acute assessment and rehabilitation services within the public sector, rather than competition. However, in the private nursing homes and residential sectors there is a health care market and, if subsidized by the state or insurer, it can be regulated by licensing and contracts, thus potentially getting the efficiency and quality benefits induced by competition. However, this situation is far from perfect if there is income, territorial or need inequities reducing consumer choice. Furthermore, when there is a fixed resource, subsidies for the residential sector have significant opportunity costs in forgone community care packages (Challis and Henwood, 1994) thereby reducing variety of choices.

Technical and allocative efficiency

For the clinician, efficiency is maximum effect or outcome for minimum waste of effort. The economist would add, for lowest possible cost. Economic efficiency can be technical, allocative, or social. Technical efficiency occurs when the costs for a given output are minimized or output maximized for a given cost. Laparoscopic surgery is a good example of a highly efficient technical medical procedure that benefits many for a reasonable cost. However, technical efficiency may increase the number of people likely to benefit thus increasing overall costs (Maynard, 2001) but reduce allocative efficiency because of lost opportunity to fund other services or interventions. When it is not possible to make any individual better off without making someone worse off a state of allocative efficiency exists. Economic theory predicts that a perfect market will lead to the maximization of technical and allocative efficiencies for an initial endowment of resources. Social efficiency is the maximization of value of all total outputs produced. This is a utilitarian concept that accepts there will always be winners and losers to some degree and determining who these should be requires society to decide.

Cost-benefit analysis

Cost-benefit economical appraisal (CBA) is an objective tool used to assist in the determination of social efficiency and equity. The analyses are complex but basically they reduce all tangible benefits and costs, including future benefits and costs, to monetary terms. Cost-benefit analyses do not include costs and benefits accruing to others because of the intervention under study. The cost-benefit model assumes there is a perfect market with a well-informed consumer making the decisions. When benefits outweigh costs, the intervention or service is socially efficient. The cost-benefit approach allows the comparison of different services or interventions for the same cost and allows society to see how many hip replacements for older people can be bought for the same cost as a heart transplant, or the cost of a cholesterol lowering programmed versus acetyl cholinesterase inhibitor treatment of Alzheimer's disease. There are problems with the cost-benefit approach, as assumptions (for example, discounting future benefits and risks, proxy measures such as shadow pricing and utilization) are needed to determine the costs of some of the risks and benefits. These can be tested using a sensitivity analysis (varying the inputted data to see if the relationships hold) but if the assumptions are wrong then the CBA will be incorrect. A major problem with CBA is that people are often quite uncomfortable with the concept of putting monetary value on human life (Kaplan and Groessl, 2002). Cost-benefit analysis is most useful when there are few constraints on alternatives (McGuire *et al.*, 1988). Cost-benefit analyses can help decide if there should be a particular health programme; or no programme; for older people only; for only those over 70 years; for all adults; in one city; in several cities; nationwide; this year; next year; or in five years.

Cost-effectiveness

A cost-effectiveness analysis (CEA) works by organizing all inputs to production in the most technically efficient way, choosing a combination that minimizes costs (Donaldson *et al.*, 2002; Kaplan and Groessl, 2002). Some benefits of a service or intervention cannot be reduced to monetary terms, e.g. relief of carer stress, or benefit of having depression or hallucinations relieved. However, these can be included in a cost-effectiveness analysis (CEA). A CEA can be conducted from various perspectives, most commonly societal, and includes all health benefits, tangible and intangible regardless of who would experience those, including people who are not the intended recipients of the intervention. Costs include all resources used, whether or not money changes hands (Russell *et al.*, 1996). A CEA should always be compared with something similar, for example, an alternative way of treating the same disease. Thus, in contrast to cost-benefit analyses, cost-effectiveness analyses compare interventions in similar patients with the same health problems. They do not address issues of equity (Ubel *et al.*, 1996) or allocative efficiency (Donaldson *et al.*, 2002).

A major problem with CEA studies is that many lack standardization. To address the issue, the US Public Health Service convened a consensus panel to look at the role of cost-effectiveness in health and medicine and to recommend standards (Russell *et al.*, 1996). The panel's findings were published in a book (Gold *et al.*, 1996). They recommended that CEA studies take the societal perspective, that a standard set of methods be used between studies, and that cost-effectiveness studies of health interventions are compared to the cost effectiveness of alternatives so that differences can be observed. The cost-utility measure Quality-Adjusted-Life-Year (QALY) was their preferred socially appropriate comparator.

Cost-utility

Cost-utility analysis (Gold *et al.*, 1996) is a form of cost-effectiveness analysis that uses a composite measure of morbidity and mortality outcomes that represent the total impact of the assessment or programme. The quality-adjusted life year (QALY) is a cost utility composite measure of life expectancy with adjustments for quality of life expected after an intervention. Essentially, this is an attempt to measure health status so that a cost per QALY can be assessed. There are various methods used to calculate QALYs. A stratified random sample of the population is given various health scenarios to study, subsequently undertaking an interview with a researcher in which they are asked to rate their preferences using a reference rating between good health rated as one, and death rated as zero. Interesting techniques used to elicit the preferences from subjects include the *time trade-off* and the *standard gamble*. In the time-trade-off technique, the subject is asked to trade off the certainty of living with a chronic illness for t years against good health for a shorter period of x years, when the end of each period is death. The time x is varied until the subject is indifferent between the two and this measurement 'h' is the valuation (h = x/t) of the health condition in QALYs. In the standard gamble, the subject is asked to make a trade-off between certainty of the chronic health condition of interest for t years and a gamble between good health for t years as one alternative and death as the other. The probability of the gamble is varied again until the point where the subject is indifferent giving the QALY valuation (McGuire *et al.*, 1988).

Whilst QALYs may have face validity as a neat objective measure, there are some problems with the derivation methodology. The different techniques used to determine preferences can give very different answers. Subjects sometimes consider the health condition under study to be worse than death, for example depression or paralysis. A subject working with a hypothetical scenario may make different decisions than they would have done if they had to deal with the situation in real life. QALY valuations have tended to be unidirectional from good health to poor and do not take improvements in health status into account. QALYs are limited in that they do not take intangible benefits beyond the subject into account, such as relief of carer stress. For administrators, many QALYs have intuitive appeal as a socially significant guide for resource allocation because of the quality of life aspect (Kaplan and Groessl, 2002). The use of QALYs as a statistic to use in arbitration for resource allocation has attracted criticism as being too simplistic and inflexible (Ubel *et al.*, 2003). For geriatric services, QALYs discriminate against the aged, as the number of years potentially gained by health interventions is considerably lower in older people compared to the general population (Donaldson *et al.*, 1988; Avorn, 1984).

QALYs only measure health outcomes and do not measure process outcomes such as waiting times or service location that have importance for patients in the total delivery. Recently, health economists have introduced a new technique of cost utility analysis that goes beyond the restrictions of the QALY model in the form of discrete choice experiments, which investigate trade-offs between process outcome (effects of waiting lists, location of services, health professional assessing etc) and health outcome attributes (Ryan, 2004). Whether use of this technique will answer the critics of QALYs or will be less discriminatory towards older people remains to be seen.

Cost offset

This is the value of money saved by an intervention independently of any health benefits, for example, if there is reduced health care utilization and care costs. It is often included in cost-benefit or cost-effectiveness analyses (Kaplan and Groessl, 2002).

Evaluating cost-effectiveness studies

It is important to interpret and evaluate cost-effectiveness studies carefully if they are used in health service planning.

The following checklist for evaluating or planning a cost-effectiveness study is adapted from Kaplan and Groessl (2002).

1. Which perspective will evaluate the study (i.e. consumer, clinician, administrative, societal)?

2. What systematic experimental design used to evaluate the treatment? A randomized clinical trial, an observational study, or some other design?

3. What will be the comparator for the analysis?

4. Will all costs of treatment accounted for?

5. Does the analysis consider costs of treatment for patients who do not get the intervention or disease in question?

6. What is the unit of outcome? Cost? Health Status? Mental Health Status? QALYs?

7. Will future outcomes be measured and discounted to current value?

8. Will uncertainty be evaluated through a sensitivity analysis?

Evidence

Archie Cochrane has been one of the most influential figures in the medical world in the last thirty years. His groundbreaking book *Effectiveness and Efficiency: Random Reflections on Health Services* (1972) stated a simple, yet until then not particularly evident, premise that services and medical interventions would be a lot more effective if based on '*evidence*'. The gold standard of evidence is the randomized controlled trial. Everyone in the health field likes to think that they are improving standards of health care and the concept of evidence has appeal for clinicians, researchers, journal editors, clinical teachers, health economists and health planners. After Archie Cochrane's death in 1988, the idea has proven to be remarkably robust and has become a movement of almost evangelical fervour. Its progeny are numerous and include the Cochrane Collaboration, 'an international organization that aims to help people make well informed decisions about health care by preparing, maintaining and promoting the accessibility of systematic reviews of the effects of healthcare interventions' (Chalmers *et al.*, 1997, p. 247). Other progeny are evidenced-based medicine journals, and numerous clinical trials units in universities all over the world. The concept of 'evidence-based medicine' is important in textbooks (including this one), recommendations on

Table 4.2 Economic analyses and geriatric psychiatry service delivery

Analysis	Assesses	Implications for geriatric psychiatry
Cost-benefit	Social efficiency, equity	Disadvantageous
Cost utility e.g. QALY	Allocative efficiency	Disadvantages older people
Cost-effectiveness	Technical efficiency	Useful tool in geriatric psychiatry

Table 4.3 Levels of evidence

Level	Description
I	Evidence from meta analyses of properly conducted and similar randomized controlled trials
II	Evidence from at least one properly conducted randomized control trial
III	Evidence from other controlled studies, before and after, multiple baseline, matched trials
IV	Evidence from descriptive studies or expert opinion

access to health care interventions by organizations such as the National Institute for Clinical Excellence (NICE) (Raftery, 2001), and the Scottish Intercollegiate Guidelines Network (SIGN) in the UK. Evidenced-based studies are increasingly informing health planning, fulfilling Archie Cochrane's aim. Systematic reviews of evidence are even enlightening health economics (Byford *et al.*, 2003; Jefferson *et al.*, 2002)!

Levels of evidence are important to planners. The problem with the evidenced-based approach in planning is that planners would much rather have evidence from level I and II. Randomized controlled trials lend themselves well to the investigation of single interventions with clear cut outcomes such as the drug treatment of depression, or outcomes where there is a clear difference between caseness versus non caseness, but are less easy to apply to the evaluation of service delivery when there are complex social and psychological variables, as in geriatric psychiatry. Many studies evaluating geriatric psychiatry services are uncontrolled and lose weight as evidence, at least in the eyes of planners. Nevertheless, some good studies provide evidence of effectiveness of geriatric psychiatry services (Burns *et al.*, 2001; Draper, 2000). These will be discussed in further detail in Chapter 5.

Evidence-based medicine, as a tool in service purchasing planning, is not without its critics. Clinicians often see randomization in social interventions as unethical. This presupposes that the intervention withheld from the control group *is* effective and that the normal service *is* completely fair and equitable. Such assumptions are problematic. Some social determinants of health such as income, poverty and housing are impossible to randomize yet may be crucial to health outcomes. Control groups are difficult to recruit, yet research funding is often withheld for non-randomized studies (Thomson *et al.*, 2004). Evidence from experimental studies might not be generalizable to real world clinical situations. Complex management problems generating a range of outcomes are particularly difficult to evaluate. Some interventions such as psychotherapies are challenging to research in randomized controlled trials (Kisely, 1999). Evidence based medicine also attracts criticism for its lack of considerations of equity and cost-effectiveness, something that would have been an anathema to Archie Cochrane (Maynard, 1996).

Health planners may discount lower levels of evidence whilst acknowledging they may be the only levels available. This is a real problem that could hinder the development of services, in the current climate of 'evidence-based medicine'. There is an urgent need for well-designed controlled studies to provide more rigorous evidence than is currently the case.

Operationalizing planning

Much of the planning process is taken up in determining the need for service development and establishing the principles. Once service development is considered fair and just, there is a demand, economically it is cost-effective, cost-beneficial and there is a clinical evidence base, the process may move on to operationalization. It is beyond the scope of this chapter to describe operational planning in any detail apart from some basic principles discussed below. Each locality will have its own implementation policies and priorities. The components of service required and the issues to be addressed are discussed in detail in Chapters 15–22 of this book.

Audits

An audit or stocktake is usually a priority but even if not, then it is still a very useful exercise. Amazingly, health departments often don't know what services are available in different regions under their control. A recent audit of Australasian services (O'Connor, personal communication, 2003) indicated that some services could not define their population catchments or caseloads accurately. The survey revealed major inequities in service provision for parts of both Australia and New Zealand. A separate stocktake of all New Zealand geriatric services by the Ministry of Health (Cornwall and Fletcher, 2003) requested information on geriatric and geriatric psychiatry services in each health district, how many services such as inpatients, outpatients, specialized clinics, rural outreach were provided and what were their staffing levels. Again, this survey showed marked inequities across the country. A stocktake mapped against demographic profiles and epidemiological predictions can be a very useful starting point to highlight deficiencies, reveal inequities, and indicate where to prioritize development. Repeating the exercise at intervals can review progress in development of services.

Strategies and frameworks

An OECD study by Jacobzone et al. (1998) noted the usefulness of an 'active' strategy towards population ageing in relation to the need for long-term care services. Strategies set out the policy direction and principles for future service development and addresses issues such as equity and access. They should also include population-based mental health initiatives in addition to primary and secondary illness and disability services. Frameworks and guidelines generally provide directions and advice for operationalizing a strategy. Sometimes, as in the UK National Service Frameworks for Older People, these functions are combined. As health care organizations have decentralized, there seems to be a move away from explicit prescription by health departments to guiding principles and expectations for local administrators. Local planners are expected to adhere to these principles or standards to ensure access to services but have a certain amount of freedom to interpret them appropriately for their populations. For example, in the UK, standard seven of the National Service Frameworks For Services For Older People is 'Older people who have mental health problems have access to integrated mental health services, provided by the NHS and councils to ensure effective diagnosis, treatment and support, for them and their carers' (Department of Health, 2001).

In New Zealand, the Health of Older People Strategy (New Zealand Ministry of Health, 2002b) set out a series of principles for health care of older people, the key ones being an emphasis on patient-centred care and patient ability to access an integrated spectrum of services responsive to complex medical and psychiatric needs. The New Zealand Guideline for Specialist Health Services for Older People (New Zealand Ministry of Health, 2004) set out a set of expectations and goals that health districts will:

1. Improve the process and outcome for specialist geriatric and geriatric psychiatry health services for older people,

2. Build linkages to ensure a continuum of care between specialist hospital-based services, general practice, community providers, medical and surgical hospital services and

3. Address quality issues in the provision of care.

It is up to the local planners to decide exactly how these goals will be achieved. These strategic documents are useful for:

- Articulating the policies behind the strategic direction
- Highlighting the issues that need to be addressed
- Presenting the evidence for the developments, the rationale
- Indicating the guiding principles behind service development
- Stipulating the objectives and expectations
- Highlighting problem areas
- Suggesting a methodology for prioritizing developments
- Rationalizing funding arrangements and contracts
- Addressing quality issues

Addressing workforce issues

Geriatric psychiatry services are labour intensive, in that it is health professionals that deliver effective interventions. Service development is contingent on there being a skilled, educated workforce. A workforce development plan needs to consider which disciplines are required, their availability, recruitment and retention policies, morale and job satisfaction and, very importantly, training issues.

Summary

Like Alice in the opening metaphor of this chapter, getting 'somewhere' in planning health services for a population requires 'walking long enough'. Some, with few services, may have the opportunity to start from scratch. Others have to progress along pathways already taken, hopefully improving matters as they go. An unfortunate few may have had their efforts hampered by changing political ideologies, multiple reforms and restructuring and have to retrace their steps and try another approach.

Identifying the key principles is crucial to planning. How will the society deal with its most disadvantaged, the old, the frail, and the mentally ill? A society needs to decide whether its values support utilitarian, difference principle, or other theories of allocative distribution. A development plan needs to define how it will deal with inequities of access, geography age, gender, and ethnicity, and how it will remove any barriers. Planning needs to acknowledge that the twenty-first century consumer has unprecedented ability to get information, and that they are more articulate and assertive. Older people and their carers want to be more involved in both health care planning and personal care plans and it is important to include them in the process. It is unethical to set up ineffective services and it is socially responsible to determine clinical and cost-effectiveness in recognition that there are limited resources. An operational plan should articulate all the principles and main objectives underpinning the development and also set the limitations so that public and professional expectations of service delivery are unambiguous. Then might the Cheshire Cat smile!

References

Andrews, G., Henderson, S., and Hall, W. (2001a) Prevalence, comorbidity, disability and service utilisation: Overview of the Australian National Mental Health Survey. *The British Journal of Psychiatry,* **178**, 145–53.

Andrews, G., Issakidis, C., and Carter, G. (2001b) Shortfall in mental health service utilization. *The British Journal of Psychiatry,* **179**, 417–25.

Avorn, J. (1984) Benefit and cost analysis in geriatric care: turning age discrimination into public health policy. *New England Journal of Medicine,* **310**, 1294–301.

Beauchamp, T.L. and Walters, L. (1989) *Contemporary issues in Bioethics,* 3rd edn. Wadsworth Publishing Company, Belmont California.

Bowling, A. (1996) Health care rationing the publics debate. *BMJ* **312** (7032), 670–4.

Brannigan, M. (1993) Oregon's experiment. *Health Care Analysis,* **1** (1), 15–32.

Burns, A., Dening, T., and Baldwin, R. (2001) Mental health problems. *BMJ* **322** (7289), 789–91.

Byford, S., McCrone, P., and Barrett, B. (2003) Developments in the quantity and quality of economic evaluations in mental health, *Current Opinion in Psychiatry,* **16** (6), 703–7.

Campbell, A., Gillett, G., and Jones, G. (1992) *Practical Medical Ethics.* Oxford University Press, Oxford, Auckland, Melbourne, New York.

Challis, L. and Henwood, M. (1994) Equity in the NHS: equity in community care. *BMJ* **308** (6942), 1496–9.

Chalmers, I., Sackett, D., and Silagy, C. (1997) The Cochrane Collaboration. In A. Maynard and I. Chalmers (eds.) *Non-Random Reflections on Health Service Research*. British Medical Journal Publishing Group, London.

Cochrane, A. (1972) *Effectiveness and Efficiency: Random Reflections on Health Services*. The Nuffield Hospitals Provincial Trust, London.

Cooper, B. and Singh, B. (2000) Populaton research and mental health policy: bridging the gap. *British Journal of Psychiatry*, **176**, 407–11.

Cornwall, J. and Fletcher, P. (2003) *National Overview Report on the Provision of Specialist Geriatric Services and Mental Health Services for Older People in New Zealand*. Ministry of Health, Wellington.

Department of Health (2001) *National Service Framework for Older People*. Department of Health, London.

Department of Health (2002) *Single Assessment Process: Guidelines for Local Implementation*. www.doh.gov.uk/scg/sap

Donaldson, C., Atkinson, A., Bond, J., and Wright, K. (1988) QALYS and the long term care for elderly people in the UK. *Age and Ageing*, **17**, 379–87.

Donaldson, C., Currie, G., and Milton, C. (2002) Cost effectiveness analysis in health care: contraindications. *BMJ* **325** (7369), 891–4.

Draper, B. (2001) Consultation liaison geriatric psychiatry. In P. Melding and B. Draper (eds.) *Consultation Liaison Geriatric Psychiatry*. Oxford University Press, Oxford, New York.

Draper, B. (2000) The effectiveness of old age psychiatry services. *International Journal of Geriatric Psychiatry*, **15**, 687–703.

Fletcher, P. (2003) A stocktake of geriatric and psychogeriatric services in New Zealand. Unpublished briefing paper. Ministry of Health, Wellington.

Gold, M.R., Siegel, J. E., Russell, L.B., and Weinstein, M.C. (1996). *Cost-Effectiveness in Health and Medicine*. Oxford University Press, New York.

Gutmann, A. and Thompson D. (2002) 'Just deliberation about health care' with Dennis Thompson. In M. Danis, C. Clancy, and L. Churchill (eds.) *Ethical Dimensions of Health Policy*, Oxford University Press, Oxford, pp. 77–94.

Ham, C. and Maynard, A. (1994) Managing the NHS Market. *BMJ* **308** (6932), 845–7.

Hornblow, A. (1997) New Zealand's health reforms: a clash of cultures. *BMJ* **314** (7098), 1892–4.

Hulka, B.S., Kupper, L.L., and Cassel, J.C. (1972) Determinants of physician utilization: approach to a service-oriented classification of symptoms. *Medical Care*, **10**, 300–9.

Jacobzone, S., Cambois, E., and Chaplain, E. (1998) *The Health of Older People in OECD Countries: Is it improving fast enough to compensate for population ageing?* Labour Market and Social Policy, Occasional Papers, No 37. Paris: Organization for Economic Co-Operation and Development.

James, V. (1995) Health care provision: the six key players. *Nursing Standard*, **9** (39), 30–2.

Jefferson, T., Demicheli, V., and Vale, L. (2002) Quality of systematic reviews of economic evaluations in health care. *Journal of the American Medical Association*, **287** (21), 2809–12.

Jones, D. and Gill, P. (1998) Breaking down language barriers: The NHS needs to provide accessible interpreting services for all. *BMJ* **316** (7143), 1476.

Kaplan, R.M. and Groessl, E.J. (2002) Applications of Cost-Effectiveness Methodologies in Behavioral Medicine. *Journal of Consulting and Clinical Psychology*, **70** (3), 482–93.

Kisely, S. (1999) Psychotherapy for severe personality disorder: exploring the limits of evidence based purchasing. *BMJ* **318** (7195), 1410–12.

Kronick, R., Goodman, D.C., and Wennberg, J. (1993) The marketplace in health care reform – the demographic limitations of managed competition. *New England Journal of Medicine,* **328** (2), 148–52.

Maynard, A. and Sheldon, T.A. (1997) Health economics: has it fulfilled its potential? In A. Maynard and I. Chalmers (eds.) *Non-Random Reflections on Health Service Research.* British Medical Journal Publishing Group, London.

Maynard, A. (1996) Evidence-based medicine: cost effectiveness and equity are ignored. *BMJ* **313** (7050), 170.

Maynard, A. (2001) Limits to demand for health care: rationing is needed in a national health service. *BMJ* b (7288), 734.

McGuire, A., Henderson, J., and Mooney, G. (1998) *The Economics of Health Care. An Introductory Text.* Routledge, London.

Mooney, G.H. (1983) Equity in health care: confronting the confusion. *Effective Health Care,* **1**, 179–85.

New Zealand Ministry of Health (2002a) *Health of Older People in New Zealand. A Statistical Reference.* Ministry of Health, Wellington.

New Zealand Ministry of Health (2002b) *Health of Older People: Health sector action to 2010 to support positive ageing.* Ministry of Health, Wellington.

New Zealand Ministry of Health (2004) *New Zealand Guideline for Specialist Health Services for Older People.* Ministry of Health, Wellington.

O'Connor, D. (2003) *A Binational Survery of Aged Psychiatry Services in Australia and New Zealand.* Presentation to Faculty of Psychiatry of Old Age, RANZCP, Annual Scientific Meeting, Brisbane.

Raftery, J. (2001) NICE: faster access to modern treatments? Analysis of guidance on health technologies. *BMJ* **323** (7324), 1300–3.

Rawls, J. (1971) *A Theory of Justice.* Cambridge, Mass: Harvard University Press.

Richards, T. (1999) Australia's consumer champion. *BMJ* **319** (7212), 730.

Richmond, D., Baskett, J., Bonita, R., and Melding, P.S. (1995) *Care of Older People in New Zealand.* National Health Committee, Wellington.

Robinson, J.C. (2001). The end of managed care. *Journal of the American Medical Association,* **285** (20), 2622–8.

Russell, L.B., Gold, M.R., Siegel, J.E., Daniels, N., and Weinstein, M.C. (1996) The role of cost-effectiveness analysis in health and medicine. *Journal of the American Medical Association,* **276** (14), 1172–7.

Ryan, M. (2004) Discrete choice experiments in health care. *BMJ* **328** (7436), 360–1.

Smith, R. (1996) Rationing happens all the time. *BMJ* **313** (7060), 722.

Thomson, H., Hoskins, R., Petticrew, M., Ogilvie, D., Craig, N., Quinn, T., and Lindsay, G. (2004) Evaluating the health effects of social interventions. *BMJ* **328** (7434), 282–5.

Ubel, P.A., Hirth, R.A., Chernew, M.E., and Fendrick, A.M. (2003) What is the price of life and why doesn't it increase at the rate of inflation? *Journal of the American Medical Association,* **163** (14), 1637–41.

Ubel, P.A., DeKay, M.L., Baron, J., and Asch, D.A. (1996) Cost-effectiveness analysis in a setting of budget constraints – is it equitable? *New England Journal of Medicine,* **334** (18), 1174–7.

Wasson, J., Stuckel, T., Weiss, J., Hays, R., Jette, A., and Nelson, E. (1999) A randomized trial of the use of a patient self administered data to improve community practice. *Effective Clinical Practice,* **2** (1), 1–10.

Chapter 5

Evidence-based psychogeriatric service delivery

Brian Draper and Lee-Fay Low

Over the last 15 years it has become apparent that old age psychiatry services need to provide evidence of their effectiveness to health administrators, whether it be in terms of patient outcomes, acceptability to consumers, or economic considerations (Draper, 1990, 2000a). The most widely accepted model of multidisciplinary, comprehensive, integrated service delivery to a defined catchment area was based on the experiences of geriatric medicine in the UK, pragmatism, advocacy and available resources rather than on formal evaluation (Banerjee, 1998). The Geriatric Psychiatry Section of the World Psychiatric Association and WHO, with the collaboration of the International Psychogeriatric Association, jointly produced a consensus statement on the organization of care in the psychiatry of the elderly (see Chapter 2) that supported this type of model (Wertheimer, 1997). In this chapter, we shall examine the effectiveness of old age psychiatry services by evaluating the quality of the available evidence that allows an appraisal of this model of care.

Evidence-based medicine in psychogeriatrics

Evidence-based medicine (EBM) is a paradigm that employs the use of contemporaneous, appraised, research findings as the basis for clinical decisions (Evidence-Based Medicine Working Group, 1992; Schmidt *et al.*, 1996). It is claimed that the best evidence of effectiveness of old age psychiatry services comes from well-designed randomized controlled trials (RCTs) (Cole, 1988). According to Cole (1988), RCTs of specific disorders in old age psychiatry should focus on five issues:

1. The need for specialized old age psychiatry services

2. The effectiveness of specific services

3. The effectiveness of different types of old age psychiatry services

4. The outcomes of care from different types of healthcare professionals in old age psychiatry services, and

5. The location of the services.

These evaluations should include measures of psychopathology, physical illness, functional disability, social functioning, quality of life and costs (Cole, 1988).

However, the applicability of RCTs to everyday care cannot be determined without the regular measurement of outcomes in daily practice as well because they cannot address every evaluative issue, especially when interventions are not uniform or are liable to be influenced by a multitude of real life extraneous factors (Marks, 1998; Knapp, 1998). It is also acknowledged that there are many areas of clinical practice that can never be adequately tested for ethical reasons (Evidence-Based Medicine Working Group, 1992). Further, the application of EBM to psychiatry is controversial, as concern has been expressed that where evidence is scant, EBM may facilitate cost-cutting exercises (Schmidt *et al.*, 1996).

For this reason, it has been argued that the evaluation of old age psychiatry services is 'best achieved by the construction of relatively simple models from an array of complex knowledge' (Harrison and Sheldon, 1994). It should encompass both summative evaluation based on quantitative measures of health care outcomes (for example, the routine use of scales to measure symptomatic change) and formative evaluation based on qualitative measures of health care processes (for example, consumer satisfaction) (Harrison and Sheldon, 1994). Medical audit, a process of review of medical records, has emerged as an effective method of evaluating the outcomes of old age psychiatry services, for example, by measuring adherence to simple clinical guidelines such as for psychotropic medication (Harrison and Sheldon, 1994; Jones, 1987). To be effective, medical audit ought to employ explicit criteria in order to compare patterns of clinical practice and to identify actions required to resolve any discrepancies (Shaw, 1990). Medical audits in old age psychiatry have increasingly been published over the last decade and provide data for EBM in areas where RCTs are not possible.

Formative evaluation has a more important role in old age psychiatry, where the processes of service provision may be valued for their own sake, for example, the quality of the therapeutic relationship (Harrison and Sheldon, 1994). The perspective from which the service is being evaluated determines the goals of evaluation. For patients, carers and referring agents the main domain may be satisfaction with the service provided; for staff job satisfaction and morale are key issues (Dening and Lawton, 1998; Kirby and Cooney, 1998; Nolan and Grant, 1993). For managers, the main issue may be the efficient use of services without compromising the quality of care (Harrison and Sheldon, 1994). Equity may be a key issue for those involved in health policy, so a comparison between health care needs and the services provided would also be required (Hamid *et al.*, 1995; Harrison and Sheldon, 1994).

Models of service delivery

There has been very limited evaluation of different models of psychogeriatric service delivery, and yet major changes have been occurring in service delivery in developed countries through deinstitutionalization and a focus on community care. This has been driven through a mix of consumer demand for improved care and cost pressures in meeting the needs of an ageing population. Extrapolation of data from studies that have focused primarily on the care of frail and/or institutionalized older people provides some guidance for models of psychogeriatric service delivery.

Johri et al. (2003) systematically reviewed the international literature on demonstration projects that tested innovative models of care for the elderly in OECD countries. They reviewed seven projects from Italy, the UK, Canada and the USA. Each of these projects aimed to create comprehensive integration of acute and long-term care. Common features of an effective system of care were identified including a single entry point system; case management; geriatric assessment and a multidisciplinary team and use of financial incentives to encourage less expensive community-based care (Johri et al., 2003). Apart from the use of financial incentives, each of these features are also mentioned in the consensus statement on the organization of care in the psychiatry of the elderly, providing some support for this approach (Wertheimer, 1997).

One of the shortcomings of clinical models of mental health care is that they rely upon the identification of the problem by the older person, their carer or a primary care health worker. In clinical models, detection and treatment of both syndromal and subsyndromal mental disorders are poor (Burns and Taube, 1990; Cole and Yaffe, 1996). Cole (2002) suggested the use of a 'public health model' of care that targets mental health of all older people in a defined population by systematic case identification, facilitation of access to treatment, delivery of quality care and assessment of outcomes. Additionally, this model has a strong health promotion and disease prevention focus. While there have been a number of studies that have utilized elements of the public health model in the community (Banerjee et al., 1996; Hinchliffe et al., 1997), general hospitals (Inouye et al., 1999) and residential care (Brodaty et al., 2003b, Llewellyn-Jones et al., 1999, 2001), the feasibility of its broader application that includes health promotion and disease prevention is questionable as it may not be cost-effective.

Few countries have widespread comprehensive psychogeriatric services able to provide the full range of services mentioned in the consensus statement (Reifler and Cohen, 1998). Even in OECD countries, rural and regional areas have relatively little service development. A recent survey in the state of New South Wales, Australia found that only 10 per cent of psychogeriatric services were located in rural areas (Draper et al., 2003), although 42.3 per cent of persons aged over 65 in the state reside in non-capital city areas. In many countries, mental health care for older people is provided by a range of different health professionals and services (Banerjee, 1998). Unfortunately there are few data that allow valid comparisons of the effectiveness of mental health service provision to older people by psychogeriatric services and by other types of services.

While there has been limited evaluation of the overall model of service delivery, a body of literature has developed on the evaluation of service delivery to older people in different settings and by a range of services. A search to May 2003 was undertaken of Medline, PsycINFO, CINAHL, EMBASE and Cochrane Collaboration databases of English language papers on service delivery evaluation. Keywords entered were

Table 5.1 Designation of levels of evidence (National Health and Medical Research Council, 2001)

I	Evidence obtained from a systematic review of all relevant randomized controlled trials.
II	Evidence obtained from at least one properly designed randomized controlled trial.
III-1	Evidence obtained from well-designed pseudo-randomized controlled trials (alternate allocation or some other method).
III-2	Evidence obtained from comparative studies (including systematic reviews of such studies) with concurrent controls and allocation not randomized, cohort studies, case-control studies, or interrupted time series with a control group.
III-3	Evidence obtained from comparative studies with historical control, two or more single arm studies, or interrupted time series without a parallel control group.
IV	Evidence obtained from case series, either post-test or pretest/post-test.

Source: *How to Use the Evidence: assessment and application of scientific evidence*. National Health and Medical Research Council (2000) copyright Commonwealth of Australia. Reproduced by permission.

'old age psychiatry' or 'psychogeriatrics' or 'geriatric psychiatry' combined with 'acute care' or 'long-term care' or 'general hospital' or 'nursing home' or 'consultation-liaison' and 'evaluation' or 'audit' or 'intervention' or 'service delivery'. This was supplemented by a manual search of references from relevant literature. All controlled trials and audits of the outcomes of care of older people by mental health services were included.

The authors independently assessed data quality of individual outcome studies using a revised version of the Methodological Quality Instrument (Cho and Bero, 1994). Scores on this instrument range from 0.00–1.00, with higher scores representing better quality studies. As inter-rater reliability between authors was high (Kendall's W = 0.896, p = 0.000), only the mean quality rating is presented. The overall quality of the evidence for the effectiveness of old age psychiatry service delivery in specific domains was rated on an evidence hierarchy that has four levels of evidence (Evidence-Based Medicine Working Group, 1992) (Table 5.1).

These data are supplemented by studies from the same search that focused on the processes of care. These studies were not rated for quality and have been included to assist in the interpretation of the outcome data.

Summaries of individual studies are included in Tables 5.1 to 5.11. If there were more than two controlled trials in a particular area of service delivery only those are presented in the tables. Otherwise all studies meeting a minimum quality rating of 0.60 are included in the table for that area of service delivery. An overall summary of studies in each area is presented in Table 5.12.

Community-based service delivery
Old age psychiatry day hospitals

There has been debate about the effectiveness of day hospitals in old age psychiatry, particularly in acute care (Fasey, 1994; Howard, 1994). A confounding issue in the

Table 5.2 Studies of psychogeriatric day hospitals

	Bergener et al. (1987) (Germany)	Plotkin and Wells (1993) (USA)	Corcoran et al. (1994) (UK)
Design	Retrospective concurrent controlled study	Retrospective case series	Prospective case series
Sample size	352	100	237
Age	Not stated	72.6	78
Psychiatric morbidity	Mixed psychiatric diagnoses, 55.4 per cent with depression	Mixed psychiatric diagnoses, not cognitively impaired	Mixed functional psychiatric and organic diagnoses
Intervention and/or Comparison Group	Medical treatment, individual and group therapy, occupational and creative therapy, physical therapy and counselling. Day hospital compared with acute psychogeriatric wards	Intensive treatment (3 months) followed by modified treatment (3 months) then open-ended maintenance 1 day a week Group therapy and individual attention from case manager	Acute psychiatric treatment, physical investigation and treatment Psychotherapy, counselling, reality orientation, reminiscence Carer support groups
Outcomes	Mean LOS = 46.5 days Virtually all discharges from day hospital and 75 per cent inpatient discharges returned to pre-admission environment At 2-year follow-up (FU), 53.3 per cent discharges from day hospital and 43.7 per cent discharges from an open ward were not readmitted	After intensive phase: 31 per cent moderately or markedly improved, 57 per cent showed some clinical improvement After modified phase: 25 per cent improved in clinical status	40 per cent functional disorder patients improved and discharged (mean LOS 5 months) 52 per cent dementia patients (mean LOS 8 months) deteriorated Lower than average psychogeriatric hospitalizations in the area
Quality rating	0.61	0.64	0.65

Continued

Table 5.2 Studies of psychogeriatric day hospitals—Cont'd

	Collier and Baldwin (1999) (UK)	Ashaye et al. (2003) (UK)
Design	Concurrent controlled study	Randomized controlled trial (of assessment process but not treatment)
Sample size	20 from day hospital, 64 attending day care	112
Age	Majority in age band 70–74	76.4
Psychiatric morbidity	Behavioural problems causing management difficulty	Psychological, physical and physical symptoms and social needs
Intervention and/or Comparison Group	1 day hospital and 7 day care facilities in one UK health authority	All patients assessed using the Camberwell Assessment of Need for the Elderly (CANE). CANE results defining areas of unmet needs were given to key workers of the experimental group but not the controls.
Outcomes	Day hospital attenders scored higher on restlessness, friction, sexual disinhibition, memory and motility compared to day care attenders	Follow up at 3 months or discharge (whichever first) Decrease in total number of unmet needs in both groups with no significant difference between them HoNOS scores decreased in both groups Behaviour problems and dependency increased in both groups
Quality rating	0.60	0.82

evaluation of day hospitals is that there is often a blurring of roles between assessment and treatment of the patient and provision of respite for the carer. The former is traditionally seen as being the primary concern of day hospitals (often funded by health authorities), while the latter is usually regarded as being the primary concern of day care centres (often funded by social/welfare agencies). But in many cases, facilities provide a mix of both functions. One study has shown that National Health Service day hospital attenders showed more behavioural disturbances, memory impairment and mobility restriction than those attending non-NHS day care (Collier and Baldwin, 1999, quality 0.60).

Studies of the outcome of day hospital treatment are listed in Table 5.2. The only RCT of day hospital treatment compared the three month outcomes of 112 older people who received a standardized needs assessment before psychiatric day hospital admission with those who did not receive such an assessment (Ashaye *et al.*, 2003, quality 0.82). No significant differences were noted between the two groups. Both groups had significant improvement in their Health of the Nation Outcome Scales (HoNOS) 65+ scores and reduction in their unmet needs. While this study does not address the fundamental issue of the effectiveness of day hospitals compared with other types of care, it does provide good quality evidence that those attending the psychiatric day hospital had significant improvements on well-accepted standard outcome measures.

In a retrospective concurrent control study, Bergener *et al.* (1987, quality 0.61) extensively evaluated their psychogeriatric day hospital in Cologne and compared the psychopathology, social circumstances and psychological strain of patients treated in the day hospital with those who were fully hospitalized. Contrary to their expectations, they could not detect any significant differences between the two groups. Further evaluation using cluster analysis of a second sample based upon the primary treatment location found that day hospital patients tended to be in better physical health, have less severe symptoms of mental illness and require less assistance with financial issues than patients fully hospitalized. The day hospital was found to be more efficient in the post-hospital discharge rehabilitation of schizophrenia, endogenous depression and organic psychoses than neurotic depression.

A number of uncontrolled case series have also examined treatment outcomes. Bramesfeld *et al.* (2001, quality 0.57) studied 44 depressed older patients who attended a gerontopsychiatric day clinic for a mean of 11 weeks. At discharge the patients showed a significant reduction in depressive symptoms on the Hamilton Depression Scale and improvement in cognition on the Mini Mental State Examination. Overall, 45.5 per cent of the patients were deemed to have fully recovered. Plotkin and Wells (1993, quality 0.64) retrospectively reviewed the charts of 100 day treatment patients, most of whom had a depressive disorder, and found that 57 per cent experienced clinical improvement over an approximate three month period. Patients with mood disorders, better initial functional status, greater initial social support, fewer stressful events during treatment and longer duration of treatment had better outcomes.

The outcome of depression following consultation by a psychiatrist in a geriatric medical day hospital showed that 64 per cent were well at 6 months and 50 per cent at 12 months (Agbayewa, 1990, quality 0.57). Other studies have shown an effect on the reduction of carer stress (Rolleston and Ball, 1994, quality 0.44; Rosenvinge et al., 1994, quality 0.48). It has been suggested that day hospitals may reduce the need for psychogeriatric unit (PGU) admissions, but the evidence is poor (Corcoran et al., 1994). One study of the effects of moving a day hospital from a community location to an inpatient site found that admissions were actually increased (Rosenvinge et al., 2001, quality 0.43).

From the available evidence, the part that day hospitals can play effectively in acute care remains unresolved, largely because studies comparing day hospital treatment with either community treatment or inpatient treatment are lacking. However, there is mounting evidence that they are effective in improving mental health outcomes, particularly for depression. The quality of the available evidence is level IV on the evidence hierarchy.

Community old age psychiatry services

There have been six RCTs of treatments provided by old age psychiatry services, four of which demonstrated that the community old age psychiatry service was more effective than the control intervention (see Table 5.3). Banerjee et al. (1996, quality 0.94) used a RCT to examine the efficacy of an intervention by a multidisciplinary community psychogeriatric team coordinated by a psychiatrist that developed individualized packages of care for depressed frail elderly living at home. They found that significantly more of the intervention group (58 per cent) had recovered after six months as compared to the general practitioner-(GP) managed control group (25 per cent). These results were not explained by the use of antidepressant medication alone.

Blanchard et al. (1995, quality 0.89) assessed the efficacy of psychiatric community nurse management of depression in community dwelling older people in a RCT and demonstrated that seven hours face-to-face time over a three month period was sufficient to improve the patient's depression scores compared to GP-managed controls. Greatest effect was noted in cases with longstanding depressive symptoms and this was maintained at longer term (6–23 month) follow-up (Blanchard et al., 1995, 1999, quality 0.89).

A RCT of treatment of depression in older GP clinic attenders by a multidisciplinary community old age psychiatry team found no significant difference at nine month outcome compared with GP managed patients (Jenkins and Macdonald, 1994, quality 0.81). There was a trend toward greater improvement in the intervention group but the study was under-powered to demonstrate an effect. Another RCT of older people identified through routine health checks in a large general practice as having significant depressive symptoms compared those allocated to community mental health team follow-up to routine GP care. Again a small sample size of 34 meant that the study had low power to detect effects and no significant differences were found at 18 months' follow-up (Arthur et al., 2002, quality 0.85).

Table 5.3 Controlled studies of community old age psychiatry services

	Jenkins and McDonald (1994) (UK)	Cole et al. (1995) (Canada)	Hinchliffe et al. (1995) (UK)
Design	Randomized controlled trial	Randomized controlled trial	Randomized controlled trial
Sample size	65	32	38
Mean age	73	75.2	81
Sample characteristics	General practice patients > 64 years of age who screened positive for depression	Outpatient clinic referrals who screened positive for depression and negative for cognitive impairment	Community-dwelling persons with DSM-III-R diagnosed dementia with behavioural problems and their carers who screened positive for psychological morbidity
Intervention and/or Comparison Group	Intervention group received a home assessment by a psychiatrist and tailored multidisciplinary treatment plan that was executed for 9 months Control group received usual GP care	Home assessment group received a psychiatric assessment at home and FU in clinic by study psychiatrist Clinic assessment group assessed and followed up in clinic by study psychiatrist	Intervention group received a 16-week individualized care package including medication, psychological techniques and social measures Control group acted as wait list controls receiving the intervention package between weeks 16 and 32
Outcomes	9 month FU No significant difference between groups on improvement in depression Inadequate sample size	12 weeks FU Significant improvements in both groups on depression and overall psychopathology measured by the SCL-42, social resources, patient rated evaluation of change scale and cognition No significant differences between groups	16 and 32 week FU Significant improvements on patient behaviour and caregiver stress in the intervention group compared to wait-list controls in the first 16 weeks Improvements were maintained at 32 week FU
Quality rating	0.81	0.86	0.85

Continued

Table 5.3 Controlled studies of community old age psychiatry services—Cont'd

	Blanchard et al. (1995, 1999) (UK)	Banerjee et al. (1996) (UK)	Rabins et al. (2000) (USA)
Design	Randomized controlled trial	Randomized controlled trial	Randomized controlled trial
Sample size	112	69	945 in 6 sites
Age	75.4 (intervention group) 76.5 (control group)	80.4 (intervention group), 80.1 (controls)	73.1 (intervention group), 72.0 (comparison group)
Sample characteristics	Community cohort screened positive for pervasive depression	Population cohort screening positive for depression	Population sample of city housing residents
Intervention and/or Comparison Group	Management plan formulated by multidisciplinary team before randomisation. GPs given an estimate of depression severity Intervention group – the study nurse, working closely with GP, attempted to implement the management plan Control group – usual GP care	Intervention cases presented at multidisciplinary team meeting where a management plan was formulated Control group received usual GP care	3 sites randomly assigned to the nurse-co-ordinated intervention programme, supervised by geriatric psychiatrists, assessments in residents' apartment and care provided when indicated 3 sites randomly assigned to the control group and received usual care
Outcomes	At 3 month FU intervention group improved on depression scores compared to controls At longer-term FU no significant differences between groups on depression scores but the intervention did have long term benefit for the chronically depressed	6 month FU 19 (58 per cent) of intervention group recovered compared to 9 (25 per cent) of control group	26 month FU Psychiatric cases in intervention sites had significantly lower depression and psychiatric symptom and behavioural disorder scores than controls.
Quality rating	0.89	0.94	0.91

Continued

Table 5.3 Controlled studies of community old age psychiatry services—Cont'd

	Arthur et al. (2002) (UK)
Design	Randomized controlled trial
Sample size	93
Mean age	Median 82 in intervention group, 79 in control group
Sample characteristics	Population sample of elderly patients screening positive for depression
Intervention and/or Comparison Group	Mental health assessment by community mental health team. A report with recommendations was sent to the patient's GP. Control group patients received usual care
Outcomes	12–18month FU: A greater proportion (non-significant) proportion of the control group had reduced GDS scores. Inadequate sample size
Quality rating	0.85

A nurse-based mobile outreach programme to seriously mentally ill older people (PATCH programme) was found to be more effective than usual care at 26 month follow-up in diminishing levels of depression and psychiatric symptoms in a RCT in public housing in Baltimore (Rabins *et al.*, 2000, quality 0.91). The PATCH model intervention included educating staff of the public housing to be case finders, home-based assessments, and providing care where indicated. On average, patients were seen five times by the nurses in sessions that most frequently involved counseling and education. Coordination of care amongst the housing staff members, patient's carers and their primary care providers were important features of the model (Robbins *et al.*, 2000).

There has been one RCT using a cross-over design by a multidisciplinary old age psychiatry team of the community treatment of behavioural disturbances associated with dementia (Hinchliffe *et al.*, 1995). Improved patient behaviour and reduced carer stress were achieved with individualized care packages during a 16 week trial that occurred in the patient's home, particularly if the intervention was implemented without delay, i.e. before the cross-over.

Uncontrolled community case series have also shown positive outcomes. Wasylenki *et al.* (1984, quality 0.54) reported a six month follow-up of a community programme in Canada and found that 82 per cent of referring doctors were satisfied with the consultation and that 25 per cent of patients had improved mental functioning, while 55 per cent had maintained their level of functioning. Another Canadian evaluation of an old age psychiatry outreach programme based on a community development model that emphasized caregiver education, found that 90 per cent of referred cases were able to be managed at a similar or lower level of care (Stolee *et al.*, 1996, quality 0.66). Depression outcomes obtained by a community psychogeriatric service reported that at 20–38 month follow-up, 45 per cent had fully recovered and a further 40 per cent had made a moderate improvement. These outcomes compared favourably with those obtained by the local adult mental health service (Hickie *et al.*, 2000, quality 0.59). Significant improvements have also been reported between assessment and discharge on the HoNOS 65+ in a West Australian multidisciplinary psychogeriatric service that was predominantly (85 per cent) community-based and included a diverse range of psychiatric disorders (Spear *et al.*, 2002, quality 0.67). Homebound mentally ill older people in the United States were also noted to benefit from a multidisciplinary community psychiatric team that utilized intensive case management with significant improvement on the Global Assessment of Function Scale (Kohn *et al.*, 2002, quality 0.61).

How the process of care impacts upon clinical outcome is increasingly the focus of investigation. One issue is whether initial assessment is best located in the patient's home or in an outpatient clinic. A RCT comparing initial home assessment with clinic based assessments in the treatment of depression in late life found no significant differences in treatment outcome or useful clinical information that was elicited (Cole *et al.*, 1995, quality 0.86). However, improvement of accessibility to psychogeriatric services is one of the major reasons that home assessment is advocated, and this was not addressed in the RCT. A community old age psychiatry service to a public housing complex proved successful in averting risk of eviction by providing continuing care to residents, two-thirds of whom were unwilling to attend clinics (Roca et al., 1990, quality 0.58). More recently, the rate of non-attendance of new referrals at a hospital-based clinic (21 per cent) was much higher than in a home-based clinic (2 per cent) (Anderson and Aquilina, 2002, quality 0.67). Two studies that have examined the costs of home-based clinics as compared with hospital-based clinics in the United Kingdom have found the home-based clinics to be marginally cheaper and hence more cost-effective (Aquilina and Anderson, 2002, quality 0.67, Shah, 1994, quality 0.60).

There is ongoing debate about the added value of consultant home visits in the UK (Jolley, 1999; Orrell and Katona, 1998), where it has been seen as a way of bypassing waiting lists and as an additional source of income to the consultant (Baldwin, 1998). A prospective study of home visits in the UK found that 81 per cent of GPs were satisfied with the outcome. However, GPs' expectations were not well matched by the services offered for inpatient admission, community psychiatric nurse input and outpatient follow-up (Orrell et al., 1998).

There is agreement that a multidisciplinary team member should visit the patient at home. Initial assessments can be effectively undertaken by non-medical staff without reducing diagnostic accuracy (Collighan et al., 1993, quality 0.66). The multidisciplinary approach has also been shown to increase the frequency of continuing care by the service as compared to that provided by a consultant psychogeriatrician domiciliary service (Coles et al., 1991, quality 0.58). Referring GPs have been shown to discriminate the roles of medical and non-medical staff by referring patients with treatment-resistant problems to medical staff and patients requiring specific therapies to nursing staff (Ball et al., 1996, quality 0.65). However some have expressed concern about this approach (Ginsburg et al., 1998; Jolley, 1993).

A second issue is that of community case management. Two quasi-experimental studies of models of community case management of dementia have been reported. Challis et al. (2002, quality 0.73) found that a case management scheme for dementia located in a community psychogeriatric service was more effective at maintaining the patient at home (51 per cent) than standard community psychogeriatric care (33 per cent) by the end of the second year. Also carer stress and unmet need were reduced and social contacts and level of researcher-rated risk in the domains of activities of daily living, health, behaviour, environment and carer distress were improved. Features of the scheme thought important to this outcome included long term contact with older people and their carers, small caseloads and access to a significant range of other resources. Woods et al. (2003, quality 0.78) examined a specialist mental health nursing service that focused on providing information and practical and emotional support to carers of people with dementia on a long term basis, even after placement or patient death. This was compared with conventional patient-focused services, where disorders other than dementia are also treated, and discharge occurs at death or placement.

Some of these conventional services only provided assessment without long term input to the patients or carers. No significant differences were noted on the primary outcome measure for carer stress or on community survival after 8 months. However, 'assessment only'-style services that provide no long term input have significantly worse outcomes (Woods *et al.*, 2003). The problem with the consultative style of service was illustrated by a Canadian study that reported only 31 per cent of referring physicians had followed the consultant's advice (Teitelbaum *et al.*, 1996, quality 0.57).

In summary, there is good evidence from a systematized review (Draper, 2000a) and RCTs that multidisciplinary community psychogeriatric teams are more effective than usual care in the management of depression and other mental disorders in late life (level I on the evidence hierarchy). Important components of community treatment are multidisciplinary teams, an individualized case management approach with ongoing care (rather than just assessment), home-based assessments to improve attendance and carer education (level III-2 on the evidence hierarchy). There is limited evidence (level IV) that management of depression for the elderly by a psychogeriatric service is more effective than that by an adult mental health.

Integrated hospital and community care

Home assessment before hospitalization is often recommended but there is little formal evaluation. One retrospective Irish study of 205 first admissions found that pre-admission home assessment was feasible, defined criteria that clarified reasons for hospitalization and ensured appropriate admission (Freyne and Wrigley, 1997, quality 0.55).

Community care after discharge from acute hospitalization may be an important factor in the prevention of readmissions. But a systematic review of the impact of geriatric medicine post-discharge services on mental state from controlled trials found that there was little evidence that they were beneficial (Cole, 2001).

The Unified Psychogeriatric Biopsychosocial Evaluation and Treatment (UPBEAT) study identified older veterans with previously unrecognized psychiatric conditions during medical and surgical hospitalization in 9 VA sites. Subsequent comprehensive psychogeriatric assessment and management was arranged post-discharge in a randomized trial. At 12-months' follow-up, the intervention group had lower inpatient costs, though this was due to fewer bed days rather than lower rate of readmissions (Kominski *et al.*, 2001, quality 0.71). Another study found that the post-discharge interpersonal counselling of older hospitalized medically ill patients with subdysthymic depression by community psychiatric nurses was more effective than usual care in reducing depressive symptoms after 6 months (Mossey *et al.*, 1996, quality 0.82).

In a study of late life depression, Philpot *et al.* (2000, quality 0.67) found lower rates of readmission where there was aftercare by community mental health teams or through an outpatients department, though the authors note that they were unable

Table 5.4 Controlled studies of integrated hospital and community care

	Kominski *et al.* (2001) (USA)	Mossey *et al.* (1996) (USA)
Design	Randomized controlled trial	Randomized controlled trial
Sample size	1687	76
Mean age	69.4	71
Sample characteristics	Screened positive for depression or anxiety, or alcohol abuse	Hospitalized medically ill elderly with subdysthymic depression scoring >10 on the Geriatric Depression Scale (GDS) and not meeting DSM-III-R criteria for major depression or dysthymia
Intervention and/or Comparison Group	UPBEAT intervention involved in-depth psychogeriatric assessment and proactive mental health care coordination by a multi-disciplinary team compared with usual care	The intervention group received up to 10 interpersonal psychotherapy sessions The control group received usual care
Outcomes	12 month FU Mental health and general health improved in both groups UPBEAT resulted in overall savings of $1,856 per patient by reducing inpatient bed use	At 3 months, the intervention group showed greater improvement than controls on the GDS, health ratings and physical and social functioning At 6 months, the intervention group improved significantly more over time than the control group
Quality rating	0.71	0.82

to control for illness severity. Earlier, it was noted that the initial positive discharge outcomes for 52 patients had largely dissipated by around 30 months post-discharge in the absence of community follow-up (Sadavoy and Reiman-Sheldon, 1983, quality 0.80).

Although there have been few studies in this area (see Table 5.4), integrated post-discharge services appear to be an important component of care. The quality of available evidence is level II for mental health services and there is no evidence of effectiveness of geriatric medical services (level I). There is level IV evidence of the effectiveness of community assessment before hospital admission.

Primary care collaborations

Most authorities agree that collaboration between primary and specialist care is desirable to improve treatment outcomes. It has been estimated that about 80 per cent of older people with moderate-severe depression consult a GP, although the depression may only be detected in about 25 per cent of these cases with fewer being treated and even less being referred for specialist advice (Cole and Yaffe, 1996). Simple educational approaches for GPs may be ineffective, particularly if implemented by non-medical staff (Livingston *et al.*, 2000, quality 0.61).

Two RCTs have now demonstrated benefits of the collaborative approach in the treatment of late-life depression (Table 5.5). Llewellyn-Jones *et al.* (1999, quality 0.89) evaluated the effectiveness of a population based multifaceted shared care intervention for elderly patients with depression in a residential care setting, approximately one-third of whom lived in self-care units. The intervention included multidisciplinary consultation and collaboration, training of GPs and carers in detection and management of depression, and depression-related health education and activity programmes. The control group received routine care. The intervention group at 9.5 months follow-up had significantly greater improvement on the Geriatric Depression Scale than the control group, though the clinical significance of the change was unclear.

A large multi-centre IMPACT (Improving Mood-Promoting Access to Collaborative Treatment) study randomly assigned 1801 patients aged 60 years and over to IMPACT

Table 5.5 Controlled studies of primary care collaborations

	Llewellyn-Jones *et al.* (1999) (Australia)	**Unutzer *et al.* (2002) (USA)**
Design	Randomized controlled trial	Randomized controlled trial
Sample size	220	1810 residents from 18 primary care clinics
Mean age	83.9 (control group) 84.9 (intervention group)	71.2
Sample characteristics	Depressed self-care unit and hostel patients aged ≥ 65 living in residential care facilities	Patients aged ≥ 60 with major depression and/or dysthymic disorder
Intervention and/or Comparison Group	Intervention group received multidisciplinary consultation and collaboration, training of GP and carers on management of depression and depression related health education and activity programmes Control group received usual care	Intervention group had 12 months access to a depression care manager offering support for primary care physician or brief psychotherapy for depression Control group received usual care
Outcomes	9.5 month FU Significant improvement on depression in intervention group compared to controls Intervention group significantly more likely to be taking antidepressants at FU than controls	3, 6, 12 month FU Intervention group had greater rates of depression treatment, more satisfaction with depression care, lower depression severity, less functional impairment and greater quality of life than controls
Quality rating	0.89	0.94

intervention or usual care. The IMPACT intervention involved access to a depression case manager supervised by a psychiatrist and a primary care expert. IMPACT included education, care management, and support of antidepressant management by the patient's primary care physician or brief psychotherapy by the depression case manager. The intervention patients had a significantly better outcome at 12 months with 45 per cent having a 50 per cent or greater reduction in depressive symptoms as compared to 19 per cent in the usual care group. There were also benefits in terms of quality of life and functional capacity (Unutzer *et al.*, 2002, quality 0.94).

These two studies provide good evidence (level II) that collaborations between specialist and primary care can be an effective model for the identification and management of late life depression. Whether such approaches can be effectively extended to a broader range of conditions has yet to be established.

Hospital-based acute psychogeriatric treatment

There have been few randomized controlled trials (RCTs) of acute hospital treatment of older people with mental disorders, and none controlling for either the type of ward (i.e. psychogeriatric, general adult psychiatry or geriatric medicine) or for actual hospitalization (i.e. hospital versus community care). This reflects the methodological and ethical challenges posed by such studies e.g. hospital versus community studies would require stringent inclusion and exclusion criteria to ensure safety. Such hospital versus community studies have been run in general adult psychiatry (e.g. Hoult and Reynolds, 1984) and in geriatric medicine (e.g. Caplan *et al.*, 1999), so it does seem feasible for old age psychiatry to mount such studies.

Existing evidence regarding hospital versus community care is meagre. Community treated patients have less functional disability, less severe depression, less cognitive impairment and fewer medical problems (Pasternak *et al.*, 1998) and have lower HoNOS scores (Shergill *et al.*, 1999) than inpatients. One non-randomized Canadian study compared the two-year outcome of patients treated by a psychogeriatric outreach service with patients admitted to a psychogeriatric unit. It found that while there was less institutionalization of the community cases, older people with affective disorders managed in the community had a poorer outcome than the hospitalized group (Houston, 1983, quality 0.43). These findings should be interpreted with great caution due to the study's methodological shortcomings.

Thus published studies of treatment outcome in hospital wards are largely restricted to uncontrolled prospective and retrospective case series.

General adult psychiatry wards

Only a few prospective and retrospective case series have examined the outcomes of treatment of older people in general adult psychiatry wards (Table 5.6). Although positive outcomes in terms of global improvement at discharge were reported in 75–81 per cent of cases (Conwell *et al.*, 1989, quality 0.62; Draper, 1994, quality 0.61; Sadavoy, 1981,

Table 5.6 Studies of older people in general adult psychiatry wards

	Sadavoy (1981) (Canada)	Conwell et al. (1989) (USA)	Draper (1994) (Australia)
Design	Retrospective case series	Prospective case series	Retrospective case series
Sample size	52	168	489
Age	73.4	69.7	74.3
Sample characteristics	Mixed functional psychiatric and organic diagnoses	Mixed functional psychiatric and organic diagnoses	Mixed functional psychiatric and organic diagnoses
Intervention and/or Comparison Group	Pharmacotherapy, ECT and other treatments	Pharmacotherapy and/or ECT	Psychotropics prescribed for 94 per cent ECT used for 18 per cent
Outcomes	Average LOS – 48.9 days Symptom remission to level of mental and emotional functioning prior to illness onset in 78.9 per cent	Mean LOS – 53.3 days 81.7 per cent discharged home 57.4 per cent had a good response to somatic treatments	Global clinical outcome – 81 per cent considered significantly improved 52 per cent discharged home 5 per cent readmitted within 30 days of discharge
Quality rating	0.61	0.62	0.61

Continued

Table 5.6 Studies of older people in general adult psychiatry wards—Cont'd

	Heinik et al. (1995) (Israel)
Design	Retrospective concurrent controlled study
Sample size	79 in one hospital A, 133 in hospital B
Age	72.6; 74.24 in the groups respectively
Sample characteristics	Mixed functional psychiatric and organic diagnoses
Intervention and/or Comparison Group	Hospital A has 2 psychogeriatric wards with chronic beds slowly transforming into acute beds Psychogeriatric patients in hospital B are admitted to general psychiatry wards
Outcomes	No significant differences between groups on outcomes: Mean LOS 58.3 days and 47.1 days respectively Death rates 5.1 per cent and 1.5 per cent respectively Independent at discharge: 69.6 per cent and 83.5 per cent respectively Discharged home: 74.7 per cent and 97.0 per cent respectively
Quality rating	0.67

quality 0.61), the extent to which these findings can be generalized is unclear. It is notable that the case mix of these studies was heavily biased toward depression with relatively few dementia cases complicated by behavioural disturbances. Thus the limited evidence may not be applicable to dementia. Also, three of the four general hospital ward studies included an old age psychiatrist in the staffing (Conwell *et al.*, 1989; Draper, 1994; Sadavoy, 1981).

The only comparison of the outcomes of care in a general hospital psychiatry ward with an acute psychogeriatric unit (PGU) was a retrospective concurrent control study from Israel. It found no significant differences on the outcome measures of length of stay (LOS), functional status, mortality and placement, though no psychiatric outcome measures were included (Heinik *et al.*, 1995, quality 0.67). The two main differences between the units were the higher admission rates and closer links with geriatric medicine noted in the PGU.

Additionally, it has been reported that the introduction of a psychogeriatric clinical nurse specialist into general psychiatric wards was effective at reducing LOS and costs while improving nurses' job satisfaction and patient outcomes (Mathew *et al.*, 1994, quality 0.51). A comparison of psychogeriatric services provided by specialist old age psychiatrists and those provided by 'non-specialist' consultants in the UK found that the 'specialist' services had more acute and long stay beds for older people, staffing, teaching and research (Wattis, 1989, quality 0.51). The limited evidence of effectiveness of treatment in general hospital psychiatry wards suggests that the involvement of specialist psychogeriatric staff may be an important factor. On the evidence hierarchy, the quality of evidence for the effectiveness of adult psychiatry wards is level IV.

Acute psychogeriatric units

Although there have been no controlled trials, numerous uncontrolled prospective and retrospective case series have examined discharge outcomes of acute psychogeriatric units (PGUs) and some have also reported long-term outcomes (see Table 5.7). Overall, the majority of patients are reported to make significant symptomatic improvement during hospitalization.

Significant improvements on standardized depression scales at discharge have been reported in depressed patients (Djernes *et al.*, 1998, quality 0.63; Riordan and Mockler, 1996, quality 0.65). Between 38–69 per cent of depressed patients are reported to be fully recovered at discharge, while 51–96 per cent having at least partial recovery (Baldwin and Jolley, 1986, quality 0.62; Cole, 1983; Heeren *et al.*, 1997, quality 0.65; Rubin *et al.*, 1991, quality 0.63; Zubenko *et al.*, 1994, quality 0.65). Better response both at discharge and in the medium term is associated with more intensive treatment, including the use of electroconvulsive therapy (Draper and Luscombe, 1998, quality 0.67; Heeren *et al.*, 1997; Philpot *et al.*, 2000; Zubenko *et al.*, 1994).

Few studies have examined long-term outcomes. In one study, 69 per cent were non-depressed at three months post discharge (Casten *et al.*, 2000, quality 0.59).

Table 5.7 Studies of older people in acute psychogeriatric units

	Baldwin and Jolley (1986) (UK)	Rubin et al. (1991) (USA)	Zubenko et al. (1992) (USA)
Design	Retrospective case series	Retrospective case series	Prospective case series
Sample size	100	101	120
Age	74	76.0	79.6
Sample characteristics	Hospitalized patients over 65 years of age with severe, non-neurotic depression	Hospitalized patients on a geropsychiatric unit with major unipolar depression meeting DSM-III criteria	All Alzheimer's disease meeting DSM-III-R criteria All had problem behaviours
Intervention and/or Comparison Group	45 per cent received antidepressants 48 per cent received ECT	Patients received psychiatric care from their private physician, specialized social service and activity therapy services as well as weekly or twice weekly assessment.	Physical environment designed to facilitate care of frail elderly Pharmacotherapy
Outcomes	58 per cent were recovered at 1 year, 22 per cent depression free at 3–8 years 39 per cent had further episodes with full recovery at 3–8 years 32 per cent had further episodes with incomplete recovery at 3–8 years	58.4 per cent of patients were judged globally by their physician to have shown major improvement ie symptoms diminished to baseline levels 37.6 per cent of patients were judged globally to have some improvement	Significant improvements at discharge from admission in domains of cognition, mood, behaviour and global assessment that varied according to presence of delirium, depression or psychosis. 53.8 per cent of patients who could no longer be managed at home before admission were discharged home
Quality rating	0.62	0.63	0.70

Continued

Table 5.7 Studies of older people in acute psychogeriatric units—Cont'd

	Zubenko et al. (1994) (USA)	Moss et al. (1995) (Australia)	Simpson et al. (1995) (UK)
Design	Prospective case series	Prospective case series	Case series
Sample size	205	110	41
Age	71.1	74	Not Stated
Sample characteristics	All had major depression meeting DSM-III-R criteria	Mixed functional psychiatric and organic diagnoses	Randomly selected caregivers of elderly mentally ill inpatients
Intervention and/or Comparison Group	Comprehensive psychiatric and medical review Pharmacotherapy, ECT, individual, group and milieu psychotherapy Families given educational counselling and supportive care	Physical therapies, depression treatment group, OT support groups and a dementia management programme 13.6 per cent received ECT, all depressed patients received antidepressants or lithium, all psychotic individuals received antipsychotics	8 psychogeriatric wards in Leicestershire, England
Outcomes	45.9 per cent full responders (Hamilton depression Rating score ≤10 at discharge) 5.4 per cent partial responders (HAM-D score had decreased by >50 per cent at discharge) 48.8 per cent non-responders	78 per cent returned to former level of accommodation, 22 per cent discharged to a more independent level LOS median = 129 days, range 1 to 194	Interviews post-discharge: 47.5 per cent carers thought the hospital stay was good/excellent 59 per cent were dissatisfied with some aspects of the hospital stay 85 per cent had positive comments about nursing care 50 per cent had positive comments about medical care
Quality rating	0.65	0.68	0.64

Continued

Table 5.7 Studies of older people in acute psychogeriatric units—Cont'd

	Kunik et al. (1996) (USA)	Riordan and Mockler (1996) (UK)	Heeren et al. (1997) (Netherlands)
Design	Retrospective case series	Prospective case series	Prospective case series
Sample size	41	60	225
Age	70.6	77.1	73.9
Sample characteristics	All patients admitted from nursing homes Mixed functional psychiatric and organic diagnoses	Mixed functional psychiatric and organic diagnoses	Any mood disorder meeting DSM-III-R criteria
Intervention and/or Comparison Group	Multidisciplinary treatment including pharmacotherapy, individual, family and group therapy	Inpatient admission unit for the elderly mentally ill staffed by a multidisciplinary team	Three old age psychiatry acute wards
Outcomes	Significant improvement in depression, psychiatric symptoms, agitation and global functioning scores No differences in cognition and side effects 49.8 per cent patients discharged to less restrictive environments	Patients with mood disorders improved significantly on discharge on depression measured using the GDS 2 month FU ratings of problem resolution (by service provider, carers and patients) showed the best outcomes for mood disorder symptoms and anxiety.	Post-discharge assessment (median LOS = 12 weeks): Full recovery in 40 per cent Partial recovery in 53 per cent Not recovered 7 per cent
Quality rating	0.66	0.65	0.65

Continued

Table 5.7 Studies of older people in acute psychogeriatric units—Cont'd

	Draper and Luscombe (1998, 1999) (Australia)	Djernes et al. (1998) (Denmark)	Holm et al. (1999) (USA)
Design	Prospective case series	Prospective case series	Prospective case series
Sample size	73	148	250
Age	77.8 ± 6.86	Not stated	81
Sample characteristics	Mixed functional psychiatric and organic diagnoses	Psychogeriatric inpatients with principle diagnosis of major depression (54 per cent), dementia (23 per cent), delirium (18 per cent) or psychosis (5 per cent)	All had dementia and behavioural disturbance
Intervention and/or Comparison Group	Pharmacotherapy, ECT and other treatments	Multidisciplinary team management including physiotherapy, occupational therapy and psychopharmacologic treatment	Multidisciplinary care involving comprehensive assessment, individualized care plan, pharmacotherapy, maximizing environmental and structural interventions and individual therapy
Outcomes	Average global assessment of functioning at discharge significantly higher than at admission 18 per cent fully recovered, 64 per cent improved with some residual symptoms, 11 per cent unchanged, 7 per cent worse 19 per cent died within 12 months of discharge	Significant decrease at discharge in level of: Psychopathology in depressed, demented and delirious patients Behavioural disorders, depression, intellectual performance, ADL and gait in depressed and delirious patients	Significant decrease in mean aggression scale scores with complete elimination in 38 per cent of patients Significant increase in mean cognition scores with improvement in 79 per cent Significant improvement in function scores – 92 per cent improved
Quality rating	0.67, 0.65	0.63	0.66

Continued

Table 5.7 Studies of older people in acute psychogeriatric units—Cont'd

	Neville et al. (1999) (UK)	Akpaffiong et al. (1999) (USA)	Philpot et al. (2000) (UK)
Design	Prospective case series	Prospective case series	Retrospective concurrent controlled study
Sample size	230	141 Caucasians, 56 African Americans	131 in total: 72 in service A, 59 in service B
Age	80.2	74.1 NB: only 4 females in sample	76.0 for service A, 75.3 for service B
Sample characteristics	Dementia and/or delirium, most with behavioural problems	All had dementia	All had affective disorder by ICD-10 criteria. Not significantly cognitively impaired
Intervention and/or Comparison Group	2 general hospitals and an old psychiatric hospital	Pharmacotherapy	Service A was a consultant led service with a large in-patient unit, well-staffed psychiatric team and day hospital, and a small team of community nurses. Service B was a smaller in-patient unit well-staffed interdisciplinary community mental health team
Outcomes	Mean LOS = 59 days. Of the total problems listed as reasons for admission, at discharge, 84 per cent improved, 15 per cent were unchanged, 1 per cent were worse. 33.5 per cent of subjects discharged home	Improvement between admission and discharge on agitation, depression or psychiatric symptoms	Patients at A more likely to be discharged to residential care than B. LOS lower in A (median of 80 vs 43 days). Survival time out of hospital greater in B. Survival time to death greater in B
Quality rating	0.65	0.78	0.67

Philpot *et al.* (2000, quality 0.67) in a retrospective case note study, found that over a follow-up period of 5–8 years in two neighbouring psychogeriatric services, 50 per cent of patients were readmitted. Readmissions were less likely in the service that had a community orientation, after longer index admissions, and where outpatient and community psychiatric nurse follow-up was arranged. Interestingly, mortality was also lower in the community-oriented service.

The discharge outcomes of the treatment of the behavioural and psychological symptoms of dementia (BPSD) have been reported in prospective and retrospective case series utilizing standardized behaviour scales (Akpaffiong *et al.*, 1999, quality 0.78; Kunik *et al.*, 1996, quality 0.66). Significant improvements were found in the larger better quality studies (Akpaffiong *et al.*, 1999; Kunik *et al.*, 1996; Zubenko *et al.*, 1992, quality 0.70). A prospective study employing a problem-oriented approach that mainly involved patients with BPSD, found that 84 per cent of problems were rated to have improved by discharge (Neville *et al.*, 1999, quality 0.65). Between 39–50 per cent of patients with BPSD are discharged to their pre-admission level of care (Neville *et al.*, 1999; Zubenko *et al.*, 1992). Mortality rates during admission range from 0–9 per cent (Akpaffiong *et al.*, 1999; Kunik *et al.*, 1996; Neville *et al.*, 1999; Zubenko *et al.*, 1992).

Overall, global measures of outcome irrespective of diagnosis indicate that 82–86 per cent of patients have improved at discharge (Draper and Luscombe, 1999, quality 0.65; Grant and Casey, 2000, quality 0.50; Moss *et al.*, 1995, quality 0.68). Other outcomes have also been considered. Functional capacity is reported to improve in some but not all studies. Studies that have reported functional improvement in dementia patients (Holm *et al.*, 1999, quality 0.66; Zubenko *et al.*, 1992) have had larger sample sizes than one that failed to demonstrate improvement (Djernes *et al.*, 1998). Cognitive outcomes are also variable. Some studies report significantly improved cognition in dementia (Holm *et al.*, 1999; Zubenko *et al.*, 1992), but most do not (Akpaffiong *et al.*, 1999; Djernes *et al.*, 1998; Kunik *et al.*, 1996; Wattis *et al.*, 1994). Improved cognition has also been reported in depression (Djernes *et al.*, 1998) and delirium (Djernes *et al.*, 1998; Zubenko *et al.*, 1992).

Outcomes that encompass the views of patients and carers are also important but few pluralistic evaluations have been published. While studies in this area have found that carers are generally satisfied with the service received, their perceptions of improvement are more conservative than those of service providers (Riordan and Mockler, 1996; Simpson *et al.*, 1995, quality 0.64; Wattis *et al.*, 1994).

Length of stay (LOS) is often used as an outcome measure because it is a proxy for service efficiency. There is no consistent evidence that links LOS with other outcomes of care (Draper 2000a), though longer LOS has been found to predict better depression outcomes in terms of readmissions (Philpot *et al.*, 2000). The investigation of factors contributing to LOS have yielded contradictory findings, with medical, social and psychiatric variables being implicated (Draper and Luscombe, 1998).

Cost containment has also been examined in other ways. Clinical pathways have been successfully used to reduce LOS and hence costs (Bultema *et al.*, 1996, quality 0.47), but no other outcomes were reported so it is unclear whether there were detrimental effects. Another approach has been the use of less expensive intermediate care, often located in a local authority home, as an alternative to hospitalization or admission to long-term care. The only study, which was uncontrolled and descriptive, provided very limited evidence that this could be feasible but insufficient to recommend it as a specific form of care (Ackermann *et al.*, 2003, quality 0.43).

In summary, there is only one non-randomized comparison study of acute care in PGUs and this is a major gap in evidence. Uncontrolled case series from centres in the US, Australia, the UK, Denmark and the Netherlands indicate that discharge treatment outcomes for depression and BPSD are positive in the majority of cases. Long-term outcomes are influenced by the intensity of inpatient treatment and post discharge follow-up arrangements. On the evidence hierarchy, the quality of evidence for the effectiveness of acute psychogeriatric units is level III-2 for depression, level IV for BPSD.

Mental health services provided by hospital medical services

Controlled studies of mental health outcomes achieved by geriatric medical services have been reviewed by Cole (1993) who concluded that there was little evidence that they had an important measurable impact upon cognitive function and depression. In a large retrospective medical chart audit in the US, the quality of care for depressed elderly inpatients was better on a range of criteria in psychiatric wards compared with general medical wards (Norquist *et al.*, 1995, quality 0.75). The psychiatric ward patients had better overall psychological assessments, received more psychological services, their clinical status at discharge was better but they had more medical complications. One caveat to these studies is that mental health may have been a secondary outcome measure.

Few studies based in medical wards have a primary mental health objective (see Table 5.8). A randomized trial of geriatric liaison intervention by a multidisciplinary team led by a geriatrician trained in old age psychiatry, focused on the detection of depression and cognitive dysfunction (Slaets *et al.*, 1997, quality 0.88). The intervention resulted in improved physical functioning, shorter LOS and fewer nursing home transfers. However, no mental health outcomes were reported. Thus it is unclear whether the intervention was specifically beneficial for depression or cognition.

Some retrospective case series have suggested a positive impact of medical services when mental health outcomes are primary measures. A psychogeriatric ward run by a geriatrician, with consultations from a psychiatrist, and with 94 per cent patients having organic mental disturbances, had 'improved' outcomes in 47 per cent of cases (Prinsley, 1973, quality 0.57). A Dutch geriatric assessment team that included a psychologist was found to reduce the impact of BPSD upon the carer (Gerritsen *et al.*, 1995, quality 0.43).

Table 5.8 Studies of psychogeriatric services provided by hospital medical services

	Cole *et al.* (1994) (Canada)	Slaets *et al.* (1997) (Netherlands)
Design	Randomized controlled trial	Randomized controlled trial
Sample size	88	237 (from 2 different general medicine wards)
Age	86.8 (intervention), 85.4 (controls)	82.8
Sample characteristics	Delirium meeting DSM-III-R criteria	75 years of age or older
Intervention and/or Comparison Group	Intervention group received consultation within 24 hours by geriatrician or geriatric psychiatrist and daily follow-up by liaison nurse Control group received regular usual medical care	Intervention group received multidisciplinary joint management by geriatric care team in addition to usual care involving daily contact with the ward staff and patients Controls receive usual general medicine ward care
Outcomes	Improvement in intervention group in cognition at 2 weeks compared to controls, but not maintained at 8 weeks Significant improvement on behaviour over 8 weeks in intervention group compared to controls No differences on restraint use, LOS, place of discharge or mortality	Discharge and 12-month post-discharge FU: More intervention patients improved on physical functioning Mean LOS was 5 days shorter for the intervention group and fewer readmissions Institutionalization was significantly more likely in the controls
Quality rating	0.90	0.88

The prevention and treatment of delirium is one area that medical services have targeted with RCTs. In a systematic review, Cole (1999) concluded that there were modest benefits for systematic interventions to prevent delirium in elderly medical patients. Another systematic review found no evidence that delirium prevention programmes were effective when there is comorbid dementia (Britton and Russell, 2003).

In summary, delirium prevention programmes by medical services appear to be moderately effective in intermediate risk patients without comorbid dementia (level II evidence) but there is little evidence that medical services are effective in treating other mental disorders (level I).

Combined psychogeriatric and geriatric medical wards

Combined psychogeriatric and geriatric medical wards intentionally established to be jointly run by psychogeriatricians and geriatricians have been frequently described but not well evaluated (Arie and Dunn, 1973, quality 0.52; Pitt and Silver, 1980, quality 0.52; Porello *et al.*, 1995, quality 0.53). The wards are described as being particularly useful in the management of the medically unwell behaviourally disturbed patient, but apart from uncontrolled LOS, discharge and mortality data, there are no other reported outcomes. So their actual effectiveness in improving mental health and other outcomes has yet to be established (level IV on evidence hierarchy).

Consultation/liaison old age psychiatry services to medical wards

This is one area of hospital-based psychogeriatric service delivery where there have been RCTs in addition to case series (see Table 5.9). The overall results in mental health outcomes have been modest with two studies demonstrating only non-significant trends towards improvement on measures of depression and cognitive function (Cole et al., 1991, quality 0.90; Strain et al., 1991, quality 0.62). A smaller study with high attrition found no significant differences between the intervention group and controls at 10 weeks and at one year (Shah et al., 2001, quality 0.85). However, a multi-site historic controlled study of psychiatric consultation/liaison (CL) intervention with elderly hip fracture patients produced a significant reduction in LOS and hospital costs (Strain et al., 1991) as did an earlier natural experiment (Levitan and Kornfeld, 1981, quality 0.59).

It is important to put these CL intervention studies into perspective by examining RCTs of antidepressant treatment of similar patients. Of five placebo-controlled studies of medically ill older patients in medical and rehabilitation wards, only two found that antidepressants were significantly better than placebo and both of these involved chronic illnesses (Draper, 2000b). Recruitment difficulties and high dropout rates combined to leave small sample sizes with insufficient power to determine antidepressant efficacy. Thus it is unsurprising given that the efficacy of antidepressant therapy for depression in acute physical illness is not firmly established, that the effectiveness of CL interventions is also unclear.

Uncontrolled case series provide some additional outcome data. The establishment of a formal psychogeriatric unit in one Italian centre was associated with increased consultation rates, the frequency of follow-up consultations, use of psychological interventions, implementation of psychiatric prescriptions by referring agents and a reduction length of stay (de Leo et al., 1989, quality 0.61). The presence of a formal old age psychiatry CL service may also increase the recognition of depression by referring agents (Scott et al., 1988). Three months' follow-up of a CL intervention showed an increased utilization of community services and community nursing, while 54 per cent had further psychiatric contact and 14 per cent a psychiatric admission (Loane and Jefferys, 1998, quality 0.67). A study from Italy found that 60 per cent of consultations reported that they felt better 3–5 months post-consultation (Rigatelli et al., 2001, quality 0.57). There have been no studies directly comparing outcomes of service delivery by CL psychiatry and CL old age psychiatry. One review noted that published cohort studies tend to suggest that CL old age psychiatry services are more likely to consider

Table 5.9 Studies of CL psychogeriatric service delivery

	Cole et al. (1991) (Canada)	Strain et al. (1991) (USA)	Shah et al. (2001) (UK)
Design	Randomized controlled trial	Historical control study	Randomized controlled trial
Sample size	80	452	47
Age	86.3 (intervention group) 82.4 (control group)	83.7 (site 1), 80.3 (site 2)	Median age 85
Sample characteristics	Hospitalized patients referred to the multidisciplinary geriatric team screening positive for either cognitive impairment, depression or anxiety	Aged 65 and older admitted to one of 4 orthopaedic units for surgical repair of fractured hips	Patients admitted to 3 acute geriatric medicine wards screening positive for depression
Intervention and/or Comparison Group	Treatment group received geriatric psychiatry consultation involving comprehensive assessment and treatment recommendations Control group did not	The psychiatric liaison intervention comprised evaluation of every consenting patient and treatment as necessary, weekly ombudsman rounds and nursing and discharge meetings, family and social work conferences At site 1, usual care in year 1 compared to psychiatric liaison intervention in year 2. At site 2, all units received usual care in year 1, 1 unit received psychiatric liaison intervention while 2 received usual care in year 2	Intervention group received detailed formal psychogeriatric consultation within 24 hours Control group received standard care
Outcomes	Significant improvement on anxiety scores in intervention group compared with controls at 8 weeks Trend towards greater improvement in intervention group on cognition, depression and behavioural disturbance Twice as many intervention patients discharged home	Patients in the intervention group had higher consultation rates than controls Mean LOS was reduced from 20.7 to 18.5 days in site 1, and from 15.5 to 13.8 days in site 2, resulting in reduced hospital costs No difference between groups in discharge placement	Discharge, 10 week, 1 yr FU Both groups improved in depression over time No difference between groups on change in depression scores or interventions received Poor concordance between recommended interventions and implementation by geriatricians in the control group
Quality rating	0.90	0.62	0.85

post-discharge follow-up and community services as treatment options than pure CL services (Draper, 2001).

In summary, there have been several RCTs that have shown a significant benefit for CL services, though not on mental health outcomes. The overall quality of evidence for the effectiveness of interventions by CL services on non-mental health outcomes such as LOS and costs is level II, while the evidence for mental health outcomes is level IV. There are no outcome studies that address whether CL interventions for older people should be provided by CL or old age psychiatry.

Long-term institutional care

Psychogeriatric outreach to long-term residential care

There have been nine controlled trials of psychogeriatric service interventions in long term care (see Table 5.10). Overall, the results are mixed. One interpretation of the evidence suggests that liaison-style services that employ educational approaches including treatment guidelines and ongoing involvement are more effective than a pure case-based consultative approach. Rovner *et al.* (1996), Lawton *et al.* (1998), Proctor *et al.* (1999) and Ballard *et al.* (2002) exemplify good examples of studies of the liaison approach.

Rovner *et al.* (1996, quality 0.94) undertook a RCT of a dementia care programme consisting of activities, guidelines for psychotropic medications and educational rounds and found that the prevalence of behaviour disorders: use of antipsychotic medication and restraints were all reduced at 6 month follow-up. Lawton *et al.* (1998, quality 0.79) used a stimulation-retreat intervention that included staff training, inter-disciplinary care planning with a psychologist, activity programming, and family support by a social worker in a special care unit. Apart from some significant effects on positive behaviours and affects, there were few measurable differences at 12 months when compared with the routine care group. Proctor *et al.* (1999, quality 0.91) provided staff training and psychosocial management of behavioural problems in a RCT involving 12 long-term care facilities. After 6 months, significant improvements were noted in levels of depression and cognitive functioning in the intervention group but there were no significant differences in behavioural disorders. Finally, Ballard *et al.* (2002, quality 0.81) performed a non-randomized trial involving weekly visits to six long-term care facilities by a community psychiatric nurse with support from a consultant psychiatrist and a clinical psychologist to develop care plans with medication review as compared with usual care in three long-term care facilities. While there were no differences detected in levels of behavioural disorders or well-being after 9 months, the intervention group were prescribed fewer neuroleptic drugs, had fewer GP contacts and used fewer inpatient beds. Staff training alone to recognize and manage behavioural disturbances may be ineffective, as found in one study after 3 and 12 months (Moniz-Cook *et al.*, 1998, quality 0.78).

Table 5.10 Controlled studies of psychogeriatric outreach to long-term care

	Ames et al. (1990) (UK)	Abraham et al. (1992) (USA)	Rovner et al. (1996) (USA)
Design	Randomized controlled trial	Randomized controlled trial	Randomized controlled trial
Sample size	93	76	89
Mean age	82.3	84.4	82.0 (intervention group) 81.2 (control group)
Sample characteristics	Nursing home patients screening positive for significant depressive symptoms without severe dementia	Non-cognitively impaired nursing home residents screening positive for depression	Nursing home residents meeting criteria for dementia on DSM-III-R and with behavioural disturbance
Intervention and/or Comparison Group	Intervention group visited by psychogeriatrician and social worker throughout the 3 month intervention. Advice given to GPs, senior care staff and relevant agencies Wait list controls received treatment after 3 months Non-intervention controls were from homes not visited until 3 month FU	Cognitive behavioural group therapy Focused visual imagery group Control subjects participated in education discussion groups	The intervention group participated in a day activity program, psychotropic management and weekly education rounds for staff by the psychiatrist The control group received usual care except for an increase in the nurse-to-patient ratio during the day
Outcomes	3 and 12 month FU No significant differences on depression between groups at 3 months and on rate of recovery at 12 months Only 28 per cent of patients reassessed at 12 months showed evidence of recovery from depression	Assessment at −4, 8, 20 and 28 weeks No significant changes in depression, hopelessness or life satisfaction in any of the three groups Cognitive-behavioural and visual imagery groups showed a significant improvement on cognition after 8 weeks	At 6 month FU, significantly fewer intervention patients exhibited behaviour disorders compared with controls Intervention patients were significantly less likely to receive antipsychotics, be restrained during activity times and more likely to participate in activities
Quality rating	0.73	0.78	0.94

Continued

Table 5.10 Controlled studies of psychogeriatric outreach to long-term care—Cont'd

	Lawton et al. (1998) (USA)	Moniz-Cook et al. (1998) (UK)	Proctor et al. (1999) (UK)
Design	Cluster randomized study	Cluster randomized study	Cluster randomized study
Sample size	97	84 residents, 83 staff from 3 nursing homes	120 residents from 12 nursing homes
Mean Age	Not stated	83.4 at follow-up	83.1
Sample characteristics	All nursing home residents in the units studied living there for at least 6 months	All residents included, the majority had dementia	Nursing home residents with difficult to manage behavioural problems
Intervention and/or Comparison Group	Experimental unit provided both high and low stimulation areas for residents (n = 49) Control residents received usual care (n = 48)	Intervention homes received weekly 3-hour training sessions for 5 weeks for all staff. Sessions consisted of a formal talk, small-group work, feedback and a homework task based on person-centred approaches to dementia care (n = 2) The control home received no extra training (n = 1)	Intervention homes received staff training from an outreach team and weekly visits for 6 months from a psychiatric nurse to assist with psychosocial management of behavioural problems using a 'goal planning' strategy (6 homes, 60 residents) Control homes received usual services (6 homes, 60 residents)
Outcomes	Baseline, 6 and 13 month FU No significant effect on cognition, function, negative behaviours and affect Marginally significant effect on positive behaviours and affect	3 and 12 month follow-up Frequency of behavioural problems reported increased in all homes At 3 months, experimental homes reported significantly less difficulty managing behavioural problems than controls At 12 months, no differences between homes on behavioural problem frequency or ease of management	6 month FU The intervention group was significantly improved on depression and cognition but not on behaviour or function
Quality rating	0.79	0.78	0.91

Continued

Table 5.10 Controlled studies of psychogeriatric outreach to long-term care—Cont'd

	Opie et al. (2002) (Australia)	Ballard et al. (2002) (UK)	Brodaty et al. (2003b) (Australia)
Design	Randomized wait-list controlled trial	Non-randomized controlled trial	Randomized controlled trial
Sample size	99	330 residents from 9 care facilities	86
Mean age	84.1 (intervention) 83.7 (control)	83.0 (intervention group) 82.0 (control group)	82.9
Sample characteristics	Nursing home residents with a diagnosis of dementia and moderately disruptive behaviour	Nursing home residents with dementia	Nursing home residents with dementia meeting DSM-IV criteria and depression and/or psychosis
Intervention and/or Comparison Group	The intervention group received 4 weeks of multidisciplinary consultancy including individually tailored plan with strategies targeting specific behaviours The control group received the intervention after 4 weeks	Intervention care facilities received 9 month psychiatric liaison delivered by a psychiatric nurse who visited weekly providing review 24 hours after referrals, help developing tailored care plans using psychological interventions as a first line approach, psychiatric evaluation and medication review (6 homes, 208 residents) Control facilities received usual services (3 homes, 125 residents)	Case management patients received multidisciplinary team intervention for 12 weeks Consultation patients had management plans sent to the nursing home and GP Controls received standard care
Outcomes	1 month FU Significant decrease in challenging behaviours in the intervention group compared with controls	9 month follow-up Significant decrease in neuroleptic usage in intervention group Significantly fewer GP contacts in intervention group and 3 × reduction in psychiatric in-patient bed usage No differences between groups in behavioural and psychological symptoms or wellbeing	12 week FU All three groups improved on depression scales and psychosis scales No significant differences between groups over time
Quality rating	0.84	0.81	0.95

Two consultation-style controlled trials of BPSD found that both intervention and usual care control groups improved significantly on measures of behaviour and psychopathology over the course of the intervention. Both sets of authors speculated that this may be due to the Hawthorne effect and 'leakage' of intervention strategies to control subjects (Brodaty *et al.*, 2003b, quality 0.95; Opie *et al.*, 2002, quality 0.84) as in both studies, intervention subjects and control subjects resided in the same nursing home. The interventions were extensive with multidisciplinary research teams being present in the facilities for many months. In effect, while the interventions were essentially consultative, the prolonged involvement of research staff in facilities mimicked a liaison-style intervention.

Two pure consultation-style controlled interventions failed to demonstrate significant differences on measures of depression. Ames (1990, quality 0.73) recommended psychiatric, medical and social interventions after consultation by a psychiatrist and social worker in 12 local authority residential homes. Relatively few of the recommended interventions were carried out and only 28 per cent of the surviving subjects had improved at 12 months. Abraham *et al.* (1993, quality 0.78) compared three group approaches to the treatment of depression in seven nursing homes – cognitive-behaviour therapy, visual imagery and education/discussion. While some cognitive improvements were noted, no effect on depression was found at 24-week follow-up.

There have also been a number of uncontrolled evaluations of outreach services to nursing homes. A South Australian psychogeriatric outreach team reported significant improvement in the behavioural disturbances of nursing home and hostel residents, although outcomes for those with depression were not as good. Eighty-seven percent of referring agents and 80 per cent of carers rated the service as being 'helpful' or 'very helpful' (Seidel *et al.*, 1992, quality 0.62). Regular visits from psychogeriatric nurses and psychogeriatricians have been reported to decrease hospital admissions, improve communication, increase the frequency of therapeutic programmes and to improve staff understanding and acceptance of emotional problems and behaviours (Goldman and Klugman, 1990, quality 0.55; Tourigny-Rivard and Drury, 1987, quality 0.41).

These studies suggest that old age psychiatry services are capable of providing effective outreach services to long-term residential care. This is best delivered by a liaison model of care with a strong educational component that includes treatment guidelines and possibly emotional support and/or supervision of the nursing staff. The quality of available evidence for this type of service is level I on the evidence hierarchy, while for consultation only service, the quality of evidence is level II.

Long stay psychogeriatric wards and community residences

In many countries, long stay psychogeriatric wards were the traditional location of long-term institutional care of older patients with dementia and chronic mental illnesses. Over the last thirty years a combination of deinstitutionalization and transinstitutionalization policies has resulted in a marked reduction in long stay psychogeriatric beds in many countries including the US (Bartels *et al.*, 1999), the UK (Simmons and Orrell, 2001), the Netherlands (Pijl and Sytema, 2003) and Germany (Wormstall and Guenthner, 2002). These changes have been driven by a mix of economic and care issues. Many patients in traditional long stay psychogeriatric wards were managed in less restrictive, less expensive community settings (Bartels *et al.*, 1999; Wills and Leff, 1996).

There have been no RCTs and few evaluations of long term psychogeriatric care that focus on non-economic issues (see Table 5.11). The best available data are derived from well-designed service evaluations such as the TAPS project in the UK, which was set up to evaluate the closure of Freiern and Claybury Hospitals from the early 1980s until the early 1990s. In this project, psychogeriatric wards at Freiern Hospital were compared with community residences that had been developed as part of the transinstitutionalization programme (Wills and Leff, 1996, quality 0.69; Wills *et al.*, 1998, quality 0.70). Patients in the community residences were found to have a better quality of life, more social contacts and more privacy. Schizophrenic patients in the community residences tended to stabilize or improve slightly, while those in the hospital wards deteriorated over three years. The community residences were superior to the hospital wards in terms of family satisfaction, equipment and safety features. The more 'home-like' environment of the community residences was particularly noted. These advantages need to be interpreted with some caution because the patients selected for the community residences were more highly functioning than those who remained.

A second evaluation of transinstitutionalization involved the use of domus units that are purpose built 12-bed residential facilities that have a philosophy of maintaining residents' independence and residual capacities as far as possible through active participation (Dean *et al.*, 1993, quality 0.57; Lindesay *et al.*, 1991, quality 0.70). Two facilities were prospectively evaluated – one for dementia residents requiring intensive nursing care and the other for 'graduate' patients with chronic schizophrenia. At 12 months, improvements were noted in cognition, communication, self-care skills, activity participation, interpersonal interactions and on measures of resident choice, privacy and control.

A nationwide survey from France compared 110 residents from 10 cantou and 242 long stay psychogeriatric ward residents with dementia (Ritchie *et al.*, 1992, quality 0.69). Cantou are an innovative form of communal non-medical care for dementia residents, housed in a separate enclosed area with 12–15 rooms organized around common living areas. The cantou have a home-like atmosphere and encourage family participation. The cantou group residents had fewer depressive symptoms, improved communication skills, better quality of life and greater mobility in the first year. Families expressed greater satisfaction with the cantou than with hospital wards.

One model of long-term care-service provision has proposed that there is a small group of older patients with very severe intractable behavioural disturbances, usually aggression, due to dementia and other mental disorders that require care in a secure mental health psychogeriatric facility (Brodaty *et al.*, 2003a). While this view seems to be in keeping with many expert opinions, there have been no evaluations.

Table 5.11 Studies of long term psychogeriatric care

	Lindsay et al. (1991) (UK)	Ritchie et al. (1992) (France)	Dean et al. (1993) (UK)
Design	Concurrent controlled study	Concurrent control with case-controlled subsample	Prospective historical controlled study
Sample size	72	352 (27 case-controlled pairs directly observed)	12 dementia, 12 'graduate elderly' with chronic schizophrenia
Age	77.1 (domus), 78.5 (ward 1), 78.1 (ward 2)	81.3 (cantou), 85.3 (hospital)	75.8 (dementia), 74.1 'graduate elderly'
Sample characteristics	Most with dementia, some with functional psychiatric disorders	Most with dementia, some with functional psychiatric disorders	Two domuses – one for dementia, one for 'graduate elderly' with chronic mental illness, mainly schizophrenia
Intervention and/or Comparison Group	Domus unit in which resident and staff well-being are both important, and the emphasis is on maintaining residents' independence and residual capacities through active participation Two typical long-stay psychogeriatric wards	10 cantou care facilities offering communal non-medical care with individual rooms and activities centred around tasks of daily living 25 long-stay hospitals	Prospective evaluation over 12 months of the residents of the two domuses in comparison with baseline assessment in long stay psychogeriatric ward
Outcomes	No differences on resident mortality, cognition, and depression between groups Significantly higher levels of activities and staff-resident interaction on domus compared to hospital wards	Significant differences in populations at admission Cantou group significantly less dependent, less depressed and more mobile with better and more frequent communication abilities	Domuses offered more policy choice, resident control, provision for privacy, and availability of social and recreational activities Improvement in resident cognition, and communication skills Higher levels of activities and interpersonal interactions compared with baseline
Quality rating	0.70	0.69	0.58

Continued

Table 5.11 Studies of long term psychogeriatric care—Cont'd

	Wills and Leff (1996) (UK)	Wills et al. (1998) (UK)	Trieman et al. (1999) (UK)
Design	Concurrent controlled study	Concurrent controlled study	Longitudinal cohort study
Sample size	174	168	71
Age	Not stated	Not stated	78.3 (hospital group); 79.6 (community group)
Sample characteristics	Psychogeriatric patients with mixed functional psychiatric and organic diagnoses	Professional care staff working in: 7 psychogeriatric wards (n = 79) 4 community-based psychogeriatric facilities (n = 89)	Hospitalized psychiatric patients for at least 1 year aged 70 or older without dementia (most with schizophrenia)
Intervention and/or Comparison Group	Hospitalized patients resided in 6 psychogeriatric wards. Community-dwelling patients resided in 4 units designated for their continuing care	Average staff-patient ratio similar between hospital and community settings The largest proportion of unqualified staff was in hospital compared to the community but in general community staff had fewer years of experience in working with psychogeriatric patients	'Hospital group' remained in hospital 'Community group' discharged to 6 new specialized community psychogeriatric wards
Outcomes	The average time spent in social contact, having drinks between meals and being with relatives was significantly greater in the community sample. Relatives perceived the community residents in more positive ways than hospital wards.	Community facilities were better equipped with physical amenities and safety features, provided more privacy and were more encouraging of independence. Hospital care staff were more likely to express dissatisfaction with pay, working conditions and social status.	3 year FU The behaviour of community patients was stable over time whereas hospital patients became more disturbed Community patients declined less cognitively than hospital patients
Quality rating	0.69	0.70	0.71

Table 5.12 Level of evidence and study quality for each area of service delivery

Area	No of studies	No of controlled trials	Quality range*	Mean rating*	Level of evidence of effectiveness
Psychogeriatric day hospitals	10	0	0.43–0.82	0.57	Level IV
Community old age psychiatry services	24	7	0.79–0.94	0.87	Level I for multidisciplinary psychogeriatric teams, Level IV for adult psychiatry teams
Integrated hospital and community care	4	2	0.71–0.82	0.76	Level II for psychogeriatric services post-discharge care, no evidence for geriatric medical services (level I)
Primary Care collaborations	3	2	0.89–0.94	0.92	Level II
Older people in general adult psychiatric wards	6	0	0.51–0.67	0.59	Level IV
Acute psychogeriatric wards	23	0	0.43–0.78	0.61	Level III-2 for depression, level IV for BPSD
Hospital medical services	6	2	0.82–0.90	0.89	Level II for prevention of delirium without dementia, no evidence for other mental health outcomes (level 1)
Combined psychogeriatric and medical wards	3	0	0.52–0.53	0.52	Level IV
Hospital-based CL psychogeriatric service delivery	7	3	0.62–0.90	0.79	Level II effectiveness for reducing costs and length of stay, level IV for mental health outcomes
Long-term psychogeriatric care	6	0	0.58–0.71	0.66	Level III-2
Psychogeriatric outreach to long-term care	16	9	0.73–0.95	0.84	Level I for liaison style outreach services, Level II for consultation style
Overall	108	25	0.62–0.95**	0.85**	

*If ≥ 2 controlled trials in service area, quality range and mean rating reported for controlled trials only, otherwise reported for all studies; ** overall mean and range reported for controlled trials only

In summary, purpose built community-based residential facilities have advantages over long stay psychogeriatric wards for less dependent patients with dementia and chronic schizophrenia, but it is unclear whether they are suited for patients with very severe behavioural disturbances. The quality of the evidence is level III-2.

Conclusion

Service delivery in different settings has been evaluated with varying levels of evidence quality (See Table 5.12). The quality of evidence is improving over time with a significant positive correlation between year of publication and quality rating (Pearson's R = 0.320, $p = 0.001$). Since the previous review (Draper, 2000a), there have been numerous published RCTs in community care and outreach to long term residential care that demonstrate the effectiveness of psychogeriatric services. Successful models involve case management styles in the community and liaison styles in long term residential care. Both options are more staff intensive than the alternative assessment only consultation service style. Integration of hospital and community care is also important in improving outcomes following hospital discharge. All the limited evidence also suggests that psychogeriatric services provide more effective mental health service delivery to older people than geriatric medical services.

One area of service delivery that only has lower quality, albeit consistently positive, evidence of effectiveness is acute inpatient care in PGUs. Controlled studies are required to determine whether alternative forms of community or hospital care are as effective. While community residences for long term institutional care appear to offer better quality care than hospitals, it is unclear whether there are particular patients who require long term psychogeriatric hospitalization.

In conclusion, there is a growing evidence of psychogeriatric service delivery effectiveness. More research is required but a firm foundation has now been established.

Acknowledgement

Parts of this chapter were published in a synthesis 'What is the effectiveness of old age mental health services?' undertaken for the World Health Organization's Regional Office for Europe and the Health Evidence Network. August 2004. www.euro.who.int/eprise/main/WHO/Progs/HEN/Syntheses/20030820_1.

References

Abraham, I.L., Neundorfer, M.M., and Currie, L.J. (1992) Effects of group interventions on cognition and depression in nursing home residents. *Nursing Research*, 41, 196–202.

Abraham, I.L., Buckwalter, K.C., Snustad, D.G., Smullen, D.E., Thompson-Heisterman, A.A., Neese, J.B., and Smith, M. (1993) Psychogeriatric outreach to rural families: the Iowa and Virginia models. *International Psychogeriatrics*, 5, 203–11.

Ackermann, E., Burnand, J., Horton, C., Jenkins, D., Joomraty, H., Pritchard, D., Rayner, F., Wedatilake, G., and Wilson, R. (2003) Two year outcomes of a multi-agency elderly mentally ill unit providing intermediate care. *International Journal of Geriatric Psychiatry,* **18**, 359–60.

Agbayewa, M.O. (1990) Outcome of depression in a geriatric medical day hospital following psychiatric consultation. *International Journal of Geriatric Psychiatry,* **5**, 33–9.

Akpaffiong, M., Kunik, M.E., Hale, D., Molinari, V., and Orengo, C. (1999) Cross-cultural differences in demented geropsychiatric inpatients with behavioral disturbances. *International Journal of Geriatric Psychiatry,* **14**, 845–50.

Ames, D. (1990) Depression among elderly residents of local-authority residential homes. Its nature and the efficacy of intervention. *British Journal of Psychiatry,* **156**, 667–75.

Anderson, D.N. and Aquilina, C. (2002) Domiciliary clinics I: effects on non-attendance. *International Journal of Geriatric Psychiatry,* **17**, 941–4.

Aquilina, C. and Anderson, D. (2002) Domiciliary clinics II: a cost minimisation analysis. *International Journal of Geriatric Psychiatry,* **17**, 945–9.

Arie, T. and Dunn, T. (1973) A 'do-it-yourself' psychiatric-geriatric joint patient unit. *Lancet,* **2**, 1313–16.

Arthur, A.J., Jagger, C., Lindesay, J., and Matthews, R.J. (2002) Evaluating a mental health assessment for older people with depressive symptoms in general practice: a randomised controlled trial. *British Journal of General Practice,* **52**, 202–7.

Ashaye, O.A., Livingston, G., and Orrell, M. (2003) Does standardized needs assessment improve the outcome of psychiatric day hospital care for older people? A randomised controlled trial. *Aging and Mental Health,* **7**, 195–9.

Baldwin, R.C. (1998) Re: Geriatric consultation and liaison service. *International Journal of Geriatric Psychiatry,* **13**, 820–1.

Baldwin, R.C. and Jolley, D.J. (1986) The prognosis of depression in old age. *British Journal of Psychiatry,* **149**, 574–83.

Ball, C., Payne, M., and Lewis, E. (1996) Doctors and nurses: referrals by general practitioners to different arms of an old age psychiatry service. *International Journal of Geriatric Psychiatry,* **11**, 995–9.

Ballard, C., Powell, I., James, I., Reichelt, K., Myint, P., Potkins, D., Bannister, C., Lana, M., Howard, R., O'Brien, J., Swann, A., Robinson, D., Shrimanker, J., and Barber, R. (2002) Can psychiatric liaison reduce neuroleptic use and reduce health service utilization for dementia patients residing in care facilities. *International Journal of Geriatric Psychiatry,* **17**, 140–5.

Banerjee, S. (1998) Organization of old age psychiatry services. *Reviews in Clinical Gerontology,* **8**, 217–25.

Banerjee, S., Shamash, K., Macdonald, A.J., and Mann, A.H. (1996) Randomised controlled trial of effect of intervention by psychogeriatric team on depression in frail elderly people at home. *BMJ* **313**, 1058–61.

Bartels, S.J., Levine, K.J., and Shea, D. (1999) Community-based long-term care for older persons with severe and persistent mental illness in an era of managed care. *Psychiatric Services,* **50**, 1189–97.

Bellelli, G., Frisoni, G.B., Bianchetti, A., Boffelli, S., Guerrini, G.B., Scotuzzi, A., Ranieri, P., Ritondale, G., Guglielmi, L., Fusari, A., Raggi, G., Gasparotti, A., Gheza, A., Nobili, G., and Trabucchi, M (1998) Special care units for demented patients: a multicenter study. *Gerontologist,* **38**, 456–62.

Bergener, M., Kranzhoff, E.U., Husser, J., and Markser, V. (1987) The psychogeriatric day hospital: definition, historical development, working methods and initial efforts in research. In M. Bergener (ed.) *Psychogeriatrics – An International Handbook.* Springer: New York.

Blanchard, M.R., Waterreus, A. and Mann, A.H. (1995) The effect of primary care nurse intervention upon older people screened as depressed. *International Journal of Geriatric Psychiatry,* 10, 289–98.

Blanchard, M.R., Waterreus, A., and Mann, A.H. (1999) Can a brief intervention have a longer-term benefit? The case of the research nurse and depressed older people in the community. *International Journal of Geriatric Psychiatry,* 14, 733–8.

Bramesfeld, A., Adler, G., Brassen, S., and Schnitzler, M. (2001) Day-clinic treatment of late-life depression. *International Journal of Geriatric Psychiatry,* 16, 82–7.

Britton, A. and Russell, R. (2003) *Multidisciplinary Team Interventions for Delirium in Patients with Chronic Cognitive Impairment.* Cochrane review, the Cochrane Library. John Wiley and Sons: Chichester, UK.

Brodaty, H., Draper, B.M., and Low, L.F. (2003a) Behavioural and psychological symptoms of dementia: a seven-tiered model of service delivery. *Medical Journal of Australia,* 178, 231–4.

Brodaty, H., Draper, B.M., Millar, J., Low, L.F., Lie, D., Sharah, S., and Paton, H. (2003b) Randomized controlled trial of different models of care for nursing home residents with dementia complicated by depression or psychosis. *Journal of Clinical Psychiatry,* 64, 63–72.

Bultema, J.K., Mailliard, L., Getzfrid, M.K., Lerner, R.D., and Colone, M. (1996) Geriatric patients with depression. Improving outcomes using a multidisciplinary clinical path model. *Journal of Nursing Administration,* 26, 31–8.

Burns, B.J. and Taube, C.A. (1990) Mental health services in general medical care and in nursing homes. In B. Fogel, A. Furino and G. L. Gottlieb (eds.) *Mental Health Policy for Older Americans: Protecting Minds at Risk.* American Psychiatric Press: Washington DC.

Caplan, G.A., Ward, J.A., Brennan, N.J., Coconis, J., Board, N., and Brown, A. (1999) Hospital in the home: a randomised controlled trial. [comment]. *Medical Journal of Australia,* 170, 156–60.

Casten, R.J., Rovner, B.W., Pasternak, R.E., and Pelchat, R. (2000) A comparison of self-reported function assessed before and after depression treatment among depressed geriatric inpatients. *International Journal of Geriatric Psychiatry,* 15, 813–8.

Challis, D., von Abendorff, R., Brown, P., Chesterman, J., and Hughes, J. (2002) Care management, dementia care and specialist mental health services: an evaluation. *International Journal of Geriatric Psychiatry,* 17, 315–25.

Cho, M.K. and Bero, L.A. (1994) Instruments for assessing the quality of drug studies published in the medical literature. *JAMA,* 272, 101–4.

Cole, M.G. (1983) Age, age of onset and course of primary depressive illness in the elderly. *Canadian Journal of Psychiatry – Revue Canadienne de Psychiatrie,* 28, 102–4.

Cole, M.G. (1988) Evaluation of psychogeriatric services. *Canadian Journal of Psychiatry – Revue Canadienne de Psychiatrie,* 33, 57–8.

Cole, M.G. (1993) The impact of geriatric medical services on mental state. *International Psychogeriatrics,* 5, 91–101.

Cole, M.G. (1999) Delirium: effectiveness of systematic interventions. *Dementia and Geriatric Cognitive Disorders,* 10, 406–11.

Cole, M.G. (2001) The impact of geriatric post-discharge services on mental state. *Age and Ageing,* 30, 415–18.

Cole, M.G. (2002) Public health models of mental health care for elderly populations. *International Psychogeriatrics,* 14, 3–6.

Cole, M.G., Fenton, F.R., Engelsmann, F., and Mansouri, I. (1991) Effectiveness of geriatric psychiatry consultation in an acute care hospital: a randomized clinical trial. *Journal of the American Geriatrics Society,* 39, 1183–8.

Cole, M.G., Primeau, F.J., Bailey, R.F., Bonnycastle, M.J., Masciarelli, F., Engelsmann, F., Pepin, M.J., and Ducic, D. (1994) Systematic intervention for elderly inpatients with delirium: a randomized trial. *CMAJ Canadian Medical Association Journal*, **151**, 965–70.

Cole, M.G., Rochon, D.T., Engelsmann, F., and Ducic, D. (1995) The impact of home assessment on depression in the elderly: a clinical trial. *International Journal of Geriatric Psychiatry*, **10**, 19–23.

Cole, M.G. and Yaffe, M.J. (1996) Pathway to psychiatric care of the elderly with depression. *International Journal of Geriatric Psychiatry*, **11**, 157–61.

Coles, R.J., von Abendorff, R., and Herzberg, J.L. (1991) The impact of a new community mental health team on an inner city psychogeriatric service. *International Journal of Geriatric Psychiatry*, **6**, 31–9.

Collier, E. and Baldwin, R. (1999) The day hospital debate: a contribution. *International Journal of Geriatric Psychiatry*, **14**, 587–91.

Collighan, G., Macdonald, A., Herzberg, J., Philpot, M., and Lindesay, J. (1993) An evaluation of the multidisciplinary approach to psychiatric diagnosis in elderly people. *BMJ* **306**, 821–4.

Conwell, Y., Nelson, J.C., Kim, K., and Mazure, C.M. (1989) Elderly patients admitted to the psychiatric unit of a general hospital. *Journal of the American Geriatrics Society*, **37**, 35–41.

Corcoran, E., Guerandel, A., and Wrigley, M. (1994) The day hospital in psychiatry of old age: what difference does it make? *Irish Journal of Psychological Medicine*, **11**, 110–15.

de Leo, D., Baiocchi, A., Cipollone, B., Pavan, L., *et al.* (1989) Psychogeriatric consultation within a geriatric hospital: a six-year experience. *International Journal of Geriatric Psychiatry*, **4**, 135–41.

Dean, R., Briggs, K., and Lindesay, J. (1993) The domus philosophy: a prospective evaluation of two residential units for the elderly mentally ill. *International Journal of Geriatric Psychiatry*, **8**, 807–17.

Dening, T. and Lawton, C. (1998) The role of carers in evaluating mental health services for older people. *International Journal of Geriatric Psychiatry*, **13**, 863–70.

Djernes, J.K., Gulmann, N.C., Abelskov, K.E., Juul-Nielsen, S., and Sorensen, L. (1998) Psychopathologic and functional outcome in the treatment of elderly inpatients with depressive disorders, dementia, delirium and psychoses. *International Psychogeriatrics*, **10**, 71–83.

Draper, B. (1990) The effectiveness of services and treatment in psychogeriatrics. *Australian and New Zealand Journal of Psychiatry*, **24**, 238–51.

Draper, B. (1994) The elderly admitted to a general hospital psychiatry ward. *Australian and New Zealand Journal of Psychiatry*, **28**, 288–97.

Draper, B. (2000a) The effectiveness of old age psychiatry services. *International Journal of Geriatric Psychiatry*, **15**, 687–703.

Draper, B. (2000b) The effectiveness of the treatment of depression in the physically ill elderly. *Aging and Mental Health*, **4**, 9–20.

Draper, B. (2001) Consultation Liaison Geriatric Psychiatry. In P. Melding and B. Draper (eds.) *Geriatric Consultation Liaison Psychiatry*. Oxford University Press: Oxford.

Draper, B., Jochelson, T., Kitching, D., Snowdon, J., Brodaty, H., and Russell, B. (2003) Mental health service delivery to older people in New South Wales: perceptions of aged care, adult mental health and mental health services for older people. *Australian and New Zealand Journal of Psychiatry*, **37**, 735–40.

Draper, B. and Luscombe, G. (1998) Quantification of factors contributing to length of stay in an acute psychogeriatric ward. *International Journal of Geriatric Psychiatry*, **13**, 1–7.

Draper, B. and Luscombe, G. (1999) The effects of physical health upon the outcome of admission to an acute psychogeriatrics ward. *Australian Journal on Ageing*, **18**, 134–9.

Evidence-Based Medicine Working Group (1992) Evidence-based medicine. A new approach to teaching the practice of medicine. Evidence-Based Medicine Working Group. *JAMA*, **268**, 2420–5.

Fasey, C. (1994) The day hospital in old age psychiatry: the case against. *International Journal of Geriatric Psychiatry*, **9**, 519–23.

Freyne, A. and Wrigley, M. (1997) Acute inpatient admissions in a community oriented old age psychiatry service. *Irish Journal of Psychological Medicine*, **14**, 4–7.

Gerritsen, J.C., van der Ende, P.C., Wolffensperger, E.W., and Boom, R.C. (1995) Evaluation of a geriatric assessment unit. *International Journal of Geriatric Psychiatry*, **10**, 207–17.

Ginsburg, L., Hamilton, P., Madora, P., Robichaud, L., and White, J. (1998) Geriatric psychiatry outreach practices in the province of Ontario, the role of the psychiatrist. *Canadian Journal of Psychiatry Revue Canadienne de Psychiatrie*, **43**, 386–90.

Goldman, L.S. and Klugman, A. (1990) Psychiatric consultation in a teaching nursing home. *Psychosomatics*, **31**, 277–81.

Grant, R.W. and Casey, D.A. (2000) Geriatric psychiatry: evolution of an inpatient unit. *Administration and Policy in Mental Health*, **27**, 153–6.

Hamid, W.A., Howard, R., and Silverman, M. (1995) Needs assessment in old age psychiatry: a need for standardization. *International Journal of Geriatric Psychiatry*, **10**, 533–40.

Harrison, S. and Sheldon, T.A. (1994) Psychiatric services for elderly people: evaluating system performance. *International Journal of Geriatric Psychiatry*, **9**, 259–72.

Heeren, T.J., Derksen, P., van Heycop Ten Ham, B.F., and van Gent, P.P. (1997) Treatment, outcome and predictors of response in elderly depressed in-patients. *British Journal of Psychiatry*, **170**, 436–40.

Heinik, J., Barak, Y., Salgenik, I., and Elizur, A. (1995) Patterns of two psychogeriatric hospitalization services in Israel: a one-year survey. *International Journal of Geriatric Psychiatry*, **10**, 1051–7.

Hickie, I., Burke, D., Tobin, M., and Mutch, C. (2000) The impact of the organisation of mental health services on the quality of assessment provided to older patients with depression. *Australian and New Zealand Journal of Psychiatry*, **34**, 748–54.

Hinchliffe, A., Hyman, I., Blizard, B., and Livingston, G. (1995) Behavioural complications of dementia: can they be treated? *International Journal of Geriatric Psychiatry*, **10**, 839–47.

Hinchliffe, A.C., Katona, C., and Livingston, G. (1997) The assessment and management of behavioural manifestations of dementia: a review and results of a controlled trial. *International Journal of Psychiatry in Clinical Practice*, **1**, 157–68.

Holm, A., Michel, M., Stern, G.A., Hung, T.M., Klein, T., Flaherty, L., Michel, S., and Maletta, G. (1999) The outcomes of an inpatient treatment program for geriatric patients with dementia and dysfunctional behaviors. *Gerontologist*, **39**, 668–76.

Hoult, J. and Reynolds, I. (1984) Schizophrenia. A comparative trial of community orientated and hospital orientated psychiatric care. *Acta Psychiatrica Scandinavica*, **69**, 359–72.

Houston, F. (1983) Two year follow-up study of an outreach program in geriatric psychiatry. *Canadian Journal of Psychiatry – Revue Canadienne de Psychiatrie*, **28**, 367–70.

Howard, R. (1994) Day hospitals: the case in favour. *International Journal of Geriatric Psychiatry*, **9**, 525–9.

Inouye, S.K., Bogardus, S.T. Jr., Charpentier, P.A., Leo-Summers, L., Acampora, D., Holford, T.R., and Cooney, L.M. Jr. (1999) A multicomponent intervention to prevent delirium in hospitalized older patients. *New England Journal of Medicine*, **340**, 669–76.

Jenkins, D. and Macdonald, A. (1994) Should general practitioners refer more of their elderly depressed patients to psychiatric services? *International Journal of Geriatric Psychiatry*, **9**, 461–5.

Johri, M., Beland, F., and Bergman, H. (2003) International experiments in integrated care for the eldery: a synthesis of the evidence. *International Journal of Geriatric Psychiatry*, **18**, 222–35.

Jolley, D. (1999) Consultant home visits: Orrell and Katona – Journal (Vol)(13, 355–357). *International Journal of Geriatric Psychiatry,* **14**, 398–403.

Jolley, D.J. (1993) Psychiatry services for elderly people. Doctors should be in the front line. *BMJ* **306**, 1411.

Jones, R.G. (1987) Evaluation and effectiveness of psychogeriatric services: an economic perspective. In M. Bergener (ed.) *Psychogeriatrics – An International Handbook.* Springer: New York.

Kirby, M. and Cooney, C. (1998) Setting up a new old age psychiatry service: general practitioner views on the priorities. *Psychiatric Bulletin,* **22**, 288–90.

Knapp, M. (1998) Making music out of noise–the cost function approach to evaluation. *British Journal of Psychiatry – Supplementum* 7–11.

Kohn, R., Goldsmith, E., and Sedgwick, T.W. (2002) Treatment of homebound mentally ill elderly patients: the multidisciplinary psychiatric mobile team. *American Journal of Geriatric Psychiatry,* **10**, 469–75.

Kominski, G., Andersen, R., Bastani, R., Gould, R., Hackman, C., Huang, D., Jarvik, L., Maxwell, A., Moye, J., Olsen, E., Rohrbaugh, R., Rosansky, J., Taylor, S., and Van Stone, W. (2001) UPBEAT: the impact of a psychogeriatric intervention in VA medical centers. Unified Psychogeriatric Biopsychosocial Evaluation and Treatment. *Medical Care,* **39**, 500–12.

Kunik, M.E., Ponce, H., Molinari, V., Orengo, C., Emenaha, I., and Workman, R. (1996) The benefits of psychiatric hospitalization for older nursing home residents. *Journal of the American Geriatrics Society,* **44**, 1062–5.

Lawton, M.P., Van Haitsma, K., Klapper, J., Kleban, M.H., Katz, I.R., and Corn, J. (1998) A stimulation-retreat special care unit for elders with dementing illness. *International Psychogeriatrics,* **10**, 379–95.

Levitan, S.J. and Kornfeld, D.S. (1981) Clinical and cost benefits of liaison psychiatry. *American Journal of Psychiatry,* **138**, 790–3.

Lindesay, J., Briggs, K., Lawes, M., MacDonald, A., *et al.* (1991) The domus philosophy: A comparative evaluation of a new approach to residential care for the demented elderly. *International Journal of Geriatric Psychiatry,* **6**, 727–36.

Livingston, G., Yard, P., Beard, A., and Katona, C. (2000) A nurse-coordinated educational initiative addressing primary care professionals' attitudes to and problem-solving in depression in older people–a pilot study. *International Journal of Geriatric Psychiatry,* **15**, 401–5.

Llewellyn-Jones, R.H., Baikie, K.A., Castell, S., Andrews, C.L., Baikie, A., Pond, C.D., Willcock, S.M., Snowdon, J., and Tennant, C.C. (2001) How to help depressed older people living in residential care: a multifaceted shared-care intervention for late-life depression. *International Psychogeriatrics,* **13**, 477–92.

Llewellyn-Jones, R.H., Baikie, K.A., Smithers, H., Cohen, J., Snowdon, J., and Tennant, C.C. (1999) Multifaceted shared care intervention for late life depression in residential care: randomised controlled trial. *BMJ* **319**, 676–82.

Loane, R. and Jefferys, P. (1998) Consultation-liaison in an old age psychiatry service. *Psychiatric Bulletin,* **22**, 217–20.

Marks, I. (1998) Overcoming obstacles to routine outcome measurement. The nuts and bolts of implementing clinical audit. *British Journal of Psychiatry,* **173**, 281–6.

Mathew, L.J., Gutsch, H.M., Hackney, N.W., and Munsat, E.M. (1994) Promoting quality and cost-effective care to geropsychiatric patients. *Issues in Mental Health Nursing,* 15, 169–85.

Moniz-Cook, E., Agar, S., Silver, M., Woods, R., Wang, M., Elston, C., and Win, T. (1998) Can staff training reduce behavioural problems in residential care for the elderly mentally ill? *International Journal of Geriatric Psychiatry,* **13**, 149–58.

Moss, F., Wilson, B., Harrigan, S., and Ames, D. (1995) Psychiatric diagnoses, outcomes and lengths of stay of patients admitted to an acute psychogeriatric unit. *International Journal of Geriatric Psychiatry*, **10**, 849–54.

Mossey, J.M., Knott, K.A., Higgins, M., and Talerico, K. (1996) Effectiveness of a psychosocial intervention, interpersonal counseling, for subdysthymic depression in medically ill elderly. *Journal of Gerontology*, **4**, M172–8.

National Health and Medical Research Council (2000) *Guidelines for the Development and Implementation of Clinical Guidelines*. Australian Government Publishing Service: Canberra.

National Health and Medical Research Council (2001) *Guidelines for the Development and Implementation of Clinical Guidelines*. Australian Government Publishing Service: Canberra.

Neville, P., Boyle, A., and Baillon, S. (1999) A descriptive survey of acute bed usage for dementia care in old age psychiatry. *International Journal of Geriatric Psychiatry*, **14**, 348–54.

Nolan, M. and Grant, G. (1993) Service evaluation: time to open both eyes. *Journal of Advanced Nursing*, **18**, 1434–42.

Norquist, G., Wells, K.B., Rogers, W.H., Davis, L.M., *et al.* (1995) Quality of care for depressed elderly patients hospitalized in the specialty psychiatric units or general medical wards. *Archives of General Psychiatry*, **52**, 695–701.

O'Connor, D.W., Pollitt, P.A., Brook, C.P., Reiss, B.B., and Roth, M. (1991) Does early intervention reduce the number of elderly people with dementia admitted to institutions for long term care? *BMJ* **302**, 871–5.

Opie, J., Doyle, C., and O'Connor, D.W. (2002) Challenging behaviours in nursing home residents with dementia: a randomized controlled trial of multidisciplinary interventions. *International Journal of Geriatric Psychiatry*, **17**, 6–13.

Orrell, M. and Katona, C. (1998) Do consultant home visits have a future in old age psychiatry? *International Journal of Geriatric Psychiatry*, **13**, 355–7.

Orrell, M., Katona, C., Durani, C., Al-Asady, M., Barker, D., and Joyce, C. (1998) Do domiciliary visits in elderly people with psychiatric problems fulfil the expectations of general practitioners? *Primary Care Phsychiatry*, **4**, 47–9.

Pasternak, R., Rosenweig, A., Booth, B., Fox, A., Morycz, R., Mulsant, B., Sweet, R., Zubenko, G.S., Reynolds, C.F., 3rd, and Shear, M.K. (1998) Morbidity of homebound versus inpatient elderly psychiatric patients. *International Psychogeriatrics*, **10**, 117–25.

Philpot, M., Drahman, I., Ball, C., and Macdonald, A. (2000) The prognosis of late-life depression in two contiguous old age psychiatry services: an exploratory study. *Aging and Mental Health*, **4**, 72–8.

Pijl, Y.J. and Sytema, S. (2003) The identification of trends in the utilisation of mental health services by elderly: a Dutch case register study. *International Journal of Geriatric Psychiatry*, **18**, 373–80.

Pitt, B. and Silver, C.P. (1980) The combined approach to geriatrics and psychiatry: evaluation of a joint unit in a teaching hospital district. *Age and Ageing*, **9**, 33–7.

Plotkin, D.A. and Wells, K.B. (1993) Partial hospitalization (day treatment) for psychiatrically ill elderly patients. *American Journal of Psychiatry*, **150**, 266–71.

Porello, P.T., Madsen, L., Futterman, A., and Moak, G.S. (1995) Description of a geriatric medical/psychiatry unit in a small community general hospital. *Journal of Mental Health Administration*, **22**, 38–48.

Prinsley, D.M. (1973) Psychogeriatric ward for mentally disturbed elderly patients. *BMJ* **3**, 574–7.

Proctor, R., Burns, A., Powell, H.S., Tarrier, N., Faragher, B., Richardson, G., Davies, L., and South, B. (1999) Behavioural management in nursing and residential homes: a randomised controlled trial. *Lancet* **354**, 26–9.

Rabins, P.V., Black, B S., Roca, R., German, P., McGuire, M., Robbins, B., Rye, R., and Brant, L. (2000) Effectiveness of a nurse-based outreach program for identifying and treating psychiatric illness in the elderly. *JAMA,* **283**, 2802–9.

Reifler, B.V. and Cohen, W. (1998) Practice of geriatric psychiatry and mental health services for the elderly: results of an international survey. *International Psychogeriatrics,* **10**, 351–7.

Rigatelli, M., Casolari, L., Massari, I., and Ferrari, S. (2001) A follow-up study of psychiatric consultations in the general hospital: what happens to patients after discharge? *Psychotherapy and Psychosomatics,* **70**, 276–82.

Riordan, J. and Mockler, D. (1996) Audit of care programming in an acute psychiatric admission ward for the elderly. *International Journal of Geriatric Psychiatry,* **11**, 109–18.

Ritchie, K., Colvez, A., Ankri, J., Ledesert, B., *et al.* (1992) The evaluation of long-term care for the dementing elderly: a comparative study of hospital and collective non-medical care in France. *International Journal of Geriatric Psychiatry,* **7**, 549–57.

Robbins, B., Rye, R., German, P.S., Tlasek-Wolfson, M., Penrod, J., Rabins, P.V., and Smith Black, B. (2000) The Psychogeriatric Assessment and Treatment in City Housing (PATCH) program for elders with mental illness in public housing: getting through the crack in the door. *Archives of Psychiatric Nursing,* **14**, 163–72.

Roca, R. P., Storer, D. J., Robbins, B. M., Tlasek, M. E., *et al.* (1990) Psychogeriatric assessment and treatment in urban public housing. *Hospital and Community Psychiatry,* **41**, 916–20.

Rolleston, M. and Ball, C. (1994) Evaluating the effects of brief day hospital closure. *International Journal of Geriatric Psychiatry,* **9**, 51–3.

Rosenvinge, H.P., Jones, D., and Martin, A. (2001) The effects of moving a day hospital. *International Journal of Geriatric Psychiatry,* **16**, 1175–80.

Rosenvinge, H.P., Woolford, J.E., and Martin, A. (1994) Evaluation of extension of a psychogeriatric day hospital to open on Saturdays. *International Journal of Geriatric Psychiatry,* **9**, 764–5.

Rovner, B.W., Steele, C.D., Shmuely, Y., and Folstein, M.F. (1996) A randomized trial of dementia care in nursing homes. *Journal of the American Geriatrics Society,* **44**, 7–13.

Rubin, E.H., Kinscherf, D.A., and Wehrman, S.A. (1991) Response to treatment of depression in the old and very old. *Journal of Geriatric Psychiatry and Neurology,* **4**, 65–70.

Sadavoy, J. (1981) Psychogeriatric care in the general hospital. *Canadian Journal of Psychiatry/Revue Canadienne de Psychiatrie,* **26**, 334–6.

Sadavoy, J. and Reiman-Sheldon, E. (1983) General hospital geriatric psychiatric treatment: a follow-up study. *Journal of the American Geriatrics Society,* **31**, 200–5.

Schmidt, U., Tanner, M., and Dent, J. (1996) Evidence-based psychiatry: pride and prejudice. *Psychiatric Bulletin,* **20**, 705–7.

Scott, J., Fairbairn, A., and Woodhouse, K. (1988) Referrals to a psychogeriatric consultation-liaison service. *International Journal of Geriatric Psychiatry,* **3**, 131–5.

Seidel, G., Smith, C., Hafner, R.J., and Holme, G. (1992) A psychogeriatric community outreach service: description and evaluation. *International Journal of Geriatric Psychiatry,* **7**, 347–50.

Shah, A. (1994) Cost comparison of psychogeriatric consultations: outpatient versus home-based consultations. *International Psychogeriatrics,* **6**, 179–84.

Shah, A., Odutoye, K., and De, T. (2001) Depression in acutely medically ill elderly inpatients: a pilot study of early identification and intervention by formal psychogeriatric consultation. *Journal of Affective Disorders,* **62**, 233–40.

Shaw, C.D. (1990) Criterion-based audit. *BMJ* **300**, 649–51.

Shergill, S.S., Shankar, K.K., Seneviratna, K., and Orrell, M.W. (1999) The validity and reliability of the Health of the Nation Outcome Scales (HoNOS) in the elderly. *Journal of Mental Health,* **8**: 511–21.

Simmons, P. and Orrell, M. (2001) State funded continuing care for the elderly mentally ill: a legal and ethical solution? *International Journal of Geriatric Psychiatry,* **16**, 931–4.

Simpson, R.G., Scothern, G., and Vincent, M. (1995) Survey of carer satisfaction with the quality of care delivered to in-patients suffering from dementia. *Journal of Advanced Nursing,* **22**, 517–27.

Slaets, J.P.J., Kauffmann, R.H., Duivenvoorden, H. J., Pelemans, W., and Schudel, W.J. (1997) A randomized trial of geriatric liaison intervention in elderly medical inpatients. *Psychosomatic Medicine,* **59**, 585–91.

Spear, J., Chawla, S., O'Reilly, M., and Rock, D. (2002) Does the HoNOS 65+ meet the criteria for a clinical outcome indicator for mental health services for older people? *International Journal of Geriatric Psychiatry,* **17**, 226–30.

Stolee, P., Kessler, L., and Le Clair, J.K. (1996) A community development and outreach program in geriatric mental health: Four years' experience. *Journal of the American Geriatrics Society,* **44**, 314–20.

Strain, J.J., Lyons, J.S., Hammer, J.S., Fahs, M., Lebovits, A., Paddison, P.L., Snyder, S., Strauss, E., Burton, R., Nuber, G., *et al.* (1991) Cost offset from a psychiatric consultation-liaison intervention with elderly hip fracture patients. [comment]. *American Journal of Psychiatry,* **148**, 1044–9.

Teitelbaum, L., Cotton, D., Ginsburg, M.L., and Nashed, Y.H. (1996) Psychogeriatric consultation services: effect and effectiveness. *Canadian Journal of Psychiatry – Revue Canadienne de Psychiatrie,* **41**, 638–44.

Tourigny-Rivard, M.F., and Drury, M. (1987) The effects of monthly psychiatric consultation in a nursing home. *Gerontologist,* **27**, 363–6.

Trieman, N., Leff, J., and Glover, G. (1999) Outcome of long stay psychiatric patients resettled in the community: prospective cohort study. *BMJ* **319**, 13–16.

Unutzer, J., Katon, W., Callahan, C.M., Williams, J.W. Jr., Hunkeler, E., Harpole, L., Hoffing, M., Della Penna, R.D., Noel, P.H., Lin, E.H., Arean, P.A., Hegel, M.T., Tang, L., Belin, T.R., Oishi, S., Langston, C., and Treatment I.I.I.M.-P.A.t.C. (2002) Collaborative care management of late-life depression in the primary care setting: a randomized controlled trial. *JAMA,* **288**, 2836–45.

Wasylenki, D.A., Harrison, M.K., Britnell, J., and Hood, J. (1984) A community-based psychogeriatric service. *Journal of the American Geriatrics Society,* **32**, 213–18.

Wattis, J.P. (1989) A comparison of 'specialized' and 'nonspecialized' psychiatric services for old people in the United Kingdom. *International Journal of Geriatric Psychiatry,* **4**, 59–62.

Wattis, J.P., Butler, A., Martin, C., and Sumner, T. (1994) Outcome of admission to an acute psychiatric facility for older people: a pluralistic evaluation. *International Journal of Geriatric Psychiatry,* **9**, 835–40.

Wertheimer, J. (1997) Psychiatry of the elderly: a consensus statement. *International Journal of Geriatric Psychiatry,* **12**, 432–5.

Wills, W. and Leff, J. (1996) The TAPS project. 30: quality of life for elderly mentally ill patients–a comparison of hospital and community settings. *International Journal of Geriatric Psychiatry,* **11**, 953–963.

Wills, W., Trieman, N. and Leff, J. (1998) The Taps Project 40: quality of care provisions for the elderly mentally ill–traditional vs alternative facilities. *International Journal of Geriatric Psychiatry,* **13**, 225–34.

Woods, R.T., Wills, W., Higginson, I.J., Hobbins, J., and Whitby, M. (2003) Support in the community for people with dementia and their carers: a comparative outcome study of specialist mental health service interventions. *International Journal of Geriatric Psychiatry,* **18**, 298–307.

Wormstall, H. and Guenthner, A. (2002) The psychogeriatric health care system in Germany. *International Journal of Geriatric Psychiatry,* **17**, 786–87.

Zubenko, G.S., Rosen, J., Sweet, R.A., Mulsant, B.H., *et al.* (1992) Impact of psychiatric hospitalization on behavioral complications of Alzheimer's disease. *American Journal of Psychiatry,* **149**, 1484–91.

Zubenko, G.S., Mulsant, B.H., Rifai, A.H., Sweet, R.A., *et al.* (1994) Impact of acute psychiatric inpatient treatment on major depression in late life and prediction of response. *American Journal of Psychiatry,* **151**, 987–94.

Section 2

Chapter 6

Psychogeriatric services: current trends in the USA

Soo Borson, Christopher Colenda and Mary C. Lessig

Psychogeriatrics in the USA was founded twenty-five years ago on the pioneering contributions of old age psychiatrists in the UK. The development of the field, assessed two decades later in a cross-national study (Reifler and Cohen, 1998), was ranked by US practitioners as second only to the UK in dissemination of training programmes, emergence of national leadership, and achievement of formal certification. Rankings of service delivery were less favourable, reflecting lack of available services in many practice settings and locales. As in the rest of the world, the older population of the USA has grown rapidly in the last century, now representing 13 per cent of a population of over 282 million (US Census, 2002). Today, more than 35 million Americans are 65 years old and older, and 4.5 million are 85 or older. Here we examine current trends in US psychogeriatrics, seen from the perspectives of workforce and research development, service delivery models and payment for care, advocacy, and obstacles and opportunities for future improvement.

Trends in workforce development

Psychogeriatrics was inaugurated with the convening of the American Association for Geriatric Psychiatry (AAGP) in the late 1970s, concurrent with the first clinical training fellowships, initially funded by the National Institute of Mental Health (NIMH). Subspecialty examinations were first offered in 1992, conferring certification for 10 years. As of 2002, 2595 geriatric psychiatrists had been certified (Juul and Scheiber, 2003), most 'grandfathered' in without formal fellowship training. Since 1996, a one-year residency has been a prerequisite. Although the number of accredited training programmes has continued to increase (now numbering 92), the number of new psychogeriatricians certified each year has been generally less than 50, and only 61 per cent of residency posts were filled during 2001–2002 (Lieff *et al.*, 2003). Many currently certified geriatric psychiatrists will reach the age of retirement over the next decade, and many whose certification came up for renewal after ten years have allowed it to lapse. As a result, a net loss in qualified providers is expected by the year 2010. By 2030, older adults will comprise 20 per cent of the total population and one in five will have a mental disorder (excluding dementia; estimated from Jeste *et al.*, 1999), turning an undersupply of psychogeriatricians into a critical shortage. Workforce expansion will have to come from outside the field, including general psychiatry, geriatric medicine, psychology, nursing, and social work. Some efforts are being made to expand the pool of minimally qualified practitioners: as of 2002, all general psychiatry residents are required to complete at least one month of training in a psychogeriatric setting; fellowships in geriatric medicine offer limited cross-training. However, the numbers of psychologists, nurses, and social workers with sufficient background in mental health and ageing are also far below those required to meet minimal needs, and it is clear that massive changes in education, training, and health policy are required if better outcomes for mental disorders of ageing are to be realized (Shea, 2003).

Trends in research

Recruitment of new investigators to replace those nearing retirement is as urgent as it is for clinical practice. Active discussion is underway regarding ways to attract, develop, and retain new investigators for long-term investment in research (e.g. Olin *et al.*, 2003; Bruce, 2003). An innovative partnership of the AAGP and NIMH, the Summer Research Institute in Geriatric Psychiatry (Halpain *et al.*, 2001), has helped to improve the odds of success for junior investigators, yet a dwindling number of fellowship-trained practitioners choose research as a career. At the same time, funding for ageing research has grown several-fold within the National Institutes of Health, and some private foundations such as the Hartford have begun to venture, on a limited basis, into psychogeriatric target areas, particularly from the perspective of integrating epidemiological, clinical, and practice-based research for improved outcomes of late life depression. The most notable success of a population-based approach thus far has been achieved in the IMPACT study, a multi-site test of a collaborative primary-specialty care management model (Unützer *et al.*, 2002). A broader psychogeriatric research agenda has been proposed to enhance research training and knowledge development, explicitly in the area of mental health services for common, high risk, and high cost problems for which few services programmes currently exist (Borson *et al.*, 2001).

Trends in service delivery and payment for care

US psychogeriatrics has been largely a practitioner- and insurance-driven specialty. The role of practitioner initiative is well illustrated in a book describing a variety of approaches to care (American Psychiatric Association, 1993). However, the scarcity of trained specialists, problems in reimbursement for care provided in private office practice, home and long-term care settings, and the importance of accessible general medical and social service providers have discouraged wide dissemination of psychogeriatric care outside public and university settings.

Understanding the role of Medicare is one key to the issues in psychogeriatric service delivery in the USA. Medicare, federally funded from social security taxes and, since 1965, the principal insurer of older adults and the chronically disabled, was conceived as a means to relieve the patient and family burden of expenses for catastrophic medical illness. Eligibility for geriatric patients is based on age and an individual's (or spouse's) history of contribution to the social security fund through taxes on wages. About 95 per cent of the older population of the USA is eligible under this provision, having paid the Social Security tax for at least ten years; 5 per cent, comprising late-life immigrants and individuals whose employment and marital history exclude them, are not covered at government expense but can pay privately for Medicare coverage at relatively high premiums. Mental health benefits, barely an afterthought in the initial enabling legislation, have gradually made their way into Medicare provisions, but have been among its most controversial features. Coverage is provided for both inpatient and outpatient psychiatric treatment, but is subject to significant patient cost-sharing that is different from coverage for all other medical conditions and particularly tends to discourage use of the outpatient benefit. For example, outpatient psychotherapy and medication management services are reimbursed at substantially below market rates and require a patient contribution of 50 per cent of the covered amount, as compared to 20 per cent for medical outpatient services, and mental health expenditures now amount to about 4.9 per cent (US \$9.8 billion) of total Medicare expenditures for health care, with most paying for hospital-based services (Cano et al., 1997). Cost-sharing and uncovered benefits have created the private 'supplemental insurance' or 'Medigap' market, the premiums for which constitute the largest source of personal spending for community dwelling beneficiaries. Some Medigap policies pay part of the cost of medications; for the eligible elderly poor, Medicaid pays drug costs.

Medicare managed care programmes came into being as a response to the need to limit both governmental and patient out-of-pocket costs while preserving or even broadening the scope of benefits. Among the earliest concepts was that of the social health maintenance organization, piloted in national demonstration projects called Programmes of All-Inclusive Care for the Elderly (PACE). PACE consolidates Medicare and Medicaid funding into one financial base to provide a continuum of health care services (social case management and inpatient, outpatient and long-term care) to the elderly poor (Colenda et al., 2002). Nine states currently operate PACE programmes. Psychogeriatric services, when a need is identified, are not generally provided by psychiatrists but by case managers, social workers and primary care doctors, and neither needs of participants nor outcomes have been specifically studied. Medicare Plus Choice: Part C (M+C) programmes are more widely available than PACE (serving only a small fraction of the poor), but exist only in some locales. A lower-cost managed care programme offered by private companies and a fee-for-service plan are the two types of M+C programmes currently in operation. Programmes vary widely in specific services covered, and restricted provider panels are the norm. As of 2002, only 13 per cent of beneficiaries were enrolled in a managed care option. M+C offers opportunities to optimize population-based approaches to psychogeriatric care, but no studies have yet reported data comparing them with traditional Medicare.

The major challenges facing psychogeriatrics under Medicare currently relate to overall programme funding, repeated adjustments of payments to providers, regional inequalities in interpretation and implementation of mental health benefit policies, and vulnerability to political interests. Funds for its hospital provisions (Part A) are predicted to be exhausted by 2026 unless a radical solution is found (Center for Medicare and Medicaid Services, 2003), though funding for Part B, which is based on projected costs of physician and outpatient services, appears relatively secure. Among the most hotly debated issues are its exclusion of costs for medications and its unequal treatment of mental and general medical disorders (referred to as lack of mental health parity, an issue affecting private insurance and non-geriatric populations as well). Both houses of Congress have passed bills in 2003 calling for a Medicare drug benefit ('Part D'). In addition, two new legislative proposals – the Wellstone Mental Health Equitable Treatment Act (parity in coverage for mental and medical health services) and the Positive Aging Act (integrating mental health screening and services in primary care and providing mental health outreach to seniors) – have recently revitalized the policy discussion. The Robert Wood Johnson Foundation has independently initiated a study to improve the care of chronic conditions through integrating Medicaid and Medicare funding, a project analogous to but broader in scope than PACE. Though not specifically excluded, psychogeriatric disorders are not a featured focus.

Trends in advocacy for improving psychogeriatric services

Powerful advocacy for psychogeriatrics has come from the first-ever *US Surgeon General's Report on Mental Health* (1999), publicizing the value of diagnosis and treatment of late-life psychiatric disorders, and the Presidential New Freedom Commission on Mental Health (2003), that has moved to address the need for expansion and reform of current psychiatric services for geriatric patients. The Mental Health Liaison Group, representing over fifty national professional, research, voluntary health, consumer, and citizen advocacy organizations concerns about mental health, mental illness, and additions disorders, has urged additional federal allocations to increase mental health outreach to the elderly. Important advocacy efforts have been mounted by AAGP, through its inclusion of non-psychiatric disciplines in affiliate membership, dissemination of practice- and research-based information, efforts to improve psychogeriatric research, and increasing involvement in policy discussions at various levels of government; the American Psychiatric Association and its Council on Aging, through continuing efforts in support of Medicare reform and advocacy for high quality patient care; the Depression and Manic Depression Association, through its convening of a major conference on depression in late life (Charney *et al.*, 2003); and, among many others, the Alzheimer's Association, through its far-reaching research, education, and policy initiatives to improve the support and care of demented patients and their families. The goals of comprehensive and effective psychogeriatric care for older adults can be achieved only by collaborative efforts of many organizations and stakeholders, keeping a sharp, shared focus on developing and supporting an adequate mental health workforce, consolidating research around effective population-based care, aligning policy objectives with public health need, and sustaining pressure to secure both dollars and infrastructure to make successful models of care a permanent reality.

Summary and outlook

Psychogeriatrics in the USA is facing critical shortages of clinical manpower. Continuing challenges to funding for care, and fragmentation of general, psychiatric, and social health services for older people, remain serious problems impeding effective delivery of psychogeriatric care. Financial resources supporting research are growing faster than the supply of well-trained, qualified investigators, and there is a pressing need for post-residency research training. Though steady improvements in outcomes for some psychogeriatric disorders are being made through research, widespread implementation of these advances would require new investments in public health that are not yet on the horizon.

References

American Psychiatric Association Task Force Report (1993) *Selected Models of Practice in Geriatric Psychiatry*. American Psychiatric Press, Washington DC.

Borson, S., Bartels, S.J., Colenda, C.C., Gottlieb, G.L., and Meyers, B. (2001) Geriatric mental health services research: strategic plan for an aging population. *American Journal of Geriatric Psychiatry*, **9**, 191–204.

Bruce, M.L. (2003) Challenges to the transition to independent investigator in geriatric mental health. *American Journal of Geriatric Psychiatry*, **11**, 356–59.

Cano, C., Hennessy, K., Warren, J., and Lubitz, J. (1997) Medicare Part A utilization and expenditures for psychiatric services: 1995. *Health Care Financing Review*, **18**, 177–94.

Centers for Medicare and Medicaid Services (2003) http://cms.hhs.gov accessed 15 January 2003.

Charney, D. S., Reynolds, C. F., Lewis, L., *et al.* (2003) Depression and Bipolar Support Alliance consensus statement on the unmet needs in diagnosis and treatment of mood disorders in late life. *Archives of General Psychiatry*, **60**, 664–72.

Colenda, C.C., Bartels, S.C., and Gottlieb, G.L. (2002) The North American System of Care. In J. Copeland, M. Abou-Saleh and D. Blazer (eds.) *Principles and Practice of Geriatric Psychiatry*, 2nd edn, pp. 689–96. London, Wiley and Son, Ltd.

Halpain, M., Jeste, D.V., Katz, I.R., *et al.* (2001) Summer research institute: enhancing research career development in geriatric psychiatry. *Academic Psychiatry*, **25**, 48–56.

Jeste, D.V., Alexopoulos, G.S., Bartels, S.J., *et al.* (1999) Consensus statement on the upcoming crisis in geriatric mental health: research agenda for the next two decades. *Archives of General Psychiatry*, **56**, 848–53.

Juul, D. and Scheiber, S.C. (2003) Subspecialty certification in geriatric psychiatry. *American Journal of Geriatric Psychiatry*, **11**, 351–5.

Lieff, S.J., Warshaw, G.A., Bragg, E.J., Shaull, R.W., Lindsell, C.J., and Goldenhar, L.M. (2003) Geriatric psychiatry fellowship programs: findings from the association of directors of geriatric academic programs' longitudinal study of training and practice. *American Journal of Geriatric Psychiatry*, 11, 291–9.

Olin, J.T., Reynolds, C.F., Light, E., and Cuthbert, B.N. (2003) Career development and training in geriatric mental health: report of an NIMH workshop. *American Journal of Geriatric Psychiatry*, 11, 275–9.

Presidential New Freedom Commission on Mental Health (2003) www.mentalhealthcommission.gov accessed 15 January 2004.

Reifler, B.V. and Cohen, W. (1998) Practice of geriatric psychiatry and mental health services for the elderly: results of an international survey. *International Psychogeriatrics*, 10, 351–7.

Shea, D. (2003) Swimming upstream: geriatric mental health workforce. *Public Policy and Aging Report*, Spring: 3–7.

United States Census Bureau (2002) Table of Estimates by Age and Sex. http://eire.census.gov/popest/data/states/ST-EST 2002-ASRO-01.php. Accessed 13 November 2003.

Unützer, J., Katon, W., Callahan, C. M., *et al.* (2002) Collaborative care management of late-life depression in the primary care setting: a randomized controlled trial. *Journal of the American Medical Association*, 288, 2836–45.

US Surgeon General (1999) Older adults and mental health. In *Mental Health: A Report of the Surgeon General*, pp. 335–401. Department of Health and Human Services, Rockville, MD.

Chapter 7

Psychogeriatric services: current trends in Canada

Kenneth I. Shulman and Carole A. Cohen

Introduction

Canada will see a dramatic increase in its elderly population, rising from 13 per cent of the general population (approximately 30 million total population) in 2001 to 22 per cent in 2031, an increase due primarily to the bulge of baby boomers reaching old age. Compared to the US, where health care represents 13.9 per cent of the gross domestic product, Canada's share of health care is 9.1 per cent. Despite the difference, there is no evidence that the quality of health services in the US is any better than the Canadian system (Bravo *et al.*, 1999; Hebert *et al.*, 2001).

While there has been considerable debate in Canada regarding the contribution of the private sector with respect to the management and delivery of health care services, there are no data to support that trend as evidenced in the American experience (Deber, 2000; Relman, 2002). A disturbing trend in Canada, however, has been a steady decrease in publicly funded health expenditures per capita since 1992 (Deber, 2000). This has resulted in many problems from under-funding. However, there are indications, especially with the recent Romanow Commission (2002), that there will be a significant reinvestment in our health care system that should also translate into better psychogeriatric services. It is felt that the current public and universal health system in Canada will persist and is considered the best system to respond to the needs of the Canadian ageing population.

As of 2003, there are approximately 200 members of the Canadian Academy of Geriatric Psychiatry. The current training system for psychiatrists in Canada ensures a mandatory training period of at least three months in geriatric psychiatry. However, there is considerable variability across the country depending on the availability of supervisors and specialized geriatric psychiatric resources. This variability is reflected in psychogeriatric services nationwide, especially between rural and urban centres, a trend seen in all areas of the health care system. Because of the Canada Health Act (see below) the psychiatrist involvement in service delivery is not affected by public/private sector issues, as all psychiatrist services are publicly funded. Nonetheless, most provinces do offer additional support for geriatric psychiatrists in the form of stipends and sessional fees besides the common form of reimbursement that is fee for service.

The Canada Health Act: Should we call this a system of care?

Health services in Canada operate within the framework of the Canada Health Act, which is Canada's Federal Health Insurance Legislation. Within the federal/provincial system of government in Canada, this Act establishes the conditions that the provinces must meet in order to receive their full federal financial contribution to health care services. The aim of the Canada Health Act is to ensure that Canadians have 'reasonable access to medically necessary insured services on a prepaid basis, without direct charges at the point of service'. This includes both insured health care services as defined under the Canada Health Act as well as extended health care services, which include certain aspects of long-term residential care including nursing homes and certain health aspects of home care. Home care differs greatly across the country and is not specifically defined in the Canada Health Act.

Five programme criteria apply to insured health services:

1. *Public administration* – provincial health care insurance plans are administered and operated on a non-profit basis by a public authority and are accountable to the provincial government;

2. *Comprehensiveness* – includes all insured health services provided by hospital, medical practitioners or dentists or other health care practitioners;

3. *Universality* – all insured residents of a province remain entitled to the insured health services on uniform terms and conditions;

4. *Portability* – residents who move from one province to another must continue to be covered by insured health services;

5. *Accessibility* – all residents have 'reasonable access to insured hospital, medical and surgical-dental services … unimpeded by charges (user charges or extra billing) or any other discrimination'.

Thus, senior citizens in Canada generally have access to a full range of insured health services, which include access to extended care and residential facilities if required. The recent Romanow Commission (2002) reaffirmed Canada's commitment to the principles embodied in the Canada Health Act. While the Canada Health Act governs payment and certain principles, it does not provide for a specific system of care, which remains variable between provinces and even within provincial health care systems. Under this conceptual and policy framework, a wide range of psychogeriatric services have developed depending on available resources and specific initiatives within each provincial health system.

The influence of research on psychogeriatric services in the Canadian health care system

The Canadian Study of Health and Aging (CSHA) was undertaken in the 1990s at 18 study centres across Canada in two waves (CSHA-1 and CSHA-2) (McDowell *et al.*, 2001).

CSHA was a population based study with an overall sample of 10,250 individuals aged 65 and over divided among five geographic regions. More than a 100 journal articles have been published outlining the estimates of the prevalence and incidence of dementia, risk factors for dementia, mortality patterns, caregiver burden and economic costs and measures of disability and frailty to name a few. CSHA is one of the largest studies of dementia with excellent national data. In the future another national longitudinal study of ageing is planned to examine a host of issues related to the ageing of Canadians, which will inform the nature and extent of psychogeriatric services for dementia.

Hebert (2002) has highlighted the fact that dire predictions regarding the disproportionate use of health services by seniors in the future must be tempered by recent data that show that the health of new cohorts of seniors is expected to be much better than previous ones (Chen and Millar, 2000). These Canadian surveys show that the baby boom generation has a lower prevalence of many chronic diseases such as heart disease, hypertension and arthritis and, therefore, will arrive at retirement age in better health than previous cohorts. Moreover, disability-free life expectancy has also increased significantly (Hebert, 2002).

Projects designed to improve the effectiveness and efficiency of the Canadian health system have examined service integration, improved technology and information and the substitution of home care programmes for costly hospital-based services (Hollander and Chappell, 2001). Currently, only two to six per cent of provincial health budgets are designated for home services (Hebert, 2002). While there are some data to suggest that health reforms are resulting in a net increase in home services (Chappell, 2001), they do not appear to be benefiting the frail elderly population as much as had been hoped. This is because home care is being changed from a 'chronic care support system for seniors' to a medical support system primarily directed at post-acute care hospital discharge.

A number of experiments have taken place in Canada with regard to the development of integrated service networks, which range from simple linking to complete integration. Complete integration has shown an impact on reducing hospitalizations and emergency visits (Bergman et al., 1997). The success of these integration models appears to be related to use of standardized needs assessment tools for seniors and the rapid transition of information using computerized clinical records.

The creation of the Canadian Institutes of Health Research with a specific institute devoted to ageing research (Institute of Aging) has been an important development. It has the potential to 'bring research into line with the health priorities of Canadians and promote the translation of research findings into better services, products, programs and policies' (Hebert, 2002).

Best practices

The Guidelines for Comprehensive Services for the Elderly with Psychiatric Disorders (Health and Welfare Canada, 1988) emphasized that 'An integrated approach combining behavioural, and medical knowledge and skills ...' (p. 32) is necessary to ensure adequate services for seniors with mental health problems. These principles have guided the development of services at a local level across the country, but little progress has been made in operationalizing these at the important provincial level. Recently there has been renewed interest in these guidelines (MacCourt *et al.*, 2000). In regions where there is a regional health authority, such as the province of British Columbia, best practices for the mental health care of older adults have been developed (Donnelly, 2002). The B.C. document highlights six principles to guide the development of psychogeriatric services: client and family-centred, goal oriented, accessible and flexible, comprehensive, specific services for the elderly and accountable. The National Advisory Council on Aging (MacCourt *et al.*, 2002) has also published this document and it may serve as a template for development of provincial guidelines in other jurisdictions.

In addition, the Canadian Coalition for Seniors' Mental Health was established in 2002 in an attempt to improve the mental health of seniors through a coordinated national strategy. The Coalition includes representatives from many seniors, mental health and medical associations including the Alzheimer Society of Canada, the Canadian Academy of Geriatric Psychiatry, the Canadian Geriatrics Society, the Canadian Mental Health Association, and the College of Family Physicians of Canada. This multidisciplinary coalition is targeting its first goal as 'improving the mental health of the elderly in long-term care through education, advocacy and collaboration'. The focus on the needs of seniors living in long-term care facilities reflects the concern that nursing homes in North America have become 'the modern mental institutions for the elderly'. A study of long-term care facilities in Ontario (Conn *et al.*, 1992) showed that a vast majority of nursing homes receive five hours or less per month of psychiatric care for the entire institution.

One can only hope that the diversity of provincial approaches to psychogeriatric services developing under the framework of the federal Canada Health Act will result in more creative, effective and efficient services for the elderly.

References

Bergman, H., Béland, F., Lebel, P., *et al.* (1997) Care for Canada's frail elderly population: fragmentation or integrations. *Canadian Medical Association Journal,* **157**, 1116–21.

Bravo, G., Dubois, M.-F., Charpentier, M., DeWals, P., and Emond, A. (1999) Quality of care in unlicensed homes for the aged in the Eastern Townships of Quebec. *Canadian Medical Association Journal,* **160**, 1441–5.

Chappell, N.L. (2001) Quality long-term care: perspectives from the users of home care. In L. S. Noelker and Z. Harel (eds.) *Linking Quality of Long-term Care and Quality of Life,* pp. 75–94. Springer, New York.

Chen, J. and Millar, W.J. (2000) Les générations récentes sontelles en meilleure santé? *Rapports sur la santé,* **11**, 9–26.

Conn, D.K., Lee, V., Steingart, A., and Silberfeld, M. (1992) A survey of nursing homes and homes for the aged in Ontario. *Canadian Journal of Psychiatry*, **37**, 525–30.

Deber, R.B. (2000) Getting what we pay for: myths and realities about financing Canada's health care system. Dialogue on Health Reform. Toronto, Canada.

Donnelly, M.L. (2002) The state of seniors' health in British Columbia, *Visions: BC's Mental Health Journal*, **15**, 4–5.

Health and Welfare Canada (1988) *Guidelines for Comprehensive Services to Elderly Persons with Psychiatric Disorders*. Health and Welfare Canada, Ottawa.

Hebert, R. (2002) Research on aging: providing evidence for rescuing the Canadian Health Care System. *Canadian Journal on Aging*, **21**, 343–47.

Hebert, R., Dubuc, N., Buteau, M., *et al.* (2001) Resources and costs associated with disabilities of elderly people living at home and in institutions. *Canadian Journal on Aging*, **20**, 1–22.

Hollander, M.J. and Chappell, N.L. (2001) *Final Report of the Study on the Comparative Cost Analysis of Home Care and Residential Care Services*. National Evaluation of the Cost-Effectiveness of Home Care, Victoria, BC.

MacCourt, P., Tuokko, H., and Tierney, M. (2000) Editorial: Canadian Association on Gerontology policy statement on issues in the delivery of mental health services to older adults. *Canadian Journal on Aging*, **21**, 165–74.

MacCourt, P., Lockhart, B., and Donnelly, M. (2002) Best practices for the mental health care of older adults. *Division of Aging and Seniors: NACA Writings in Gerontology on Mental Health and Aging*, **18**, 9–21.

McDowell, I., Hill, G., and Lindsay, J. (2001) An overview of the Canadian Study of Health and Aging. *International Psychogeriatrics*, **13**, 7–18.

Relman, A.S. (2002) *For-profit Health Care: expensive, inefficient and inequitable*. Presentation to the Senate Committee Looking at Health Care Reforms. Canadian Health Coalition website www.healthcoalition.ca/relman.html accessed 12 January 2004.

Romanow, R.J. (2002) *Commission on the Future of Health Care in Canada*. Canadian Government Publishing, Ottawa.

Chapter 8

Psychogeriatric services: current trends in the UK

John Wattis

> Trying to predict the future is a mug's game.
>
> *Douglas Adams, 2003*

Introduction

Old age psychiatry in the United Kingdom is a well-established specialty. The very first survey of old age psychiatry services in the UK, in 1980, found 106 consultants working in the field (Wattis *et al.*, 1981). Further surveys saw this number rising substantially (Wattis, 1988; Wattis *et al.*, 1999). Now the Royal College of Psychiatrists database shows 584 (16 per cent) consultant members of the College in the UK work in the field (personal communication). Old age psychiatry developed early in the UK as a result of changing population demographics and the commitment of the post-war NHS to provide health services from 'cradle to grave'. Currently nearly 16 per cent of a total population of nearly 59 million is over 65 years. Women slightly outnumber men and the ratio of women:men increases markedly every 5 years from 65 years upwards (National Statistics Office Census, 2001). There are now about 4 million people over the age of 75 in the UK. More than half of women aged 75 and over live alone and there are now 336,000 people over the age of 90 in England and Wales (National Statistics Office, 2003). Women in the over 75 age group are particularly vulnerable to Alzheimer's disease, presenting a challenge to NHS primary care and social services as well as old age psychiatry services.

Against this background we can identify some important trends:

+ Developments in the knowledge base
+ Changes in social political and economic background
+ Education and developing roles of different disciplines and professions.

We need not be helpless 'victims' of these trends. Leadership and proactive management can direct change (Covey, 1989). It is hard to predict how the different forces at work will interact. 'Wild card' developments in information technology or changes in the world economy may be decisive, but we can influence trends by adhering to some principles that keep services true to purpose whatever happens. These principles include a focus on the needs of older people, a commitment to good relationships between the different disciplines and organizations that work to meet these needs, and a commitment to research to underpin evidence-based practice (and policy).

Developments in the knowledge base

Expensive technologies will have a higher short-term impact in richer countries and ones that devote a higher percentage of national wealth to health care of older people. Falling relative expenditure on older people in the UK (Seshamani and Gray, 2002) means it may no longer be the world leader in service developments for older people.

Advances in the molecular biology of Alzheimer's disease mean that we may be able to identify, with increasing certainty, individuals at risk and specific interactions between genetic and environmental factors, including diet (Petot *et al.*, 2003; Puglielli *et al.*, 2003). This may lead to prophylaxis with medications to prevent or arrest various forms of dementia, more sophisticated antidepressants and anti-psychotics and even drugs for 'new' conditions like behavioural and psychological symptoms in dementia and female sexual dysfunction (Basson *et al.*, 2003). The politics of drugs pricing is likely to produce problems as drug cost inflation consistently out-strips general inflation in the NHS (Calvert, 2002). With increasingly sophisticated neuroimaging, neurophysiological tests and blood tests, psychiatrists are likely to become more dependent on technology for early, accurate diagnosis. A comprehensive service like the NHS should, subject to funding, be well placed to exploit these possibilities.

Tests of disease progression and outcomes of interventions will become more important. These may be 'objective' results from laboratory or psychological testing or more 'subjective' measures of improvement and well-being from the patient's point of view. Despite reservations, global measures like the Health of the Nation Outcome Scales for over 65s (Burns *et al.*, 1999) may be pushed by commissioners under pressure from the Department of Health.

Research into service delivery and management is in its infancy. Most of the management changes introduced in the NHS have been based on political theory rather than evidence. Many of the service models we use have simply 'evolved' from earlier patterns of service. Nevertheless, evidence is beginning to accumulate (see Chapter 5). It would be pleasant if one day we could have evidence-based policy and evidence-based management as well as evidence-based practice (Ham *et al.*, 1995).

Social and political background

Community care for people with mental illness in the UK has 'failed' (Coid, 1994). This failure probably related to inadequate funding and inadequate service models. Proportionately less of NHS spending goes on mental health (and, allowing for changes in age structure, older people) now than did during the asylum era. Future funding will depend upon the effectiveness of competing pressure groups and political will. Community care has been re-invented, generally by emphasis on specialist models like 'crisis intervention' and 'early intervention in psychosis'. There has been little systematic attempt to use these special interventions in older adults. Attempts to argue that these developments should be applied to all age groups without discrimination have generally met with the response that 'there is no money'.

Service delivery is moving into primary care, away from the 'secondary' hospital sector. Specialist nurses, such as 'diabetic' nurses, support general practitioners. The development of Primary Care Trusts as commissioning and providing organizations may lead to a situation where more old age specialist services are located within the primary care trust rather than in the secondary hospital sector.

The public bias towards 'talking treatments' and an increasing evidence base may lead to improved availability of psychological treatments for old people, probably delivered by nurses.

The NHS, as originally conceived in the 1940s, was tripartite. The local 'shopkeepers' of the NHS, general practitioners, opticians and dentists answered to local executive committees. Other services including maternity, public health and ambulances, answered to local government. Regional boards controlled hospitals. In mental health, the 1959 Mental Health Act liberalized the treatment of mentally ill people and opened the way for a move away from the old psychiatric hospitals into district general hospital psychiatric units, often on secondary sites.

Several major reorganizations of the NHS then occurred, including the following:

- 1974, health and social services functions were separated
- 1984, 'general management' was introduced
- 1990, the 'internal market' was introduced
- 1997, *The New NHS: Modern, Dependable* (Department of Health, 1997)

For psychiatry there was also the 1983 Mental Health Act and an anticipated new Act. A major plank of the 1997 policy was the setting up of Primary Care Groups, later Trusts (PCGs/PCTs), to provide primary care and commission secondary care services. In some areas, 'Care Trusts' provided primary care, social services and some secondary services such as mental health services. This is the usual pattern in Scotland, reflecting another trend in the UK, the devolution of health policy in Wales and Scotland where services are increasingly diverging from those in England.

Whatever the detailed local arrangements, central direction is strong. The 'quality framework' involves a three-pronged approach (Department of Health, 1998). *Clear standards of service* are set by National Service Frameworks (NSFs) and a National Institute for Clinical Excellence (NICE), which evaluates new treatments. *Clinical governance* (Department of Health, 1999a) places obligations on Chief Executives of NHS Trusts for the quality of health care. This is underpinned by the national *monitoring of standards* involving a National Performance Framework, an inspectorate (the Commission for Health Improvement, replaced in 2003 by the Commission for Health Audit and Inspection) and a National Patient and User Survey.

The NSF for Older People (Department of Health, 2001) is a ten-year plan to improve standards in eight areas:

1. Rooting out age discrimination

2. Person-centred care

3. Intermediate care

4. General hospital care

5. Stroke

6. Falls

7. Mental health and

8. Health education.

The standards for older people's mental health are unambitious, and do not compare with the detailed treatment of the NSF for mental health (Department of Health, 1999b). Despite the first standard of the NSF for older people mandating that there should be no age discrimination, there is some ambiguity about how far the detailed standards of the NSF for mental health apply to older people.

What trends can we discern in all this? The original tripartite division of the NHS attempted to balance primary care services with locally provided public health services and more centrally provided hospital services. In 1974 the first steps were taken to increase centralization of health, leaving social services to local government. Attempts were made to preserve joint planning by making health authorities coterminous with local authorities. The internal market challenged the service ethos of the NHS and shifted investment from the NHS to private provision, especially for long-term nursing facilities. The latest reforms are unparalleled in their complexity and variability and it is hard to predict what they will lead to. Joint commissioning and partnership boards try to keep the peace between the centrally dominated NHS on the one side and traditional local government services on the other. The next move may be to remove social services from local government in the formation of care trusts. Other reactions that might occur include an attempt to regain 'free market' independence by consultants or general practitioners setting up in chambers. Foundation trusts (Department of Health, 2002) are intended to be more locally autonomous but the model seems more suited to acute general hospital than mental health services. Further attempts to introduce US-style Health Maintenance Organizations (Newman, 1995) cannot be ruled out.

Trends in education and professional development

Evidence-based practice

The era of evidence-based practice (Davidoff et al., 1995) is upon us. Evidence is much easier to build in some areas than others. What is the evidence of effectiveness for psychiatric day hospitals for older people? To date most of the argument has been based on opinion rather than evidence (Fasey, 1994; Howard, 1994; Rosenvinge, 1994) and only now are we beginning to develop the evidence to support (and *rationally* change) the way we practice. Information technology, linked to developments like integrated care pathways and the electronic patient record, could potentially take us a long way and the centrally-directed NHS should be in a good position to take advantage of these opportunities (which may also be threats if poorly implemented).

Specialization

The specialty of old age psychiatry is now well established. In the UK psychiatrists spend three years in general training: most trainees will spend 6 months in old age psychiatry (though this is not mandatory) and then take the examination for the Membership of the Royal College of Psychiatrists. Once they have gained the Membership, they spend three years or more in higher professional Specialist Registrar (SpR) training (Royal College of Psychiatrists, 1998). At the SpR stage, trainees for old age psychiatry must spend at least two years in 'core' old age psychiatry jobs but may spend up to a year in other relevant training (e.g. in liaison psychiatry). This results in the award of a Certificate of Completion of Specialist Training (CCST).

Further specialization, for example in dementia care, can give a greater depth of knowledge and skills, though potentially at the expense of breadth. A specialized nurse (perhaps working under the supervision of a consultant psychiatrist) might be able to make a diagnosis of Alzheimer's disease (Seymour *et al.*, 1994) with the help of the GP to exclude other conditions if necessary. Thus anti-dementia drugs might be delegated to primary care with specialist nurse support. Doctors may specialize in types of service delivery, such as dementia services or liaison old age psychiatry, alongside colleagues from nursing and other disciplines.

Shared education and roles

Increasingly modular and continuing systems of education should create scope for more multidisciplinary learning. Insight into improving the personal care of older people with dementia has come from the Bradford Dementia Group under the former leadership of professor Tom Kitwood (Kitwood, 1993, 1997) Hopefully, all professions will adopt a bio-psychosocial model of disease aetiology and management rather than polarizing into biological, psychological and sociological camps. Increasing emphasis in the importance of spiritual issues in person-centred care will also influence practice (Froggatt, 1994).

The front cover of the millennium edition *Old Age Psychiatrist*, published by the Faculty of Old Age Psychiatry (Old Age Psychiatrist, 2000) lists five roles for old age psychiatrists:

1. Doctor

2. Academic

3. Manager

4. Therapist and

5. Scientist.

Recent shortages of medical manpower in the UK have led to a debate about the role of the consultant. Doctors have been encouraged to let go of personal responsibility for their patients: but they will only do this when they are content that the skills of those in other disciplines and the systems supporting them will deliver an adequate standard of care and treatment.

Vision and principles

Ethical standards demand that doctors make the care of their patients their first concern, but old age psychiatrists in the UK have always accepted responsibilities for defined populations of older people rather than just to those individuals who come to them personally. We need a vision that unites the provision of quality services to a population of old people and the provision of quality services to individuals. The principles upon which services should be founded include:

+ Focus on the needs of patients
+ Good relationships with patients, clinical colleagues, managers and other providers of services
+ A commitment to equitable and evidence-based services
+ Willingness to change creatively over time.

Conclusion

Trends in science are worldwide: trends in education and the development of profession roles also tend to have an increasingly international aspect. Trends in service delivery are more strongly determined by national politics, though there tends to be an increasing willingness to borrow ideas (good and bad) from other countries. Some service delivery trends, like that towards increasing specialization (linked to a tendency to devolve established treatments onto the generalist in primary care) seem to be universal. Perhaps we do well to learn from evolution about the danger of over-specialization!

Issues like the politicization of health services also seem to have an international dimension. Political 'interference' in the design and management of health services in the UK is very high. Only with a clear vision and sound principles can we help shape future services to the benefit of older people.

References

Adams, D. (2003) *The Salmon of Doubt*. Pan Books, London.
Basson, R., Leiblum, S., Potts, A., *et al.* (2003) The making of a disease: female sexual dysfunction. *BMJ* 326, 658.

Burns, A., Beevor, A., Lelliott, P., *et al.* (1999) Health of the Nation Outcome Scales for Elderly peoples (HoNOS65+). *British Journal of Psychiatry*, **174**, 424–7.

Calvert, R. (2002) Medicines management. Fit to bust. *Health Services Journal*, **112**, 24–5.

Coid, J. (1994) Failure in community care: psychiatry's dilemma. *BMJ* **308**, 805–6.

Covey, S.R. (1989) *The Seven Habits of Highly Effective People.* London: Simon and Schuster.

Davidoff, F., Haynes, B., Sackett, D., *et al.* (1995) Evidence-based medicine. *BMJ* **310**, 1085–6.

Department of Health (1997) *The New NHS – Modern, Dependable.* London: Department of Health.

Department of Health (1998) *A First Class Service: Quality in the new NHS.* London, Department of Health.

Department of Health (1999a) *Clinical Governance: Quality in the new NHS.* London: Department of Health.

Department of Health (1999b) *The National Service Framework for Mental Health.* London: Department of Health.

Department of Health (2001) *National Service Framework for Older People.* London: Department of Health.

Department of Health (2002) *A Guide to NHS Foundation Trusts.* London, Department of Health.

Fasey, C. (1994) The day hospital in old age psychiatry: the case against. *International Journal of Geriatric Psychiatry*, **9**, 519–23.

Froggatt, A. (1994) Tuning in to meet spiritual needs. *Dementia Care*, **2**, 12–13.

Ham, C., Hunter, D.J., and Robinson, R. (1995) Evidence based policymaking. *BMJ* **310**, 71–2.

Howard, R. (1994) Day hospitals: the case in favour. *International Journal of Geriatric Psychiatry*, **9**, 525–9.

Kitwood, T. (1993) Person and process in dementia. *International Journal of Geriatric Psychiatry*, **8**, 541–5.

Kitwood, T. (1997) *Dementia Reconsidered: the person comes first.* Buckingham, England: Open University Press.

National Statistics Office (2001) Census: national statistics online, http:/www.statistics.gov.uk/STATBASE/ssdataset.asp?vlnk=6832

National Statistics Office (2003) Older People: http://www.statistics.gov.uk/cci/nugget.asp?id=351

Newman, P. (1995) Interview with Alain Enthoven: is there convergence between Britain and the United States in the organisation of health services? *BMJ* **310**, 1652–5.

Old Age Psychiatrist Millenium Issue, Number 17 (2000) Royal College of Psychiatrists, London. Also available through the Royal College of Psychiatrists Website (http://www.rcpsych.ac.uk.)

Petot, G.J., Traore, F., Debanne, S.M., Lerner, A.J., Smyth, K.A., and Friedland, R.P. (2003) Interactions of apolipoprotein E genotype and dietary fat intake of healthy older persons during mid-adult life. *Metabolism*, **52**, 279–81.

Puglielli, L., Tanzi, R.E., and Kovacs, D.M. (2003) Alzheimer's disease: the cholesterol connection. *Nature Neuroscience*, **6**, 345–51.

Rosenvinge, T. (1994) The role of the psychogeriatric day hospital. *Psychiatric Bulletin*, **18**, 733–6.

Royal College of Psychiatrists (1998) *Higher Specialist Training Handbook* (Occasional Paper OP43). Royal College of Psychiatrists, London.

Seshamani, M. and Gray, A. (2002) The impact of ageing on expenditures in the National Health Service. *Age and Ageing*, **31**, 287–94.

Seymour, J., Saunders, P., Wattis, J.P., *et al.* (1994) Evaluation of early dementia by a trained nurse. *International Journal of Geriatric Psychiatry*, **9**, 37–42.

Wattis, J.P., Wattis, L., and Arie, T.H. (1981) Psychogeriatrics: a national survey of a new branch of psychiatry. *BMJ* **282**, 1529–33.

Wattis, J.P. (1988) Geographical variations in the provision of psychiatric services for older people. *Age and Ageing*, **17**, 171–80.

Wattis, J., Macdonald, A., and Newton, P. (1999) Old age psychiatry: a specialty in transition – results of the 1996 survey. *Psychiatric Bulletin*, **23**, 331–5.

Chapter 9

Psychogeriatric services: current trends in Asia

Helen Chiu

In 2000, the world's population was 6 billion, 58 per cent of which lived in Asia. The population of Asia is ageing and the percentage of people aged 65 and above will be doubled between 1960 and 2020, from 4.2 per cent to 8.8 per cent. Life expectancy will rise from 66 to 77 years between 2000 and 2050.

This region is marked by great diversity in geographic, cultural and socio-economic characteristics. Many places, such as Indonesia, India and Thailand, are still developing countries, while countries like Japan are already well developed. The demographics and pace of ageing of the population also vary in different countries in the region. For instance, the percentage of people aged 65 or above was 6 per cent for the whole region, but varies from 18.5 per cent in Japan to 2.8 per cent in Cambodia.

With the rapid rise of the elderly population in this region, development of various services for older people will assume greater importance. This chapter describes the current trend of psychogeriatric services in Asia, focusing on China and Hong Kong.

Asia

In general, psychogeriatric services in Asian countries are less well developed than in many countries in Europe, North America and Australia. Separate psychogeriatric services are beginning to be established and training programmes in geriatric psychiatry are available in some areas, including Japan, South Korea, Hong Kong, Taiwan and Singapore. With the increasing number of professionals interested or working in the field of psychogeriatrics, in recent years psychogeriatric associations have been formed in several countries and cities, including Japan, South Korea, Hong Kong, Taiwan and Indonesia. For instance, the Japanese Psychogeriatric Society was established in 1986 and currently has more than 2500 members. Two separate journals on Psychogeriatrics, *Psychogeriatrics* and the *Japanese Journal of Geriatric Psychiatry*, are published in Japan. The Korean Association for Geriatric Psychiatry was formed in 1994 and has over 250 members currently. In 2002, the International Psychogeriatric Association Asia Pacific Regional Meeting was held in Hong Kong and this provided a further boost to the development of psychogeriatrics in this region.

China

China has a population of 1.27 billion. In the year 2000, 7 per cent of the population was aged 65 or above, and this figure will rise to 13 per cent in 2025 and 23 per cent in 2050. In the last 10 years, China has changed from a planned economy to a market economy, and the society is experiencing major changes in this period of rapid financial growth and modernization. At the same time, the traditional extended family structure is breaking down, in the midst of this social change. Reasons for the increasing trend of nuclear families include: the industrialization process which means young people move away from their home town to live in cities, the family planning policy in China, as well as fading of the traditional Chinese values and filial respect (Yu and Shen, 2003).

A number of epidemiological studies on dementia and depression have been carried out in China in the last 20 years. The prevalence of dementia ranged from 0.46 per cent to 7 per cent in various studies (Chiu and Zhang, 2000). In a meta-analysis of epidemiological studies on depression in older people, the pooled prevalence of depression was 3.86 per cent while that of depressive mood was 14.8 per cent (Chen *et al.*, 1999). In spite of the Chinese traditional respect for the elderly the suicide rate is very high in older people, and this is particularly marked in rural areas where the suicide rate stands at 82.8 per 100,000 for people aged 60 to 84 (Phillips *et al.*, 2002). The fivefold difference in elderly suicide rate between the urban and rural areas, as well as the high female suicide rate, are also striking and unique features in China.

In 1997, there were 485 psychiatric hospitals in China with approximately 107,000 beds (Yu and Shen, 2003). Less than 10 per cent of the total psychiatric beds served the elderly. Around 14,000 doctors were working in psychiatric hospitals, with over 100 of them working in geriatric psychiatry part-time or full time. There are an increasing number of psychiatrists interested in the care of the elderly and several prominent psychiatrists with major research interest in dementia and suicide. The subspecialty of psychogeriatrics has begun to develop in the last few years and significant progress has been made.

Apart from outpatient clinics, there are psychogeriatric wards in hospitals in some cities, including Beijing, Nanjing, Shanghai, Changsha, Wuhan, Hangzhou, Suzhou and Jilin. Currently there are around 20 special psychogeriatric wards in China. These wards provide medical services to the elderly with dementia and functional psychiatric illness. Medical doctors and nurses are the key professionals in the care of patients and there is a lack of other professionals including occupational therapists, social workers and clinical psychologists.

Residential services include homes for retired workers, homes for the aged and nursing homes. These are available in major cities and some rural areas. However, the majority of older people wish to stay in their homes (Fung *et al.*, 1997) and are reluctant to go into these residential services.

In general, community services are still in an early stage of development. In particular, there is a big difference between the rural and urban areas in service provision and various modes of support. In some major cities a home-help service is available (Ineichen, 1998), as well as a limited service of paid carers looking after frail elderly or people with dementia in the community. Other community services available in the major cities include volunteers, elderly self-help, a hotline service and meals on wheels. A major advance is the establishment of an Alzheimer's Association in 2001.

Hong Kong

The population of Hong Kong now stands at 6.8 million, 11 per cent of whom are aged 65 or above. Hong Kong was a British colony for over 100 years and returned to Chinese rule in 1997, so the development of psychogeriatric services in Hong Kong is different from that in the rest of China and follows a British model of service delivery. Specialized psychogeriatric services started in 1991 and rapid development in the field has taken place over the years. Some of these developments have been described previously (Chiu et al., 1997). There are now 15 full-time psychogeriatricians who are Fellows of the Hong Kong College of Psychiatrists. In addition, around 30 trainee psychiatrists are working in the subspecialty. There are seven major psychogeriatric teams providing service to the whole territory. A comprehensive range of services, including inpatient, outpatient, day patient, consultation and outreach services are provided for older people with dementia and psychiatric illness. The outreach services provide services to homes for the elderly. However, domiciliary visits to older people living at home are only done selectively due to inadequate manpower. A multidisciplinary community-oriented approach is adopted and a very close working relationship is maintained with the geriatric services and other agencies involved in provision of care to the elderly. Apart from psychiatrists, there is a parallel rapid development of other professionals specializing in the field of psychogeriatrics. At present there is a psychogeriatric nursing group, and occupational therapists' group on dementia.

Specialized services for dementia started to develop in recent years. A specially designed dementia centre, the Jockey Club Centre for Positive Ageing, was established in 2000 to promote the quality of care for elderly with dementia. This centre is funded by the Hong Kong Jockey Club and provides clinical services to elderly with dementia, training for professionals and carers and also carries out research in dementia care.

The 'Elderly suicide prevention programme' was established for the whole territory in late 2002 (Chiu et al., 2003). The programme is provided by the existing psychogeriatric teams with additional funding from the government. The psychogeriatric teams have established a network with the hotline services, NGOs, centres for the elderly and general practitioners to screen for depression and those who are at risk to suicide. Elderly with suicide risk or those with severe depression would be referred to fast-track psychiatric clinics. In addition, home visit and telephone monitoring would be provided by nurses regularly. Another essential feature is the training of general practitioners in the detection and treatment of depression. The programme was inspired by the reduction of suicide rates after the training of general practitioners in the Gotland Study (Rihmer *et al.*, 1995), as well as the success of the telecheck programme in reducing the elderly suicide rate in Italy (de Leo *et al.*, 1995).

Psychogeriatrics was recognized as a subspecialty by the Hong Kong College of Psychiatrists in 1994 and the Alzheimer's Association was established in 1995. The Hong Kong Psychogeriatric Association, consisting of multidisciplinary professionals, was formed in 1998 and has over 200 members.

Seminars in psychogeriatrics are part of the undergraduate syllabus of the Medical Faculty of the Chinese University of Hong Kong, one of the two universities with a medical school in Hong Kong. In addition, there is opportunity for an elective clinical attachment to the psychogeriatric team. Postgraduate training programmes are organized by the Hong Kong College of Psychiatrists. To become a Fellow of the College, one has to undergo 6 years of post-graduate training and pass three examinations, the third of which consists of a thesis and an oral examination. Subspecialty training programmes in psychogeriatrics are integrated within the 6 years of training, and there is as yet no formal certification process for geriatric psychiatrists.

Conclusions

Common problems and challenges facing many Asian countries include the break-down of the traditional family support system, a low public awareness and high stigma of mental illness, inadequate mental health services and the lack of community facilities. With the changing demographics and ageing of the population in this region, development of psychogeriatric services will be a major task in the coming years.

Acknowledgements

The author would like to thank Professor Yu Xin of Beijing and Professor Zhang Ming Yuan of Shanghai for their help in the preparation of this manuscript.

References

Chen, R., Copeland, R.M., and Wei, L. (1999) A meta-analysis of epidemiological studies in depression of older people in the People's Republic of China. *International Journal of Geriatric Psychiatry*, **14**, 821–30.

Chiu, H.F.K., Ng, L.L., Nivataphand, R., et al. (1997) Psychogeriatrics in South-East Asia. *International Journal of Geriatric Psychiatry*, **12**, 989–94.

Chiu, H.F.K. and Zhang, M.Y. (2000) Dementia Research in China. *International Journal of Geriatric Psychiatry*, **15**, 947–53.

Chiu, H.F.K., Takahashi, Y., and Suh, G.H. (2003) Elderly suicide prevention in East Asia. *International Journal of Geriatric Psychiatry*, **18**, 973–6.

De Leo, D., Carollo, G., and Dello Buono, M. (1995) Lower suicide rates associated with a tele-help/tele-check service for the elderly at home. *American Journal of Psychiatry*, **152**, 632–4.

Fung, Q.S., Shui, H.L., and Chu, J.M. (1997) *Towards the Twenty-First Century – Analysis of the Ageing Problem*. Beijing: Chinese Literature Publishing House.

Ineichen, B. (1998) Influences on the care of demented elderly people in the People's Republic of China. *International Journal of Geriatric Psychiatry*, **13**, 122–6.

Phillips, M.R., Li, X.Y., and Zhang, Y.P. (2002) Suicide rates in China, 1995–99. *Lancet*, **359**, 835–40.

Rihmer, Z., Rutz, W., and Pihlgren, H. (1995) Depression and suicide on Gotland: an intensive study of all suicides before and after a depression-training programme for general practitioners. *Journal of Affective Disorders*, **35**, 147–52.

Yu, X., and Shen, Y.C. (2003) Epidemiology of vascular dementia in China. In J. O'Brien, D. Ames, L. Gustafson, M. Folstein, and E. Chiu (eds.) *Cerebrovascular Disease and Dementia*, 2nd edn, pp. 75–83.

Chapter 10

Psychogeriatric services: current trends in Australia and New Zealand

Brian Draper, Pamela Melding and Henry Brodaty

Although separate countries, Australia and New Zealand are linked by their location in the South Pacific, history, and in many respects, culture. The countries also share the same five-year training programme for psychiatrists run by the Royal Australian and New Zealand College of Psychiatrists (RANZCP). This programme contains a mandatory three years of basic training and two years of advanced training in whatever field of psychiatry the trainee chooses. The Faculty of Psychiatry of Old Age (FPOA) runs the two-year advanced training scheme in old age psychiatry that was commenced in 1999 (Draper and Snowdon, 1999). There is a curriculum that stipulates the areas of knowledge, skills and attitudes that need to be covered in training. The scheme requires a breadth of training experiences in settings that include acute inpatients, community, consultation/liaison in general hospitals and long-term residential care. Individual training programmes are accredited by the FPOA through a combination of site visits and self-report.

While the delivery of psychogeriatric services in Australia and New Zealand are similar, there are also significant differences.

Australia

Australia is a geographically large country, approximately the size of mainland USA, which has a relatively small population of 20 million with 12.8 per cent aged 65 years and over. Despite the size of the country, Australia is highly urbanized with very few people living in the arid interior.

Australia is a federation of six States and two Territories, with both levels of government having responsibilities in psychogeriatric service delivery. The Federal government sets the overall health policies and is responsible for the funding of residential care and community support services for the aged and disabled (including dementia), private medical practitioners through the universal health insurance scheme (Medicare), and the Pharmaceutical Benefits Scheme. State and Territory governments are responsible for the provision of mental health services, general hospital services and community aged care services.

Australia is culturally and linguistically diverse, with about a third of older Australians born overseas – approximately 20 per cent from a culturally and linguistically diverse background and approximately 13 per cent from English-speaking countries (Australian Institute of Health and Welfare, 2002). Most immigration occurred following the Second World War with cohorts from Europe, the Mediterranean, the Middle East and Asia now successively reaching old age. Often migrants who came in late life are unable to speak English fluently and those who have aged in Australia and have developed dementia lose their capacity to speak the more recently acquired language. Use of interpreter services, bilingual health professionals and 'cluster' nursing homes (where there is an attempt to encourage residents and staff from the same culture to be placed or work in the same facility) have been insufficient to meet their needs. About 2.4 per cent of the population identify themselves as of Aboriginal or Torres Strait Islander descent. As their life expectancy is at least twenty years less compared to other Australians, the age of 50 is used for planning aged care services (Australian Bureau of Statistics, 2003). Little is known about rates of dementia or other psychiatric illnesses among older members of these communities. Psychogeriatric services are not well developed for helping indigenous populations.

One of the major problems that confront psychogeriatric services in Australia is the lack of a cohesive policy about which level of government is responsible for service provision, particularly with regard to dementia care. Some States insist that dementia is 'not a mental illness' and resist efforts to provide adequate services for severe behavioural and psychological symptoms of dementia (BPSD), while others accept that this is a reasonable responsibility for psychogeriatric services. Many regions and entire States have no plan for how to deal with this group of patients. Recently a model of planning services to care for people with behavioural and psychological symptoms of dementia has been proposed (Brodaty et al., 2003). There is enormous variability between States in their preparedness to fund psychogeriatric services. For example in 1997–98, per capita expenditure on psychogeriatric services by the States varied from a low of $A76.21 in New South Wales (NSW) to a high of $A174.66 in Western Australia, with a national average of $A102.91 (Commonwealth Department of Health and Aged Care, 2000). The variability in State expenditure is reflected in the marked differences in service development between States. A survey of psychogeriatric services in Australia and New Zealand undertaken by Daniel O'Connor for FPOA in 2003 found that acute psychogeriatric beds ranged from 15.6 per 100,000 in Tasmania to 75.4 per 100,000 in Western Australia. Total psychogeriatric beds that included non-acute and residential beds ranged from 34.6 per 100,000 in NSW to 130.3 per 100,000 in Victoria (O'Connor, personal communication, 2003).

Victoria probably has the most highly developed comprehensive public psychogeriatric services in Australia, particularly in metropolitan areas. They are largely modelled on the UK system with distinct multidisciplinary community teams, acute inpatient units and facilities for the medium and long-term management of severe BPSD and other chronic mental disorders that are catchment area-based. In contrast, services in NSW and Queensland are poorly developed. For example in NSW, while catchment area-based, most services are collocated with either adult mental health services or aged care services. Few catchment areas contain the full range of service components and many components are not adequately resourced in terms of staff or beds (Draper *et al.*, 2003).

Despite this variability across the country, Federal government funding of community-based services for dementia care has improved considerably over the last 20 years, largely by redirecting funds from residential care by ensuring that only the most disabled are admitted. Aged Care Assessment Teams assess the needs of older people and act as gatekeepers for community and residential care. Various packages of community support and respite care (both day care and residential) are available but not in all regions. One of the consequences has been a decline in the per capita number of nursing home beds to such a degree that there are now inadequate bed numbers. In addition, there are also concerns that staffing of nursing homes is inadequate for quality dementia care and that planning ratios do not make provision for dementia specific care (Access Economics, 2003).

The number of psychogeriatricians in Australia varies across the states from 2 per 100,000 persons aged 65 years and over in Queensland to 5.9 per 100,000 persons aged 65 years and over in Western Australia (O'Connor, personal communication, 2003). This compares unfavourably with the overall number of psychiatrists in Australia of 11.1 per 100,000 population (Australian Institute of Health and Welfare, 2003). While nearly all Australian psychogeriatricians work in the public sector, there are a number of private psychogeriatricians and psychogeriatric inpatient and outpatient facilities across the country. Overall the provision of private psychiatric services to older people is very limited. Medicare data reveals that adults under 65 years of age received 2.7 times the number of psychiatric services per capita than patients 65 years and over and 3.6 times that of patients aged 75 years and over. Medicare funding was over four times higher for younger adults than those aged 65 years and over (Draper and Koschera, 2001).

New Zealand

New Zealand is a small island nation, of 4 million people, living in an area slightly bigger than the UK. Twelve per cent of the population is over 65 years. The majority of the population lives in the four major cities of Auckland, Wellington, Christchurch and Dunedin. Most of the country is rural agricultural farmland, which is New Zealand's main source of economic income. Fifteen per cent of the population is indigenous Maori, 6.2 per cent Pacific Island People, 6 per cent Asian and the majority is of European, mostly British, origin.

History

Psychiatric services for older people were first developed in Auckland in the mid 1970s by Dr Kingsley Mortimer. After his death in 1982 service development in New Zealand stalled for a few years, but was rejuvenated in the late 1980s in response to increasing interest in the specialty resulting from the initiation of the section of psychiatry of old age (now Faculty) of the RANZCP.

Today, services are widespread throughout New Zealand with 15 out of 21 District Health Boards providing dedicated psychiatry of old age services. New Zealand has an average of 7 psychiatrists of old age for every 100,000 population over 65 years. Most psychiatry of old age is practised within the public health system.

Model of service delivery

Most services in New Zealand use a domiciliary focused model of service delivery and patients are triaged through a multidisciplinary community assessment team. These teams assess and treat about 80 per cent of referred patients in their place of residence, with medical back-up from the base hospital services and liaison with the residential and respite care sectors (Melding and Osman-Aly, 2000). Larger services usually have dedicated teams for acute inpatient units and community service delivery, but in smaller health districts a single team will work with inpatient and community patients. Acute inpatient bed numbers average 4 beds per 10,000 elderly populations nationwide but there is great variability throughout the country (range 11/10,000–0/10,000). (Melding and Osman-Aly, 2000).

Long stay beds and respite care do not exist in the public sector, but there is a network of rest homes and private hospitals, operated by both the private for-profit and the not-for-profit religious and welfare sectors that cater for short-term respite and long-term geriatric care. Older New Zealanders requiring placement are state subsidized if their income or assets fall below a threshold level.

Less than 25 per cent of New Zealand services have geriatric psychiatry day hospitals. Many private hospitals and high level rest homes have day care facilities that non-residents needing such services can access. Specialist day clinics are provided by several services for group treatment of depression or anxiety. Outpatient clinics tend to be generic geriatric psychiatry clinics, with very few services offering specialist services such as memory clinics. New Zealand services generally are co-located, functionally or administratively linked with geriatric services.

New Zealand issues

The ageing population and the strategy for health care of older people

New Zealand's ageing population in all ethnic groups is increasing and expected to reach 18 per cent by 2020 (Richmond et al., 1995). Unsurprisingly, in the last few years the New Zealand Ministry of Health has taken considerable interest in older people's health and in 2001 the *Health of Older People Strategy. Health Sector Action to 2010 to Support Positive Ageing* (Ministry of Health, 2002a) was released. The guiding principle of this document is person- (and their family-) centred care. The objectives include provision of a range of inpatient, community geriatric and geriatric psychiatry services, residential assessment, treatment and rehabilitation and residential care to be available for patients in each District Health Area, nationwide. District Health Boards are required to develop administrative processes that enable integrated services, delivery that is needs based, services that are responsive and flexible to changing patient needs, interventions that are based on best practice, supported by research and, of course, affordable to the individual and state.

Cost and standard of institutionalized care

New Zealand has one of the highest rates of subsidized institutionalization for older people in the world. Over 6 per cent of total public health expenditure and 25 per cent of all health expenditure for the over 65s is spent on residential care subsidies for older people who can no longer be supported in their own homes (Ministry of Health, 2002b). Quality and standard of care in residential institutions can be variable, and recently the requirement that residential services have to contract with the Ministry of Health through their local District Health Authorities has enabled measurable quality standards to be included in the contracts. These include provisions for training of staff, minimal staffing levels, assessment of medications practices and restraint minimization; all of which are subject to auditing and monitoring of facilities (Lewis, 2002).

Ageing in place

Current health policy advocates 'ageing in place' (Howden-Chapman *et al.*, 1999) as the preferred option. To enable patients to stay at home, New Zealand has a system of Need Assessment Service Coordinators (NASC), attached to all older people's services who design packages of home support for older patients (meals on wheels, home assistance, district nursing, respite care etc.). These are means tested and the packages have limits. When home care is no longer viable NASC will arrange placement in a rest home or private hospital. The total number and range of services available through NASC varies throughout the country. The recent adoption of *Best practice, Evidence-Based Guideline: Assessment Process for Older People* (New Zealand Guidelines Group, 2003) and the proposed use of a common assessment tool should, in the next few years, make access to homecare services more equitable, nationwide.

Maori mental health

Maori are the indigenous people of New Zealand. In 1840 the British Crown signed the Treaty of Waitangi with the Maori tribal leaders. Fundamental to the Treaty was the protection of the 'rights' of the *tangata whenua* ('The people of the land', the indigenous Maori), in exchange for the sovereignty of the Islands being succeeded to the British Crown. The principles of the Treaty are enshrined in the New Zealand legislature. In the health sector important rights to be protected are health and access to health care.

Despite improvements over the last few decades, there are still marked disparities between Maori health and life expectancy when compared to the European population of New Zealand. Maori have been prone to vascular disease, stroke, renal disease, cancer, respiratory disease and diabetes, which result in untimely deaths, disability, mental illness and early onset dementia particularly vascular dementia. Ill health commences approximately five years before other New Zealanders and life expectancy of Maori males is 10 years less and for females 8 years less than New Zealanders as a whole (Ministry of Health, 2002b). Debate is ongoing as to whether the age at which older people's services can be accessed should be a lower age than for other New Zealanders (Maaka, 1993).

Ability to provide assessment, treatment and placement options for older Maori that are also culturally appropriate is a government priority and a major challenge for all services. Many teams have limited access to cultural advisors and there is a major shortage of Maori professional staff within teams. Maori concepts of health are more holistic than those espoused by their European treaty partners. For Maori, and particularly older Maori, health has a framework of *taha tinana* (physical health), *taha hinengaro* (emotional and psychological health), *taha whanau* (family health), and *taha wairua* (spiritual health) (Durie, 1998). Traditionally, Maori culture is rooted in the *whanau* (extended family) and in contrast to the western ethos of personal autonomy; individualism is subsumed within the whanau so that for Maori, all matters relating to a patient's health need discussing with the extended family. The whanau and not the individual make the key decisions. Whilst family conferences are essential when dealing with Maori patients, involving family and or caregivers in key clinical decision-making, and discharge planning is preferred for all older patients in New Zealand irrespective of ethnicity.

Rural issues

Much of New Zealand is rural farmland and a higher proportion of older people live in these outlying areas (20 per cent as opposed to urban 15 per cent). Whilst most base hospitals have geriatric services, geriatric psychiatry services are confined to the bigger centres and so access to services for rural people in some areas of the country can be limited. For those areas that do have geriatric psychiatry teams very few have a purely urban catchment, most have outreach services to large rural hinterland areas.

Few residential facilities exist in the rural areas, thus elderly patients with mental illness are mostly cared for by relatives who are themselves isolated. If the health of caregivers breaks down, patients needing nursing home placement have to move to urban areas with consequential separation from their families.

Academia and research

There are no academic departments of geriatric psychiatry in the country and the specialty is extremely poorly represented in academic psychiatry departments nationwide. Despite mental health and older adults being priority areas for the Health Research Foundation, very few research grants have been granted to the specialty and consequently New Zealand-based research is also lacking. On the other hand, academic gerontology is quite well represented in several universities' nursing and psychology departments.

Future directions

Psychogeriatric services have developed at a rapid rate over the past fifteen years. The New Zealand branch of FPOA, RANZCP, is active in local and national planning of future services. There is commitment to collocation with our geriatric colleagues to enable a continuum of care for older people with mixed physical and mental illness. Psychologists specializing in old age are increasing in number and have formed a national network.

References

Access Economics (2003) *The Dementia Epidemic: economic impact and positive solutions for Australia.* Access Economics Pty Ltd., Canberra.

Australian Bureau of Statistics (2003) *The Health and Welfare of Australia's Aboriginal and Torres Strait Islander Peoples.* AIHW Catalogue 1HW-11, 4704.0. Australian Bureau of Statistics, Canberra.

Australian Institute of Health and Welfare (AIHW) (2002) *Older Australia at a Glance,* 3rd edn. AIHW Cat. No. AGE 25. AIHW and DOHA, Canberra.

Australian Institute of Health and Welfare (AIHW) (2003) *Mental Health Services in Australia 2000–01,* Mental Health Series no. 4. AIHW, Canberra.

Brodaty, H., Draper, B., and Low, L.-F. (2003) Behavioural and psychological symptoms of dementia – a 7-tiered triangular model of service delivery. *Medical Journal of Australia,* **178**, 231–4.

Commonwealth Department of Health and Aged Care (2000) *National Mental Health Report 2000: Sixth annual report. Changes in Australia's mental health services under the First National Mental Health Strategy 1993–98.* Australian Government Publishing Service, Canberra.

Draper, B., Jochelson, T., Kitching, D., Snowdon, J., Brodaty, H., and Russell, B. (2003) Mental health service delivery to older people in New South Wales: perceptions of aged care, adult mental health and mental health services for older people. *Australian and New Zealand Journal of Psychiatry,* **37**, 735–40.

Draper, B. and Koschera, A. (2001) Do older people receive equitable private psychiatric service provision under Medicare? *Australian and New Zealand Journal of Psychiatry,* **35**, 626–30.

Draper, B. and Snowdon, J. (1999) Psychiatry of old age – from section to faculty. *Australian and New Zealand Journal of Psychiatry,* **33**, 785–8.

Durie, M. (1998) *Whaiora, Maori Health Development.* Oxford University Press, Auckland.

Howden-Chapman, P., Signal, L., and Crane, J. (1999) Housing and Health in older people: ageing in place. *Social Policy Journal of New Zealand,* **13**, 14–30.

Lewis, H. (2002) *Dementia in New Zealand: Improving Quality in Residential Care.* Report to the Disability Issues Directorate, Ministry of Health. Ministry of Health, Wellington.

Maaka, R. (1993) Te Ao o Te Pakeketanga: The world of the aged. In P. Koopman-Boyden (ed.) *New Zealand's Ageing Society: the implications,* pp. 216–54. Daphne Brasell, Wellington.

Melding, P.S. and Osman-Aly, N. (2000) 'The view from the bottom of the cliff'. Old age psychiatry services in New Zealand: the patients and the resources. *New Zealand Medical Journal,* **113**, 439–42.

Ministry of Health (2002a) *The Health of Older People Strategy. Health Sector Action to 2010 to support Positive Ageing.* Ministry of Health, Wellington.

Ministry of Health (2002b) *Health of Older People in New Zealand. A Statistical Reference.* Ministry of Health, Wellington.

New Zealand Guidelines Group (2003) *Best Practice Evidenced-based Guideline, Assessment Processes for Older People.* Ministry of Health, Wellington.

Richmond, D., Baskett J., Bonita, R., and Melding, P. (1995) *Care of Older People in New Zealand.* New Zealand Government Press, Wellington.

Chapter 11

Psychogeriatric services: current trends in Latin America

Sergio Tamai

Introduction

Latin America is composed of 22 countries that occupy Central America, the Andean zone, the southern cone, and the area known as the Latin American Caribbean. Political and international health agencies consider other Caribbean countries like Barbados to be part of the region. In 1999, the total population of all these countries was nearly 600 million, with a growth rate of about 40 per cent in the last 30 years (Alarcón and Aguilar-Gaxiola, 2000; Levav et al., 1989). Most of the population live in urban areas (Guzmán, 2002). The region has unique social, political, economic, and cultural characteristics, which have generated great differences in economic and health development. Demographically, the Latin American region is characterized by marked differences between and within countries. Less developed countries, such as Haiti, still show patterns of high mortality and lower life expectancy, whereas other countries such as Argentina and Chile resemble more developed countries (Levav et al., 1989).

The ageing process in Latin America

The second half of the twentieth century witnessed an acceleration of the ageing process in populations of Latin America. Countries have been experiencing rapid declines in both fertility and mortality and the majority of them are in an intermediate stage of demographic transition. Latin American life expectancy has increased from 65.3 years in 1980–1985 to a projected 75.3 years in 2020–2025 (an increase of 10 years) (CELADE, 2002). Also, it is calculated that the percentage of older Latin Americans (60 years or older) has been increasing from 6.5 per cent of the total population in 1980 (22.9 million) to 7.9 per cent in 2000 (40 million). It will further increase to 14.0 per cent in 2025 (95.8 million) (CELADE, 2002). The size of the elderly population is expected to increase at an average annual rate of 3 per cent, as compared to a rate of increase for the total population of 2.04 per cent (Alarcón and Aguilar-Gaxiola, 2000). There are differences in the proportion of elderly among the regions of Latin America. For example, it has been projected that the percentage of the older population in the year 2025 for the central America will be more than 10 per cent (Costa Rica 14.6 per cent,

Panama 15.4 per cent, Mexico 13.5 per cent), the Caribbean will be near 20 per cent (Barbados 25.2 per cent, Guadalupe 15.1 per cent, Cuba 25 per cent). The increase for the southern part of the continent will be 18 per cent (Argentina 16.6 per cent, Uruguay 19.6 per cent, Chile 18.2 per cent), whereas the northern part of the continent will be more than 10 per cent (Guyana 11.7 per cent, Colombia 13.5 per cent, Brazil 15.4 per cent, Venezuela 13.2 per cent) (Guzmán, 2002).

At the end of the last century the proportion of the population older than 65 approximated or exceeded the 10 per cent level – i.e. slightly below those attained in Canada and the United – in only five countries: Argentina, Barbados, Cuba, Martinique and Uruguay (Pan American Health Organization, 1997).

The ageing process in the continent will not follow a unique, homogeneous course. There is substantial intercountry heterogeneity in the timing, levels, and other characteristics. Brazil and Mexico will age later but in a shorter period of time than Chile and Costa Rica or Uruguay and Argentina (Pan American Health Organization, 1997).

Paucity of data on geriatric mental health in Latin America

These heterogeneous scenarios are probably responsible for lack of adequate information systems that could inform situation of mental health in elderly people (Pan American Health Organization, 1997). All available information on the mental health status of older persons consists of local studies, most of which are highly selected and isolated and so thoroughly unsuitable for drawing global inferences about current and future trends of geriatric psychiatry in Latin America.

In this context of scarce information, some initiatives to promote and improve the quality of data on mental health of elderly people have been undertaken by the World Health Organization (WHO) and International Psychogeriatric Association (IPA) and specifically as regards dementia through Alzheimer's Disease International research arm, The 10/66 Group (Prince et al., 2003). WHO launched Project Atlas in 2000 to address this lack of information about mental health resources. The objectives of this project include collection, compilation and dissemination of relevant information on mental health resources in different countries. The project was designed to obtain real information from each country rather than to extrapolate based on what is known from a few countries (World Health Organization, 2001). Based on Project Atlas's database in the year of 2001, 13 countries in Latin America had mental health programmes for elderly persons. The exceptions were Ecuador, Guyana, Peru, Venezuela, El Salvador, Haiti, Guatemala, Belize and Nicaragua.

The Latin American Psychogeriatric and Psychogerontologic Association (LAPPA) was founded in 1998. It is affiliated with the IPA to support and orient professionals in their work of therapeutic management of the psychopathological and psychosocial problems experienced by the elderly (International Psychogeriatric Association, 1999). In 2000 the IPA introduced the Latin America Initiative to bring together a diverse regional group, including current and emerging Latin American opinion leaders, to begin the major task of establishing policy and guidelines for the region (International Psychogeriatric Association, 2000).

The expectation is that the Latin American Initiative will have a major impact on defining the key issues for the region and the organization of effective clinical, research, and educational programmes (International Psychogeriatric Association, 2000).

Psychogeriatric services

Evolution of the structure of health Latin American services has been based on classical western models of health care delivery where polypharmacy is frequent (Espino *et al.*, 1998). These models rarely take into account cultural aspects of how local persons understand illness, seek medical aid, or use traditional healing methods. The emphasis has been on hospitals and curative medicine rather than on trying to address local public health needs.

In this scenario, Latin American geriatric psychiatry continues to develop. There are few geriatric psychiatrists in Latin America and, for the most part, they have obtained their geriatric training abroad in either Europe or the United States of America. Most psychiatrists who work with old people are viewed as general psychiatrists with experience in geriatric syndromes. The multidisciplinary model is also used, but limited resources place the geriatric psychiatrists in the role of case managers.

Country examples

Brazil

In Latin America, few formal postgraduate geriatric training opportunities exist. In Brazil, the Psychiatry Institute of Federal University of Rio de Janeiro has a one-year residency programme in geriatric psychiatry. The Brazilian Psychiatric Association recognized psychogeriatry as a speciality in 2002. In this country other innovative programmes encompass care and research in geriatric psychiatry. At Santa Casa de Misericórdia of São Paulo, a multidisciplinary service has been delivered care to old age people with mental disorders based on case management approach since 1996 (Almeida *et al.*, 1999). Like this service, there are many others, but in the main they are isolated experiences widespread in the Latin America.

Mexico

The private sector made a majority contribution in the assessment of the country's health situation prior to the presentation of the National Plan of Health and Mental Health by the Ministry of Health in 2001. The need to develop public policy related to the dementing illnesses, particularly with regard to old people – was urgently needed. The plan covers four major areas: service delivery, health education, research and legislation (Resnikoff, 2002).

Colombia

There are few services for the elderly in Colombia. Given the ever-increasing acute care needs and the prohibitively high costs of nursing homes and rehabilitation units faced by the national health-care system, community care and other resources such as home care, day centres, day hospitals, and meal kitchens are future alternatives for improved psychogeriatric care (Guevara, 1998; Reyes-Ortiz, 1997, 1998a). Currently, there are only a few geriatric units in cities such as Bogotá, Cali, Manizales and Barranquilla. National medical schools working with the Colombian Association of Gerontology and Geriatrics (Asociacion Colombiana de Gerontologia y Geriatria) are planning to improve geriatrics education and training at all levels of research and education (Reyes-Ortiz, 1998b).

Conclusion

The ageing process of Latin America's populations poses challenges to provide appropriate mental health services for the elderly people. Issues that will be addressed include more and better epidemiological information that help the development of innovative cost-effective health-care models that take into account cultural values.

References

Alarcón, R.D. and Aguilar-Gaxiola, S.A. (2000) Mental health policy developments in Latin America. *Bulletin of the World Health Organization,* **78** (4), 483–90.

Almeida, O.P., Ratto, L., Garrido, R., and Tamai, S. (1999) [Risk factors and consequences of polypharmacy among elderly outpatients of a mental health service], *Revista Brasileira de Psiquiatria,* **21** (3) (in Portuguese).

CELADE (Latin American and Caribbean Demographic Centre) (2002) Latin America and Caribbean: population estimates and projections 1950–2050. *Demographic Bulletin,* **69**, 37–41.

Espino, D.V., Lichtenstein, M.J., Hazuda, H.P., *et al.* (1998) Correlates of prescription and over-the-counter medication usage among older Mexican Americans: The Hispanic EPESE study. *Journal of the American Geriatrics Society,* **46**, 1228–34.

Guevara, G.M. (1998) Vida a los Anos. *Revista de la Asociación Colombiana de Gerontología y Geriatría,* **12** (90).

Guzmán, J.M. (2002) Envejecimiento y desarrollo en América Latina y el Caribe. *CEPAL SERIE Población y desarrollo,* **28**, 7–13.

International Psychogeriatric Association (1999) Latin American Psychogeriatric and Psychogerontologic Association. *IPA Bulletin,* **16** (2).

International Psychogeriatric Association (2000) IPA introduces Latin American initiative to begin establishing policy and guidelines for the region. *IPA Bulletin,* **17** (4).

Levav, I., Lima, B.R., Somoza Lennon, M., Kramer, M., and Gonzalez, R. (1989) [Mental health for all in Latin America and the Caribbean. Epidemiologic basis for action]. *Boletin de la Oficina Sanitaria PanAmericana,* **107**, 196–219 (in Spanish).

Pan American Health Organization (1997) A profile of the health conditions of older persons of Latin America and the Carribean. *Epidemiological Bulletin,* **18** (2) 1–5.

Prince, M., Acosta, D., Chiu, H., Scazufca, M., and Varghese, M. (2003) Dementia diagnosis in developing countries: a cross-cultural validation study. *Lancet*, **361**, 909–17.

Resnikoff, D. (2002) Psychogeriatrics around the world: Mexico develops a national plan to address dementia. *IPA Bulletin* **19** (4).

Reyes-Ortiz, C.A. (1997) Home visiting on geriatric patients. *Journal of the American Geriatrics Society*, **45**, S29.

Reyes-Ortiz, C.A. (1998a) Visitas domiciliarias en pacientes geriatricos. *Colombia Medica*, **29**, 138–42.

Reyes-Ortiz, C.A. (1998b) Metas de la geriatria colombiana. *Colombia Medica*, **29**, 119–20.

World Health Organization (2001) *Atlas – Mental health resources in the world*. World Health Organization, Geneva.

Chapter 12

Psychogeriatric services: current trends in Europe

Karen Ritchie, Joanna Norton, Alexander Kurz, Julia Hartmann, Tadeusz Parnowski, Catalina Tudose and Sture Eriksson

Despite being the continent with the highest proportion of older people, European countries have not widely embraced the development of comprehensive psychogeriatric services of the type described by Edmond Chiu in Chapter 2. A 1997 survey found that the Netherlands and Switzerland were the only continental European countries that had a full range of long term, hospital-based and community-based psychogeriatric services in many parts of the country (Reifler and Cohen, 1998). In this chapter we have obtained descriptions of service delivery from five countries – France, Germany, Poland, Romania and Sweden – that are representative of both Eastern and Western Europe. As can be seen, services are largely focused on dementia care rather than the full range of mental disorders.

France
Karen Ritchie and Joanna Norton
Psychogeriatrics does not exist as such in France, so care is delegated either to psychiatric or geriatric specialist centres, or in the case of the dementias, to neurological departments. This splitting of services has led to wide variability in the type of care that might be offered for a single disorder as there are still very few specialized psychogeriatric units.

The provision of psychogeriatric services in France is essentially hospital-based and can be traced back to the early eighteenth century records of the Salpetriere Hospital in Paris, which tell us that around 10 per cent of the 4000 female inmates suffered from 'extreme old age and a relapse into childhood' while others exhibited 'a vagabond state'. Conditions at this time were minimal: the main preoccupations were protection from the elements (construction of an open shelter), cleanliness (the provision of mattresses which could be cleaned of faeces instead of straw beds) and minimizing self-harm (provision of soft slippers to replace wooden clogs).

Until recently institutional care, which is predominantly long-term hospital care, was still largely oriented towards these three aims, catering principally for patients with chronic conditions and multiple pathologies, such as the dementias, confusional states, severe behavioural and affective disorders and psychoses. Today, the patient and the informal caregiver – most often spouse, daughter or daughter in law – are increasingly seen as a unique entity and are both taken into account when deciding which type of care is best adapted to the situation.

Concerning long-term hospital care for non-degenerative disorders, the length of stay is between 15 to 45 days, with around 70 per cent returning home (Tessier *et al.*, 1999). Most cases are admitted at their own request. Forced admission (the Law of June 1990) may be carried out at the request of another person acting in the interest of the patient, and two medical certificates. A single medical certificate will suffice in cases of immediate danger.

For the organization of general geriatric hospital care, the creation of geriatric sites with short-, medium- and long-term stay patients, sharing a central 'medical platform' and social team is currently underway in some of the main French cities. Geriatric patients with polypathologies, including psychiatric disorders, would no longer be transported by ambulance from one department to another and would no longer 'block' beds in specialized units. Instead the specialized doctor would visit the patients on the geriatric site.

Day hospital care for psychogeriatric patients is relatively recent in France, dating from 1975, dealing principally with anxiety and depressive disorders and relief care in early stage dementia. Duration of care ranges from 3 to 8 months, with the general practitioner being the principal coordinator of ongoing care. Community care has been organized by sectors since 1960, consisting of a hospital team headed by a psychiatrist with a nurse, psychologist and home-helpers. The team may be permanently constituted to carry out this task or put together temporarily from a hospital department specifically to follow-up a patient who has been recently released. Home help tailored to individual needs may also be provided following an evaluation of the person's social situation and degree of autonomy by a social worker. The social worker coordinates the different services provided and evaluates their efficacy.

More than half of the elderly persons in France today suffering from dementia and other chronic psychogeriatric disorders are cared for at home, partly in the belief that this is psychologically more comfortable for the elderly person, but also because of economic constraints. General practitioners and nurses carry out home visits, which are subsidized by social security. Under Napoleonic law, adult children in France are responsible for the care of their dependant parents, and in the face of the costs of long-term hospital stay many families are forced to provide care in less than ideal situations. Nursing home costs are subject to means testing and are paid by the elderly person and/or family. Since July 2001, people aged 60 and above with disability in everyday life receive an allowance (Allocation Personnalisée d'Autonomie), a financial help for everyday life whether living at home or in an institution.

Temporary relief hospital care ('hospitalisation de répit') for home patients, with help programmes for caregivers, is now available. It is geared mainly towards Alzheimer patients to cover crisis periods. Although this temporarily takes the burden off the caregiver, an evaluation study has shown that it may not be beneficial in the long term (Colvez and Joël, 2002).

The last ten years has seen the development of specialized units which provide half-way houses between home and hospital care for elderly persons with neurodegenerative disorders, which aim to promote autonomy, not just provide safe shelter. The first of these units was the 'Cantou' which provided 'homely' care shared by family and non-medical personnel (Ritchie *et al.*, 1992) in small groups living in architecturally appropriate units around a central activity area. The original concept of the 'Cantou' differed significantly from that of the traditional, most often medicalized, nursing home. Today the more common 'unités de vie' or 'living units' have replaced the original Cantou, with closer links to hospital care. However, there are too few of these units to meet present demands. Day-care centres within nursing homes or group-living units are now an alternative to long-stay care.

For Alzheimer patients, there has been a recent move towards creating specific care units within hospitals and nursing homes, adapting the structure to the patients' needs. In October 2001, the government launched a dementia prevention and care programme (Plan Demence): one of the aims is to increase the early diagnosis of Alzheimer's disease and other dementias with greater access to memory clinics.

Physical and psychological abuse of the elderly person, particularly in cases where home care has been undertaken by families due to economic constraints or lack of facilities, has only been addressed in recent years. A help network called ALMA (Allo Maltraitance des Personnes Agées) has now been created in a number of French cities, which has estimated that 32 per cent of elderly persons with psychogeriatric disorders are maltreated (Busby, 1998).

The principal difficulties facing psychogeriatric care in France are the increasing numbers of dependant elderly and a decrease in the availability of family to provide care. In the 1999 census, 21.3 per cent of the population was aged 60 or above and 7.7 per cent were aged 75 and above (Insee, Recensement de la Population, 1999). The diagnosis of psychogeriatric disorder is still most commonly in the hands of the general practitioner, who has little if any specialist training, and is reluctant to refer on to specialist units for fear of diminishing the size of the medical practice. A diagnosis is often late and/or erroneous (Ledésert and Ritchie, 1994). The concept of liaison psychiatry, or the establishment of psychiatric teams within the general hospital, is frequently invoked by French psychiatrists as a useful model for psychogeriatric practice. However, severe reductions in hospital personnel, poor communication between general practitioner and specialist services for the coordination of care, have made such projects difficult to implement.

Germany
Alexander Kurz and Julia Hartmann

In 2000 23 per cent of the German population were older than 60 years, 3.6 per cent were older than 80, and 0.6 per cent were older than 90. The 'Altenquotient' (age index) population of individuals older than 60 per 100 individuals aged between 20 and 59, was 41.3. The Federal Statistical Office (Statistisches Bundesamt) predicts a significant increase of the proportion of old and very old individuals until 2050 of 12.8 per cent (60+ years), 7.7 per cent (80+ years), and 1.5 per cent (90+ years) (Ministry of Family, Seniors, Women and Youth, 2002). In Germany there are 381,342 physicians, of whom 6,113 (1.6 per cent) are psychiatrists, 2,982 (0.8 per cent) are neurologists and 6,538 are both. Geriatric psychiatry is part of psychiatric and neurological care and is not a medical specialty in this country. In some parts – e.g. in Bavaria – there is an optional continuing medical education in clinical geriatrics. Dementia is underrepresented in continuing medical education, relative to its importance and frequency (Haupt, 2002).

Focus on ambulatory care

In Germany, most mentally ill older people receive care in the home provided by family members. In spite of societal changes informal care will remain a mainstay of psychogeriatric care. An integrated system of services capable of meeting individual needs at different levels of disease severity is required to maintain older patients in the community and to minimize hospital and nursing home admissions. As a consequence, networks of ambulatory and intermediate care psychogeriatric services have been established in many cities. Parallel with the increase in the oldest segment of the population, there is an increase in the absolute numbers of hospital and nursing home admissions. The tendency to avoid institutionalization, however, is clearly evident. For example, the capacity of day care centres has increased thirty-fold from 1988 to 1998 (Lohse, 2002).

Memory clinics have an increasingly important complementary role in the ambulatory care of older patients with dementia, with more than 70 specialty units initiated in Germany since 1985. Their structure is interdisciplinary, focusing on the early recognition, diagnosis, treatment and counselling of patients with cognitive impairment of various degrees. In addition they provide a significant infrastructure for clinical drug trials and many other research activities (Lautenschlager and Kurz, 2000).

Additional evidence for the shift of psychiatric care toward ambulatory services is the growth of community care and counselling services. The national Alzheimer's Association (Deutsche Alzheimer Gesellschaft) offers countrywide counselling services free of charge. These services have been complemented in November 2001 by a telephone hotline. This self-help initiative has been gradually developing since 1989 and now has more than 60 regional associations in addition to over 300 self-help and caregiver support groups. The association has started to act as a local and national lobby of, and for, patients and caregivers and is gradually gaining political influence (Kurz et al., 2003).

In addition to the already mentioned memory clinics there are more than ten 'psychogeriatric centres' (gerontopsychiatrische Zentren) in the country and several others are being developed. The concept of psychogeriatric centres includes three essential components: outpatient clinic, day centre, and assessment unit (Wächtler and Hofmann, 2001). The objectives of the centres are to identify individual needs for treatment and care, to refer patients to adequate services in the community, and to counsel patients and carers. Ideally, a psychogeriatric centre should be attached to a geriatric unit at a psychiatric or general hospital. The general health insurance covers diagnosis and treatment in specialized centres including memory clinics and psychogeriatric centres. There is also a growing number of special care units for depressed patients in psychiatric hospitals, but not particularly for depressed elderly. In these psychogeriatric centres patients with different pychiatric diseases of old age are being treated by multiprofessional teams. The most frequent diagnoses are depression and dementia; paranoid and neurotic disorders and personality disorders are rare. However, only a small proportion of psychogeriatric patients benefits from these specialized institutions. General physicians still provide the first and the most important medical service for the elderly. In rural areas the density of psychiatric and neurologic specialists is low. Only one out of eight patients with dementia receives treatment by a specialist psychiatrist/neurologist.

Architectural design of nursing homes and novel forms of group living

Nursing home care is provided for 28 per cent of all demented individuals in need of care but to 40 per cent of subjects with moderate to severe dementia (Lohse, 2002). From the 1980s attempts have been made to create dementia-specific architectural designs. In particular, traditional large-scale nursing homes have been turned into smaller units to allow more room for privacy. Designs including bright light and ample space provide more room for mobility. Also, they facilitate perception of the environment and orientation, thus compensating for the patients' impaired cognitive ability. It is felt that a person-centred way of institutional care and an emphasis on individual psychological as well as social needs contribute to the maintenance and improvement of the quality of life of individuals with dementia. The Gradman Haus in Stuttgart is a model for modern nursing home design which incorporates the principles of milieu therapy. The architectural concepts used in this building include public areas arranged in the style of a village street (Heeg, 2001). There is no precise information on the number of nursing homes with a model design. All over the country new architectural projects are being developed. Also, existing institutions are gradually being improved.

The spectrum of institutional care facilities is complemented by short-term care, apartments for more competent older people, and disease-specific physical and social environments designed to reduce problematic behaviours. In several hospitals, special care units have been established for patients with dementia or depression in an attempt to better meet the different needs of important diagnostic groups.

Various forms of group living have been positively evaluated, but are only rarely available. Built after the Swedish, Dutch, and French 'cantou' or the British 'domus' models these developments aim at reducing the negative effects of an institutional milieu on psychogeriatric patients.

Coordination and integration of care psychogeriatric services

Disease management programmes for patients with dementia have not yet been systematically introduced in Germany. Increasing efforts are being made, however, to better coordinate and integrate psychogeriatric services, including measures of quality control, with the aims of improving care economy and identifying shortcomings as well as deficits in communication. Steering mechanisms have been implemented to safeguard optimal individual treatment strategies. In several cities combined psychogeriatric services (Gerontopsychiatrische Verbundsysteme) have been established in an attempt to integrate ambulatory, intermediate-level, and institutional components of care (Kurz *et al.*, 2003). In other cities psychogeriatric centres have been developed which include an outpatient clinic, counselling services and day centres. These centres collaborate closely with primary physicians and specialists. The Centre for the Aged (Zentrum für Ältere) in Hamburg is a unique project which features structuring of patient flow and multiprofessional treatment teams (Wächtler and Hofmann, 2001). The Alzheimer Treatment Centre (Alzheimer Therapiezentrum) at Bad Aibling is an example for a disease-specific integrated service. The centre admits patients together with their carers who live in private apartments for several weeks. The results of the treatment programme, which combines a form of validation therapy with carer counseling and support groups, are encouraging (Romero, 2001).

Poland

Tadeusz Parnowski

In 2003, the population of Poland is about 38 million people including 4.5 million people aged 65 or over (12 per cent). The number of persons at the age of over 65 years is rapidly on the rise. In 2005, this group will constitute 16.6 per cent of the whole population, while by 2020 this figure is expected to rise to 24.5 per cent (approximately 6 million people). In 2001 the number of people aged 80 and over reached 847,000 (2.2 per cent). The increase in the number of the aged is accompanied by the increase in the incidence of numerous somatic conditions and psychiatric disturbances. Only 8.8 per cent of people at the age of over 65 years do not suffer from chronic illnesses (Pietrzykowska *et al.*, 2001).

These factors led to the increasingly frequent occurrence of short-term and chronic adaptation reactions, depressive syndromes (in 6–43 per cent); disturbances of consciousness (occurring in 19.8 per cent of hospitalized patients) and dementia occur significantly more often (Parnowski, 1995).

History

Until the 1990s, there was neither any tradition nor legal foundations to organize psychogeriatric services in Poland. Undoubtedly, social movements (which started in 1991) triggered public attention and the interest of authorities in the problems of older people, including the improvement of diagnosis and treatment of Alzheimer's disease.

Although there is a lack of precise data in Poland, it is thought that Alzheimer's disease appears in 250,000 people (Bilikiewicz and Parnowski, 2002). The Lower Silesian Association of Care for patients with Alzheimer's disease (and later the Polish Alzheimer Foundation in Warsaw) was founded in 1991 and other associations have since come into being. At present, there are more than 15 non-governmental associations of guardians of patients suffering from Alzheimer's disease. Simultaneously, from 1995, the Section of Psychogeriatrics and Alzheimer's Disease of the Polish Psychiatric Society (150 members) started active teaching in the field of psychogeriatrics for specialists and primary care physicians by printing educational materials in popular Polish journals – *Postępy Psychiatrii i Neurologii (Progress in Psychiatry and Neurology)*, *Psychiatria Polska (Polish Psychiatry)* – and in 1998 started editing its own *Rocznik Psychogeriatryczny (Annals of Psychogeriatrics)* which features the results of clinical and basic studies related to dementia, schizophrenia and depression of the elderly. Since 1995, several investigative projects have been conducted, including research concerning epidemiological, clinical and specific diagnostic problems. Basic studies and studies related to the evaluation of new drugs produced in Poland (Colostrinina®) are also underway. Since 1995, the Section of Psychogeriatrics has been organizing two symposia each year dedicated to the most important psychiatric disturbances in the elderly. In 1999, a group of experts elaborated guidelines for the diagnosis and treatment of dementia (Bilikiewicz *et al.*, 1999).

As there is no recognized specialization in the field of psychogeriatrics in Poland, in 2003 the Section of Psychogeriatrics launched certification in the field of geriatric psychiatry. Of the 3100 psychiatrists in Poland, approximately 60–80 specialize in psychogeriatrics. Alzheimer's disease was clearly the driving force for the development of psychogeriatrics in Poland and for increased social interest in diseases of the elderly.

Inpatient care

The Programme of Mental Health Protection, launched in 1995, aims to conduct integrated care for the elderly in secondary (treatment) and tertiary prevention (rehabilitation). It recommends a change in the tasks of some large psychiatric hospitals wards, to convert them, after modernization, into around-the-clock and daily psychogeriatric wards or sub-wards, where all patients aged 65 years and over with depression, disturbances in consciousness, psychosis and somatic diseases can be treated. Despite the fact that patients with Alzheimer's disease are treated in these wards, they are not solely intended for the diagnosis and treatment of dementia.

According to key objectives of the Programme, every psychiatric hospital with 400–500 hospital beds should have a separate psychogeriatric ward. Thus far, such wards have been organized in six Polish cities. Other key objectives include provision of psychogeriatric outpatient clinics and day wards for cities with more than 100,000 inhabitants. The best solution for the future would be to organize small psychogeriatric wards (20 beds) affiliated to general hospitals and residential houses accessing periodic help by social care agencies.

When organizing psychogeriatric wards, one should take into consideration the specific nature of treatment for the elderly. This includes both architecture (large spaces, bright illumination, installing devices which help in functioning, etc.) and rehabilitation equipment (for music therapy, art therapy and improvement of physical condition, e.g. treadmill training). Care of older people includes engagement of a greater number of staff than would be the more norms for other age groups, nurses, auxiliary staff, and cooperation of physicians of various specialties (psychiatrists, neurologists, geriatricians) with occupational therapists, speech therapists, social workers, neuropsychologists and physiotherapists.

In 1994, the first profiled ward of psychogeriatrics was formed in Poland at the Institute of Psychiatry and Neurology in Warsaw. Its primary tasks were to create a safe therapeutic environment for the elderly, to provide them with specialist care, including the possibility of performing all necessary investigations such as neuroimaging, and to combine hospital care with environmental care.

Due to the absence of intermediate forms of care and inadequate number of trained personnel, the mean length of stay in psychogeriatric wards in Poland is approximately one year. In 1993, for example, 40.7 per cent of patients with diagnosis of organic psychic disturbances (ICD F00-F09) stayed for more than one year in psychiatric hospitals, while in 2001 this number amounted to 42.4 per cent of patients. In 1993, 32.5 per cent of patients with chronic organic non-psychotic states were hospitalized for more than one year, while in 2001 this number amounted to 46.6 per cent of patients. The mean time of stay for patients with organic psychosis diagnoses amounted to 501 in 1993 and 403 days in 2001. Similar increases in the occurrence of these conditions were observed in ambulatory care and respite care (Jaszczuk et al., 1994; Pietrzykowska et al., 2001).

As a result of the increase in the number of elderly patients, not only were psychiatric wards transformed into psychogeriatric wards, new psychogeriatric wards were founded, connected with outpatient clinics and environmental care (home visits). Integrated centres of psychogeriatrics (currently there are three of them) mark the directions of development for psychogeriatrics in Poland.

Outpatient care

Specialist outpatient clinics, for example Clinic of Degenerative Diseases, Memory Clinics and Alzheimer's Disease Clinics, which have emerged since 1992, provide diagnosis and treatment of mental (disturbances of the elderly and active and passive care for patients from a given region. The formation of such outpatient clinics was necessitated by the low rate of accurate diagnosis in the elderly, mainly of Alzheimer's disease and depression, by primary care physicians. Outpatient clinics provide medical services to elderly patients, not only with Alzheimer's disease but also with other diagnoses. Due to better accessibility, patients mainly visit these outpatient clinics from large cities. The rate of diagnosing of Alzheimer's disease among primary care physicians amounts to approximately 4 per cent, while for depression of the elderly it is approximately 15 per cent. The reliability of Alzheimer's Disease diagnosis in psychogeriatric outpatient clinics amounts to approximately 60 per cent and in Outpatient Clinics of Memory Disturbances it reaches approximately 80 per cent. For approximately 20 per cent of patients referred to a specialist outpatient clinic with a diagnosis of dementia, depression is also diagnosed (Parnowski and Kotapka-Minc, 2000).

Heading for the integrative model

The following conclusions can be drawn from the 10 years of Polish experience in the creation of psychogeriatric services:

1. Interdisciplinary care in the elderly is necessary

2. Integrated care is necessary.

Interdisciplinary care includes participation in the treatment of the elderly patient of psychiatrists, geriatricians and neurologists. Neuropsychologists participate in diagnosing disturbed behaviour and social assistants (social workers) contribute to solve social problems. Such interdisciplinary activities result in the reduction of incidence of patient hospitalizations, better therapeutic compliance and improvement of the quality of life (Parnowski *et al.*, 1998)

Integration of care includes management of care by the interdisciplinary therapeutic team in a variety of settings such as an outpatient clinic, a hospital, home hospitalization (home visits to invalid patients by staff members – doctors and nurses), or day care centres for every patient.

Studies on the effectiveness of various models of care for the elderly show that, at present, medical and social care cannot be separated from each other (Żakowska-Wachelko, 2000). The absence of an adequately developed network of community-based services leads to significant deterioration of the quality of care and increases the burden for hospital wards and custodial institutions.

The planned further development of psychogeriatric care will take the conclusions of these studies into account.

Romania

Catalina Tudose

Historically, interest in mental health problems of older people is strongly related to the Romanian scientist C. I. Parhon, and especially that of his disciple Ana Aslan.

In 1948, Professor Aslan became the first gerontologist in Romania and in 1952 she became the head of the Institute of Geriatrics and Gerontology, the first in the world to have this profile. Since 1964, at the recommendation of WHO this institution has become a European model in the field (Bogdan, 1997).

Romania, similarly to the general European trend, is ageing: from a population of 21,698,181 (on 1st January 2002) there were 15.5 per cent elderly above 65 years

Table 12.1 The ageing process in Romania (1992–2025) (percentages of population >60)

Number of old persons	1992	2000	2010	2020	2025
Men (>60 years)	14.4	16.1	15.9	17.8	17.6
Women (>60 years)	18.3	20.2	20.4	22.7	24.6
Persons above 60 years	16.4	18.3	18.2	20.3	21.1

Annual Statistics of Romania, accessed January 2004.

in 1990, 18.3 per cent in 2000 with an expected rate of 21.1 per cent in 2025. At the beginning of this century the population of persons above 65 years is almost 3.2 million (Annual Statistics of Romania).

Puwak (1995) projected that in 2003 more than 66 per cent of the supplementary costs for health will be necessary for the care of older people who are the main users of the medical services.

There are more old people in rural areas than in urban ones and more women than men (Dumitru, 1982). At present in Romania there are approximately 1 million dependent elderly people (Tudose, 2001).

Even though the phenomenon of ageing is known and recognized, Romania has no coherent national policies and there are no strategies concerning the development of the care system for older people. This can largely be explained by the deep crises of the social system through which Romania is passing after the collapse of the communist system.

Geriatrics has been recognized as a specialty since 1993 and old age psychiatry (OAP) since 2001. There are almost 1000 psychiatrists and 27 gerontopsychiatrists in Romania.

The curriculum for education in OAP is in concordance with the consensus curriculum on Skill-Based Objectives in Old Age Psychiatry developed in 2002 at the meetings initiated by the European Association of Geriatric Psychiatry and jointly organized with the WHO. It consists of 320 hours of training, including courses and practical clinical activities carried on during one year. Consequently the certification process for

Table 12.2 The structure of the population 60 years and older in Romania

Age group	1930	1956	1966	1977	1992
60–74	77.6	73.9	81.1	79.2	75.4
75–89	14.9	23.3	18.5	20.2	23.8
90–99	6.6	12.0	3.5	5.8	7.6

Annual Statistics of Romania, accessed January 2004.

geriatric psychiatrists is in place and is accepted by the professional community (stage three in concordance with the International Survey by Reifler and Cohen, 1998). There is an increased interest on behalf of the medical professionals in psychiatric disorders in elderly. But the low economical level of Romania is impeding a more rapid development of the network of specialized services.

From this point of view Romania can be considered in stage 1–2 of the Reifler and Cohen criteria (Reifler and Cohen, 1998). There are inpatient departments included in psychiatric facilities, totalling 144 beds.

The attention of the specialists is more concentrated on cognitive disorders and dementia and less on mood, psychotic, substance abuse disorders and other conditions. In 2000 a Memory Centre was set up in Bucharest in order to achieve a correct, comprehensive and early as possible diagnosis of cognitive disorders. The Memory Centre is also conducting an epidemiological survey of Alzheimer cases in Bucharest (Tudose, 2001).

Therapeutic interventions are mainly psychopharmacological – often limited by the high costs of the modern drugs – and less often psychosocial. Therefore community-based care tends to be represented by the initiatives of non-governmental organizations set up after 1989 such as the Romanian Alzheimer Society, Geron Foundation, Association for Community Care and others that have set up the first specific facilities such as day centres, home care, respite care programmes and respite hostels (Tudose, 2001).

In recent years, the Romanian Association of Gerontopsychiatry (1999), the Romanian Scientific Society for Cognitive Studies and Alzheimer Disease (2002) and the 'Ana Aslan' International Academy of Aging have been set up, the latter editing the international journal *Brain Aging* (2002).

Romania is trying to move from isolated projects to networks of specialized services, but realistically this is unlikely to happen before 2010.

Sweden
Sture Eriksson

There have been several important trends in psychogeriatric care in Sweden during the last twenty years. One of the most important can be summarized under the concept of 'normalization'. This means that those older patients with cognitive disorders such as Alzheimer's disease and psychiatric disorders should be regarded as 'normal' citizens living in a normal apartment, seeking medical care in primary care (GP). Furthermore, from a legal point of view, they are supposed to defend their own rights in court if the social welfare system did not provide their need of social services, similar to other persons in need of social support. This is a result of transferring the care of older people from the health care system to the social welfare system. The most prominent legal expression of this trend was the ÄDEL-reformen: its main intention was to transform nursing homes and other care facilities into 'ordinary living' under the management of local authorities. An important part of this trend was 'de-medicalization', including ideas that if 'healthy aspects of the elderly' were primarily taken into account the decline in, for example, cognitive function would not be a problem.

A further expression of this trend was that if medical care was needed in the apartment provided by local authorities – called special living – this care would be provided without doctors in the organization, and the patients were often regarded as guests. Thus, legally the local authorities are not allowed to engage doctors for the medical care, the idea is that the patient will seek his or her own GP.

Formally, the legal base still exists, but during the last five years this trend is decreasing in strength. Thus, a number of press and other public reports have revealed medical care of sometimes very low quality, partly because of lack of resources and medical knowledge but to a large extent due to low interest and attention of medical care by the management ('Guests do not need medical treatment'). However, in response to reports of maltreatment, mainly in newspapers and television, and pressure from general opinion, the medical training of the staff in 'special livings' has increased. Special laws against maltreatment have been put in to force and there is increasing attention to the management of both the organization and content of the medical care.

Another important trend is that very few small group living facilities for demented persons have been initiated during the last five to seven years. The main arguments against them have been that they are too expensive and less rational, for example, when staffing the units. Several isolated group-livings have been shut down and the patients have been moved to larger units, often with the intent of having several small units in the same building, giving a small unit from the patient's viewpoint but a large unit from a staffing and education perspective.

A third important trend is that there is an increase in the number of demented patients, but no similar increase in the funding for their care. Generaly two routes have been followed to manage this situation. First, the need of care is much more prominent today compared to some years ago in order to have access to nursing home care and other forms of institutional care. Second, there are several examples of various forms of increasing home care. Examples of this are the development of dementia care teams and nurses specialized in dementia care. The introduction of pharmacological treatment in Alzheimer's disease is another important recent trend in psychogeriatrics. This has given much more focus on the early detection of memory disturbances and it is evident that the pattern of referral to specialized psychogeriatric care is more and more focused on patients with mild cognitive decline. The clinical management of mild cognitive decline has developed considerably in recent years. Furthermore, today it is not uncommon that patients seek medical attention themselves, based on general public information and awareness of cognitive disorders among relatives. Those seeking medical advice for themselves are generally younger and with much less cognitive decline compared to those who were referred to specialized psychogeriatric care ten years ago.

There is also an increasing interest in Behavioural and Psychological Symptoms in Dementia (BPSD). Clinical activities, education and some research has developed during the last ten years and many nursing homes and group livings are active both in prevention and management of BPSD. However, much is still to be done, especially in the field of BPSD since, for example, drug use is still inadequate in many dementia care settings and the levels of staff knowledge are, in many settings, still too sparse.

The trends for development of care for older people with various forms of psychiatric disorders, such as depression, psychosis and other functional disorders, generally follow trends for dementia care. However, there has been much less general awareness of these patients, resulting in for example less allocation of funding. In most parts of Sweden there are very few care facilities devoted to these patients and they are often cared for in their homes, with home service support, or in caring facilities mainly intended to care for those with dementia.

Consequently, there are no devoted care facilities for acute care of these patients. This means that if they are in absolute need of acute care, it is provide by ordinary psychiatric care facilities. This often results in a mixture of patients, which has less a favourable influence on care of the elderly.

In Sweden, there is no medical speciality primarily covering the area of psychogeriatrics. Thus, these activities are undertaken informally in the specialities of geriatrics or general psychiatry and training in psychogeriatrics is incorporated into training in these disciplines. However, the training and clinical activities in psychogeriatrics are often regarded as separate parts, sometimes organized as sections within geriatrics or psychiatry.

Dementia care in Sweden has recently been evaluated officially by the government body responsible for care and their report is published on the Internet (Socialdepartementet, 2001). In summary it states that further extensive education in dementia is mandatory and that the development of organizational cooperation is necessary. Examples are development of dementia teams, dementia nurses and cooperation with NGOs. It also highlights the need for public information about dementia.

To conclude, the development of psychogeriatrics in Sweden is affected by both general trends in the community, such as trend towards 'normalization' and budget restrictions, but also by the advent of new medical diagnostics and treatment of dementia.

References

Annual Statistics of Romania www.recensamant.ro accessed January 2004.

Bilikiewicz, A., Barcikowska, M.,Kądzielawa, D., Kotapka-Minc, S., Leszek, J., Mossakowski, M., Opala, G., Parnowski, T., Pfeffer, A., Szczudlik, A., and Żakowska-Wachelko, B. (1999) *Stanowisko grupy ekspertów w sprawie zasad diagnozowania i leczenia otępienia w Polsce (IGERO) (Statement of a Group of Experts on Standards for Diagnosing and Treating Dementia in Poland (IGERO). Rocznik Psychogeriatryczny*, **1/II**, 105–52 .

Bilikiewicz, A. and Parnowski T. (2002) *Zaburzenia psychiczne, problemy psychologiczne i społeczne związane ze starzeniem się (Psychogeriatria)*. *(Mental disturbances, psychological and social problems associated with old age)* W: Psychiatria, t.2 (red. Bilikiewicz A., Pużyński S., Rybakowski J., Wciórka J.) Urban and Partner, Wroclaw, 697–734.

Bogdan, C. (1997) Aspecte medico-sociale, Geriatrie, pp. 393–400, Editura Medicală, București.

Busby, F.R. (1998) *Maltraitances et négligences envers les personnes âgées. ALMA 1995–1997*. ALMA Editions: Paris.

Colvez, A., Joël, M. (2002) *La maladie d'Alzheimer. Quelle place pour les aidants?* Editions Masson, Paris.

Dumitru. M. (1982) *Dimensiunea socială* a *Geriatriei*, Geriatrie, pp. 36–8. Editura Medicală, București.

Haupt. M. (2002) Medizinische Aus-, Weiter- und Fortbildung. In J. F. Hallauer and A. Kurz *Weißbuch Demenz*, pp. 110–12. Thieme, Stuttgart.

Heeg, S. (2001) Pflegeheimbau mit milieutherapeutischer Orientierung – Umsetzung am Beispiel des Gradmann-Hauses in Stuttgart-Kaltental. In D. A. Gesellschaft (ed.) *Brücken in die Zukunft*, pp. 615–27. Deutsche Alzheimer Gesellschaft, Berlin.

INSEE, Paris, Recensement de la population, mars 1999, http://www.insee.fr/tr/recensement/page-accueil-rp.htm.

Jaszczuk, H., Pietrzykowska, B., Wierzbicki, S., Langiewicz, W., and Sobańska, M. (eds.) (1994) *Zakłady psychiatrycznej oraz neurologicznej opieki zdrowotnej.Rocznik statystyczny 1993 (Mental and Neurological Care – Yearbook)*. IPiN, Warszawa.

Kurz, A., Jansen, S., and Tenge, B. (2003) Gerontopsychiatrische Versorgungsstrukturen. In H. Förstl (ed.) *Lehrbuch der Gerontopsychiatrie und -psychotherpaie. Grundlagen – Klinik – Therapie*, pp. 198–214. Stuttgart: Thieme.

Lautenschlager, N. and Kurz, A. (2000) Alzheimer-Zentren (Memory-Kliniken). In H. Förstl (ed.) *Demenzen in Klinik und Praxis*, pp. 291–306. Springer, Berlin, Heidelberg, New York.

Ledésert, B. and Ritchie, K. (1994) The diagnosis of senile dementia in general practice: a study of 301 general practitioners in the Montpellier region. *International Journal of Geriatric Psychiatry*, **9**, 43–6.

Lohse, J. (2002) Stationäre Versorgung. In J.F. Hallauer and A. Kurz (eds.) *Weißbuch Demenz. Versorgungssituation relevanter Demenzerkrankungen in Deutschland*, pp. 67–71. Thieme, Stuttgart.

Ministry of Family, Seniors, Women, and Youth (2002) *Report on the Situation of the Elderly*. Bundesanzeiger Verlagsgesellschaft, Bonn.

Parnowski, T. (1995) Medyczne i psychologiczne problemy wieku podeszłego (Medical and psychological problems in old age). *Post Psych Neurol*, **2** (Suppl. 1), 1–6.

Parnowski, T. and Kotapka-Minc, S. (2000) Współwystępowanie zaburzeń procsw poznawczych i depresji-badanie pilotażowe (Association of impairment of the cognitive function with depression-a pilot study). *Rocznik Psychogeriatryczny*, **3**, 71–80.

Parnowski, T., Kotapka-Minc, S., Łączkowski, J., and Maryniak-Wiśniewska, M. (1998) Poradnie dla osób w wieku podeszłym – nowe struktury w psychiatrii polskiej. (Psychogeriatric clinics – new structures in Polish psychiatry). *Postępy Psych Neurol*, **7** (Suppl. 1)(6), 107–14.

Pietrzykowska, B., Boguszewska, L., Karolak, H., Szirkowiec, W., and Skiba, K. (2001) Zakłady psychiatrycznej oraz neurologicznej opieki zdrowotnej. Rocznik statystyczny IPiN, Warszawa, 2001.

Puwak, H. (1995) *Încetinirea ireversibilului*. Editura Expert, București.

Reifler, B.V. and Cohen, W. (1998) Practice of geriatric psychiatry and mental health services for the elderly: results of an international survey. *International Psychogeriatrics*, **10**, 351–7.

Ritchie, K., Colvez, A., Ankri, J., Ledésert, B., Gardent, H., and Fontaine, A. (1992) The evaluation of long-term care for the dementing elderly. *International Journal of Geriatric Psychiatry,* 7, 5–14.

Romero, B. (2001) Integratives Behandlungsprogramm für Demenzkranke und betreuende Angehörige. In D. A. Gesellschaft (ed.) *Brücken in die Zukunft,* pp. 67–81. Deutsche Alzheimer Gesellschaft, Berlin.

Socialdepartementet (2001) Socialtjänstlag (2001:453) http://www.notisum.se/rnp/SLS/LAG/20010453.HTM Accessed 22 April 2004.

Tessier, J-F., Clément, J-P., and Léger, J-M. (1999) *Principes d'organisation des soins en psychogériatrie. Psychiatrie du Sujet Agé.* Flammarion, Paris.

Tudose, C. (2001) *Bătrânul secolului XXI, Dementele – o provocare pentru medicul de familie.* Editura Infomedica, Bucureşti.

Wächtler, C. and Hofmann, W. (2001) Kooperation von Geriatrie und Gerontopsychiatrie – Das Zentrum für Ältere in Hamburg. In *Vortrag auf dem Symposium 'Den Wandel gestalten' der DGGG,* pp. 46–7. Kiel.

Żakowska-Wachelko, B. (2000) *Zarys medycyny geriatrycznej. (Outline of geriatric medicine).* PZWL, Warszawa.

Chapter 13

Psychogeriatric services: current trends in Nigeria and South Africa

Olusegun Baiyewu and Felix Potocnik

Nigeria

Olusegun Baiyewu

Nigeria has a predominantly young population, which has been estimated at 108.9 million, with 4.9 per cent aged 60 years and over (WHO, 2000). Psychogeriatric facilities are few, and those available are concentrated in the cities, especially in southern Nigeria. At present care of older people is primarily family care and there is limited public assistance. Older persons with dementia and other mental health disorders rarely seek help, because Nigerian caregivers see most of the symptoms as part of ageing (Hendrie et al., 1996; Sokoya and Baiyewu, 2003).

Health insurance cover is not available, so the family pays for the cost of treatment, though a bill for health insurance is in parliament. There is a paucity of funding for the health sector. Older people attend general and surgical clinics when sick, because there are no specialized clinics for them.

It is important to give a brief description of health services programmes in Nigeria. At the apex are 14 university teaching hospitals run by the Federal Ministry of Health. Next are 1,170 general hospitals located in every major city and town in the country, and at the lowest level are primary health centres located throughout the 774 local government councils (Akanji et al., 2002). State governments administer the general hospitals, while federal, state and local governments jointly run the primary health centres. In addition, there are many private medical establishments in major cities and towns that provide various grades of services for people able to pay. Referrals go from the primary health centres through general hospitals to the teaching hospitals. The private medical establishments also refer cases to the teaching hospitals. Most teaching hospitals have psychiatric units, and in addition there are eight federal psychiatric hospitals, which also receive referrals. There is a parallel alternative health service consisting of traditional healers and spiritual healers: these are often patronized by poor rural dwellers. It would appear that the mental health care of older people in Nigeria is largely the responsibility of primary health and general hospital physicians with little support from the few specialized institutions available.

The Social Policy for Nigeria (Federal Ministry of Social Development, 1989) stated that establishment of nursing homes would be discouraged and older people would be visited at home for counselling and treatment; in addition, day centres would be established. However, there has been a lag between the intentions and implementation of this policy.

Currently, there are about 10 nursing homes, run mainly by churches and other religious organizations, spread over the country but mainly in southern Nigeria. Between them, they hold less than 1,000 beds, which are often reserved for destitute older people. This is clearly inadequate for a country with over 100 million people and is not in keeping with recommendations of the World Health Organization, which advises adequate number of nursing home beds for elderly who might need them (Wertheimer, 1997). In the last few years some professionals have started their own NGOs with the specific aim of providing some care for older people, and again most of them are in towns and cities in southern Nigeria. Whilst they are mainly interested in health maintenance programmes for older people, they still look after some mental health problems. In addition an outpatient psychogeriatric service started at the University College Hospital Ibadan in 2001 and other teaching hospitals are in the process of starting similar services. Apart from these, some special programmes are available to limited populations.

The Indianapolis–Ibadan project is a joint project between the University of Ibadan and the Indiana University School of Medicine USA. The project, funded by the National Institute of Aging, provides some care for about 2,500 elders on its database and runs psycho-education programmes for caregivers of demented individuals. Ibadan is in the southwestern part of the country. In the south-eastern part, a psycho-education programme for caregivers of demented older people, which has some support from Alzheimer's Disease International, is also in place.

It is hoped that similar programmes will be established in other regions of the country and that these centres will take up training of primary health and general hospital workers in psychogeriatrics, so that they can improve on their service delivery.

South Africa

Felix Potocnik

Demographics

Of Africa's estimated 800 million people, 45 million reside in South Africa. Truly a 'rainbow nation', this figure (Census, 2001) by racial grouping represents 35.5 million black Africans, 4 million coloureds (of mixed racial origins), 1.1 million Indians or Asians and 4.3 million whites. Though there are 11 official languages, key corporate communication is in English.

Of the 45 million people 3.3 million (7.3 per cent) are 60 years and older. Within their respective population groups the elderly constitute 2.26 million black Africans

(6.5 per cent), 254,000 coloureds (6.4 per cent), 87,000 Indians or Asians (7.8 per cent) and 680,000 whites (16 per cent). On the continent, South Africa appears to have the highest proportion of older inhabitants (Kinsella and Ferreira, 1997). The diversity of ageing differs among the population groups. We thus find a pyramid-shaped population structure in black Africans resembling that of developing countries (relatively high fertility and morbidity rates), while the spade-shaped white population structure simulates that of the world's more developed countries (low fertility and morbidity rates). Health problems facing the authorities are equally diverse, and because 35 per cent of the population are in the 0–15 year age group, a high percentage of resources have been shifted to maternal and child care.

Life expectancy and health

The World Health Organization Survey of healthy life expectancy in 191 countries around the world in 1999 has been reviewed in the South African context (Walker and Wadee, 2002). Mainly due to the impact of HIV/AIDS, figures dropped sharply for sub-Saharan Africa with Gabon ranking 143rd (48 years), South Africa 160th (40 years), Zimbabwe 184th (33 years) and Sierra Leone in 191st position achieving a healthy life expectancy of only 26 years. Provided a person survives to the age of 60, the years of remaining life expectancy are quite similar, regardless of race. This translates into some 16 years for males and 20 years for females (Kinsella and Ferreira, 1997).

Prior to the rapid spread of the HIV/AIDS epidemic South Africa was in the midst of an epidemiologic transition from the prominence of infectious diseases to chronic diseases, with different health patterns emerging among population groups. Among the elderly the non-communicable diseases remain the largest contributors to mortality, morbidity and disability, accounting for 84 per cent of deaths (Bradshaw *et al.*, 2003). There are no statistics available describing the range and types of psychiatric illness prevalent in South Africa. Though some psychiatric illnesses in the elderly are culture bound, influenced by nutrition or otherwise associated with harmful lifestyle patterns, the range appears to be similar to that of the rest of the world.

Socio-economic, educational and financial status

South Africa has no official 'national poverty line' (HSRC, 2003). In practice the poorest 40 per cent of individuals are classified as poor. Half of South Africa's elderly are urbanized, with rural-dwellers roughly three times more likely to be poor than their urban counterparts.

The percentage of elderly deemed functionally literate, having successfully completed seven years of schooling ranges from black Africans (17 per cent), coloureds (41 per cent), Indians or Asian (43 per cent) to whites (87 per cent). This not only affected the individual's earning capacity in working life but also determined the quality of life and the available resources on retirement. A further problem arises in that educational status determines compliance with medication management. Because the elderly have been part of the economically active population and have stored up some wealth, the distribution of elderly (household per capita) income is not very different to the overall distribution (HSRC, 2003).

Social services and health care

More than 80 per cent of the total national budget is spent on social services, namely education (40 per cent), health (24 per cent) and welfare (19 per cent) (HSRC, 2003).

South Africa is an exception among African countries in its formal economic support for older citizens. Women aged 60 years and older and men aged 65 years and older are eligible for a means-tested general social pension of R740 (USD 105) per month. Some 20 per cent of the population still travel more than an hour to get to a health care facility, and in a recent survey (HSRC, 2003), 25 per cent of the respondents indicated the unavailability or inaccessibility of services as a barrier to obtaining health care.

Staff, beds and patient ratios

The recent South African Mental Health Act emphasizes a community-based rehabilitation model of mental health care within a comprehensive integrated health service. This process has led to deinstitutionalization with a shift in human resources in psychiatric care. Numerous teething problems have emerged – many avoidable – such as those arising from the dismantling of existing facilities prior to the establishment of effective community services (Bateman, 2002; Ncayiyana, 2003).

Staff/bed and staff/patient ratios provide a useful indicator for assessing the adequacy of mental health care (Lund and Flisher, 2002a). For the public sector mental health services the staff/bed ratio for the country as a whole was 0.3 staff per bed. This figure is considerably lower than that of developed countries. The national mean nurse/bed ratio being a quarter of that in UK psychiatric hospitals who in 1986 reported a 1:1 nurse/bed ratio (DHSS, 1988).

In assessing the existing staff/population ratios per 100,000 population in the South African public sector mental health services the ratio was 19.5. Relative to international settings, this is low (Lund and Flisher, 2002b). Compared with South Africa's 0.4 psychiatrists per 100,000 population, developed countries such as Sweden rate 12.5 and the US 16.0; while developing countries such as Brazil rate 4.4. This is, however, higher than India at 0.23 and other African countries such as Botswana 0.3, Egypt 0.3, Kenya 0.1, Nigeria 0.1 and Zimbabwe 0.1.

Challenges faced by psychogeriatricians

Elderly psychiatric patients enjoy a dedicated outpatient facility at only seven university-associated psychiatric hospitals in South Africa. There are two psychogeriatric inpatient units of which only one has an integrated service with a geriatrician in attendance. While the subspeciality of geriatrics is recognized by the Health Professions Council of South Africa, there is as yet no recognition for psychogeriatrics. Within a medical school's 'big five' recognized specialties of surgery, medicine, obstetrics and gynaecology, paediatrics and psychiatry, the latter usually fares worst in both status and allocated resources. Within the discipline of psychiatry, psychogeriatrics in turn takes the back row. Since two of the universities share an inpatient psychogeriatric facility, training in this speciality is available to three registrars at a time on a six monthly rotation period.

Public sector psychiatric hospitals operate within severe budgetary restraints. A psychiatric hospital patient bed costs R350 (US$ 50) per day. The average inpatient medication cost amounts to R210 (US$ 30) per month while that of an outpatient amounts to R110 (US$ 16) per month. While the Department of Health funds the hospitals, the Department of Social Development assists in the funding of frail care at nursing homes. At present the minimum basic cost of keeping a patient in a nursing home is R2100 (US$ 300) per month. The state subsidy for these homes, currently less than R1400 (US$ 200) per month, is however gradually being reduced, as nursing homes are largely to be replaced by community outreach programmes. This bodes ill for indigent, impaired elderly patients whose current monthly pension of R740 (US$ 105) will not allow for nursing home care when the need arises.

The public service doctor is poorly paid and carries great responsibilities, with long working hours and often inadequate supervision (Bateman, 2002; Ncayiyana, 2003). A quarter of doctors have left the public service over the last three years, some to join the private sector while many have gone overseas. As such 565 doctors left the country in 2002, 54 per cent more than for the whole of 2001 (Noticeboard, 2003). The 2002 South African Health Review revealed that the number of doctors planning to leave the country on completion of their community service year has risen from 34 per cent in 1999 to 43 per cent in 2001; while the number planning to remain in the public service had fallen from 42 per cent in 1999 to 38 per cent in 2001. Factors cited for leaving related to economics, safety and security. Psychogeriatrics is thus pushed into the background as disciplines compete for remaining resources. Recruitment for psychiatry has also become an issue in that many doctors cite the envisaged costs incurred by specialist training (through loss of net earnings) as too high.

The South African Society of Psychiatrists notes that there are currently 91 state psychiatrists, each responsible for about 440,000 patients. This is an estimated third of the number required to run the public sector service. The private health sector in turn has 234 psychiatrists at a ratio of one:33,000 patients.

The scientific infrastructure has also been affected by these changes. The Centre for Research and Technology at the University of Stellenbosch states that the South African scientific workforce is ageing, the system attracting few young replacements. While 20 per cent of those who published peer reviewed articles were older than 50 in 1990, this proportion had increased to 49 per cent in 2000. Our share of the world's scientific output (measured in ISI-linked articles) has similarly declined from 0.7 per cent in 1987 to less than 0.4 per cent currently (Centre for Research on Science and Technology, 2003). This impacts on teaching and the future competence of our doctors.

A further challenge with major impact on psychogeriatric services is HIV/AIDS. The current prevalence of HIV in South Africa is estimated at 24 per cent. Some 600 people die of AIDS each day in South Africa, and in big city hospitals at least half of the patients now have HIV-related diseases (Walker and Wadee, 2002). Because the illness afflicts mainly the young and middle tier of the population, the resulting burden in terms of family care and costs falls largely on the elderly. Approximately 40 per cent of households in South Africa are headed by an older person and it is they who will be looking after an estimated 2 million orphans by 2010.

The Department of Social Development is currently responding by scaling down nursing homes and implementing outreach programmes to community home carers. The aim is to help persons with AIDS in the community and, as the elderly will be the primary caregivers, to assist them financially in turn. Maintenance grants such as care dependency, foster care and grant-in-aid are continually being upgraded. A home facility would thus emerge which not only acts as hospice and foster home, but also accommodates the elderly.

References

Akanji, B.O., Ogunniyi, A., and Baiyewu, O. (2002) Healthcare for older persons, a country profile: Nigeria. *Journal of the American Geriatrics Society*, **50**, 1289–92.

Bateman, C. (2002) Tertiary doctors draw the battle lines. *South African Medical Journal*, **92** (11) 844–6.

Bradshaw, D., Groenewald, P., Laubscher, R., Nannan, N., Nojilana, B., Norman, R., Pieterse, D., and Schneider, M. (2003) *Initial Burden of Disease Estimates for South Africa, 2000*. Medical Research Council Technical Report, Cape Town.

Census 2001 (2003) *Census in Brief*. Pali Lehohla Statistician-General, Statistics South Africa, Pretoria.

Centre for Research on Science and Technology (2003) Stellenbosch University Centre's repositioning marks new era for the study of science. *University of Stellenbosch Kampusnuus*, http://www.sun.ac.za/news/NewsItem.asp?ItemID=4745&Zone=A05 accessed November 23 2004.

Department of Health and Social Security (DHSS) (1988) *Comparing Health Authorities: Health Service Indicators 1983–1986*. DHSS, London.

Federal Ministry of Social Development (1989) *Social Policy for Nigeria*. DSC Unit Eleme, Enugu, Nigeria.

Hendrie, H.C., Baiyewu, O., Eldermire, D., and Prince, C. (1996) Behavioral disorders in dementia, cross-cultural perspectives: Caribbean Native American and Yoruba. *International Psychogeriatrics*, **8** (Suppl. 3), 483–6.

HSRC 2003 (2003) *Ageing in South Africa. Report on the Minimum Data Set on Ageing, March 2002*. Human Sciences Research Council, Pretoria.

Kinsella, K. and Ferreira, M. (1997) International brief. Ageing trends: South Africa. *US Bureau of the Census*. August, 1–6.

Lund, C. and Flisher, A.J. (2002a) Staff/bed and staff/patient ratios in South African public sector mental health services. *South African Medical Journal*, **92** (2), 157–60.

Lund, C. and Flisher, A.J. (2002b) Staff/population ratios in South African public sector mental health services. *South African Medical Journal*, **92** (2), 161–4.

Ncayiyana, D.J. (2003) Longing for Egypt – the Transkei dilemma. *South African Medical Journal,* **93** (2), 1.

Noticeboard (2003) Doctors on the Move. Medical Protection Society. *Africa Casebook 3,* August, 4.

Sokoya, O.O. and Baiyewu, O. (2003) Geriatric Depression in Primary Care Attendees. *International Journal of Geriatric Psychiatry,* **18**, 505–10.

Walker, A.R.P. and Wadee, A.A. (2002) World Health Organisation: healthy life expectancy in 191 countries, 1999. What of the future? *South African Medical Journal,* **92** (2), 135–7.

Wertheimer, J. (1997) Psychiatry of the elderly: a consensus statement. *International Journal of Geriatric Psychiatry,* **12**, 432–5.

World Health Organization (2000) *World Health Report 2000. Health systems: improving performance.* Geneva, WHO.

Section 3

Chapter 14

Core service components – acute care

Ajit Shah and Shirish Bhatkal

Introduction

Old age psychiatry is recognized as an important sub-speciality of psychiatry and in some countries, like the United Kingdom (UK), it enjoys specialty status. The core components of an acute old age psychiatry service are described here.

Planning the core components of acute care

Definition of the service

An old age psychiatry service ought to cater for a well-defined geographical catchment area (Jolley and Arie, 1978; Draper, 1990; Clement and Leger, 2000; Bragason, 2003). The UK Royal College of Psychiatrists has recommended an ideal catchment area size of 10,000 older people to be serviced by a community team including one old age psychiatrist. The Norwegian Psychiatric Association recommends a catchment area size of 15,000–30,000 older people (Bragason, 2003). The traditional cut-off age for service users is 65 years (Arie, 1970; Lennon and Jolley, 1991): however, this should be flexible. For example, patients with presenile dementias are best managed by old age psychiatry services (Lennon and Jolley, 1991; Baldwin and Murray, 2000) as they have greater expertise in dementia. The recent *National Service Framework (NSF) for Older People* (Department of Health, 2001) in the UK recommends development of services for presenile dementia within the rubric of old age psychiatry services. All types of mental illness can be catered for by an old age psychiatry service. However, in practice this may be unrealistic due to resource constraints and under those circumstances there may be a need for clear local protocols for transfer of graduate patients (defined as patients who developed mental illness early in life that has become complicated by ageing) from services catering for those under 65 years (Shah and Ames, 1994). It has previously been suggested that poorly resourced services should solely focus on dementia or functional illness (Shah and Ames, 1994); however, a dementia-only or a functional illness-only service may lead to poor staff morale and job satisfaction and ideally should to be avoided.

Sources of new referrals

Patients can be referred by medical (closed model) and non-medical personnel (open model) (Banerjee, 1998; Challis *et al.*, 2002a). Medical personnel include general practitioners (GPs) (otherwise known as primary care physicians) and virtually all specialists from any other medical discipline including geriatricians, general psychiatrists and neurologists. Non-medical personnel include professionals from other disciplines (social workers, district nurses, domiciliary care staff, residential home staff, nursing home staff) and lay people (relatives, friends, neighbours and patients themselves).

There is controversy over the use of open and closed referral systems (Tym, 1991; Dening, 1992; Coles et al., 1991; Challis et al., 2002a). The advantages of receiving referrals from GPs include (Shah and Ames, 1994):

1. Avoidance of duplication and substitution of the GP's role;

2. Allowing GPs to treat patients they feel confident to treat and are able to do so;

3. Allowing GPs to continue longer term management in the community;

4. GPs filtering medically ill patients by referring to geriatricians or other physicians; and

5. Allowing GPs to be the central focus of the patients care, which would help with avoiding polypharmacy and potential drug interactions.

This approach may be appropriate and satisfactory in countries with a well-developed primary care system and where the majority of older people are registered with one GP. There are potential pitfalls with this approach in countries where not every one has a GP, where older people may have more than one GP (for example in Australia), where general practice services are on a fee for service basis, and where payment methods dictate short consultations that discourage mental state examinations (Flynn et al., 2000).

Whilst an open referral system may be expected to attract inappropriate referrals (Banerjee, 1998; Challis et al., 2002a), formal evaluation of such service models has not found this to be the case (Macdonald et al., 1994; Gupta et al., 1996). Indeed, open models may attract patients who otherwise may not be referred and thus denied access to services (Macdonald et al., 1994).

Factors influencing the type of referral system adopted include the availability and accessibility of GPs, staffing complement of the old age psychiatry service, the personalities and known skills of people employed in the service, availability of other agencies involved with older people, and the needs and views of consumers (Shah and Ames, 1994). If an open referral system is adopted then the GP needs to be kept fully informed (Coles et al., 1991; Dening, 1992).

Mode of referral

The different methods of referral include the traditional letter sent through the postal system, a letter sent over the fax, telephoned referral, and a letter through electronic mail. The new UK NSF (Department of Health, 2001) requires development of a referral protocol from primary care and a single assessment process, both of which will facilitate standardization of the method of referral and the type of information required from the referrer.

Referrals should ideally be seen within few days of referral (Jolley and Arie, 1978; Arie and Jolley, 1982; Lennon and Jolley, 1991; Seidel *et al.*, 1992; Doyle and Varian, 1994) to avoid waiting lists and routine referrals turning into emergencies (Lennon and Jolley, 1991). This can be facilitated by using a triage process whereby the urgency of the requested assessment of each referral is determined on the basis of identified risk. An ideal service would be accessible round the clock. However, due to financial constraints, most services operate during the working week and hospital-based services cover emergencies at other times. Any developing service should give consideration to provision of some community staff at the weekend and in the early evening for emergencies.

Where should new referrals be assessed?

Many authorities believe that the initial assessment should occur in the patient's home (Jolley and Arie, 1978; Arie and Jolley, 1982; Wasylenki *et al.*, 1984; Roca *et al.*, 1990; Challis *et al.*, 2002a) except for patients already in non-psychiatric hospital beds (i.e. liaison referrals). One advantage is that the consultation rate at home approaches 100 per cent (Benbow, 1990; Shah, 1994; Anderson and Aquilina, 2002). Also, the home environment can be observed first hand (Benbow, 1990; Banerjee, 1998; Anderson and Aquilina, 2002) and this may help avoid unnecessary occupational therapy and social work assessments that may otherwise be ordered from the outpatient clinic (Shah, 1994). There is ready access to family members, other informants (e.g. neighbours) and possibly log books kept at the patient's home by home care, home help and district nursing services for a collateral history (Benbow, 1990; Shah, 1994; Banerjee, 1998). In addition, there is easy access to medication and it is therefore possible to make a better assessment of polypharmacy, poor compliance, drug interactions, dependence on benzo-diazepines and hoarding for overdose (Shah and Ames, 1994; Banerjee, 1998). However, one small Canadian study failed to demonstrate differences between home-based and clinic-based assessments in terms of gathering clinically useful information (Cole *et al.*, 1995). Home assessment avoids the stigma of attending a psychiatric clinic, the indignity of lengthy ambulance rides, irregularities in the timing and availability of ambulance and related modes of transport, and the personal costs of any trip to the clinic incurred by the patient or their families (Benbow, 1990; Shah and Ames, 1994). Finally, many older patients with hearing and visual deficits, cognitive impairment, reduced mobility and physical illness or disability may not be able to travel to the clinic (Banerjee, 1998). Conversely, some patients may object to professionals intruding on their privacy.

Although successful models of home visiting in rural areas in the US have been developed (Abraham *et al.*, 1993; Neese and Abraham, 1997), they can be difficult to implement in a huge rural areas because time spent travelling can add vastly to the cost (Anderson and Aquilina, 2002). Moreover, home visiting has been difficult to achieve in the US due to the reimbursement and pay structure of psychiatrists (Reifler, 1997).

Visiting patients at home in the UK is no more expensive than seeing them in hospital-based clinics, and this is largely due to the compact nature of the catchment area and a significant non-attendance rate in the hospital-based outpatient clinic when compared to home visits (Shah, 1994, 1997a; Aquilina and Anderson, 2002).

Nature of the initial assessment

A 'core' multidisciplinary team comprising of psychiatrists, clinical psychologists, community psychiatric nurses, occupational therapists and social workers can receive the referral (Abraham et al., 1993; Reifler, 1997; Ginsburg et al., 1998); other disciplines like physiotherapists, speech therapists, dietetics and neuropsychology usually support this core team and in some countries (for example the UK and Australia) the first three of these disciplines are often available from the geriatric medicine team. This core team should review referrals and decide on the two most appropriate disciplines to assess the patient. Two members are ideally needed to assess the patient for safety reasons (staff safety and possibility of inaccurate allegations) and to enable comprehensive assessment from the perspective of two disciplines (Shulman et al., 1986; Shah and Ames, 1994). Where possible, one member should be a psychiatrist so a mental state and physical examination can be performed (Seidel et al., 1992; Shah and Ames, 1994). However, there is evidence that an accurate diagnosis can be reached after assessment by appropriately trained members of the multidisciplinary team, particularly nurses, by using standardized assessments and subsequent team discussion (Collighan et al., 1993; Dennis et al., 1998; Seymour et al., 1994; Ball et al., 1996). Such assessments by any member of the team can also result in a speedier response (Challis et al., 2002a) and better staff morale (Challis et al., 2002b). However, this approach requires highly motivated staff, well-designed protocols, appropriate training, and professional and clinical supervision (Collighan et al., 1993). This option is also helpful where there are medical staff shortages (Dening, 1992; Ginsburg et al., 1998).

In less well-resourced and emerging services the luxury of two staff members assessing the patient will not be available. There is evidence that with good supervision and training management decisions made by the non-medical members of the team are similar to those made by the medical members (Lindesay et al., 1996; Ball et al., 1996).

The initial assessment should be discussed with the multidisciplinary team in a meeting similar to the traditional ward round (Cole et al., 1991; Dening, 1992; Abraham et al., 1993). The purpose of such a meeting is to facilitate liaison between team members, to allow discussion of the clinical management of patients, cross-refer cases between team members, to provide mutual support, and to discuss new plans, ideas and problems (Tym, 1991; Shah and Ames, 1994). The new UK NSF (Department of Health, 2001) directs development of such teams and they are well-established in parts of the UK, Australia, New Zealand and Canada. Such multidisciplinary teams have been difficult to organize in some parts of the US because of reimbursement and pay structure of doctors that do not recognize the need for reimbursement of time spent in team meetings (Reifler, 1997).

The broad principles of case-management should be the framework for subsequent management (Dening, 1992; Abraham *et al.*, 1993; Casten and Rovner, 2000; Von Abendorff *et al.*, 1994). The case manager will provide professional assistance from his/her discipline and also coordinate other aspects of the patient's management strategies (Casten and Rovner, 2000). This model has been successfully used in the UK, Australia and the US (Flynn *et al.*, 2000; Casten and Rovner, 2000). When individual disciplines are particularly short-staffed, it is perhaps wise to free them up from case-management so that they can focus on their area of expertise. Intensive case-management of dementia sufferers has been shown to allow patients to remain at home for longer, improve social contacts, reduce carer stress and improve activities of daily living (Williams *et al.*, 1997; Challis *et al.*, 2002b).

The patient, referrer, GP, carers, and any other interested parties need to be kept fully informed of progress at all stages. In the UK this has been formalized with the Care Programme Approach, whereby a formal written care plan is required to be issued to all interested parties in order to ensure that everyone is aware of the care plan and the action to be taken in a crises.

Safety of staff working in the community is paramount and adequate policy and protocols to ensure safety are essential. Staff should have access to both mobile tele-phones and long-range pagers (Shah and Ames, 1994). The team base ought to be aware of the whereabouts of staff members and the times they are visiting a given patient. Adequate transportation or reimbursement of travelling expenses is required for staff (Jolley and Arie, 1992). Calculation of staffing levels should account for 'dead time' lost in travelling (Shah and Ames, 1994); this will depend on the geographical size of the catchment area, local traffic conditions and the rural or urban nature of the catchment area.

The need for subsequent follow-up after initial assessment

Some patients may not require further follow-up after the initial assessment, as advice to the referrer may suffice. Further follow-up should be for specific well-defined rea-sons and if these cease the patient can be discharged. Good reasons to continue follow-up are further assessment, treatment, rehabilitation, monitoring of drug and other treatment side-effects, monitoring of mental state, support for patients and carers and advocacy (Shah and Ames, 1994).

Outpatient clinics

Outpatient follow-up includes home visiting clinics, hospital- or primary care-based outpatient clinics and specialist memory clinics (Shulman *et al.*, 1986; Benbow, 1990; Lennon and Jolley, 1991; Shah, 1994, 1997a). Any team member can offer these clinics. The feasibility of such clinics will depend upon the geographical size of the catchment area, the travelling time involved, local clusters of patients and the availability of adequate establishment of staff (Shah and Ames, 1994).

Home visiting can be complemented by outpatient clinics and specialist memory clinics with more detailed assessment including neuropsychometry, blood and radio-logical investigations (see Chapter 17). They are best provided in a general hospital set-ting with access to all their facilities (Tym, 1991; Jolley and Arie, 1992). Outpatient clinics based in primary care (general practice health centres) are also fashionable because they are in a location familiar to patients and relatives, closer to the patients' home, are no more costly than hospital-based clinics and there is ready access to general practice case notes and GPs (Shah, 1995).

Due to paucity of efficacy, effectiveness and comparative studies of different types of outpatient clinics there are no recommended norms for the number of outpatient clinic sessions and staffing levels for a given catchment area size. Planning is generally based on experience, availability of multidisciplinary staff, flexibility and revisions with further experience (Shah and Ames, 1994).

Day hospitals

Day hospitals can be a useful component of an old age psychiatry service (Howard, 1995; Brown et al., 2000). However, day hospitals need to be clearly distinguished from day centres run by the voluntary sector, social services or welfare services, where patients receive social activities and carers receive respite. Day hospitals allow the patient to receive treatment and at the same time remain at home (Weyerer and Schaufele, 2000; Casten and Rovner, 2000), are clinically effective (Plotkin and Wells, 1993; Rolleston and Ball, 1994) and may reduce usage of inpatient beds (Corcoran and Wrigley, 1994). The primary functions of the day hospital include: assessment, treat-ment, rehabilitation, short and medium-term support, development of social networks and initial support for carers (Brown et al., 2000; Clement and Leger, 2000; Casten and Rovner, 2000). It is useful to define the function of the day hospital and the broad indi-cations for admission in an operational protocol that reflects availability of resources.

An ideal day hospital could cater for all types of mental illness in older people. There is a debate about mixing or segregating 'organically' and 'functionally' ill patients in a day hospital (Tym, 1991) because the clinical features, disabilities, needs and manage-ment strategies may be different for the two groups. The day hospital could ideally be located with the rest of the old age psychiatry service in a general hospital setting for similar reasons to those for outpatient clinics. Models of travelling day hospitals have been described, particularly in rural areas (Hettiaratchy, 1985; Tym, 1991). Innovative models of intensive nursing at home, almost like a travelling day hospital in the patient's home, have been developed (Williams et al., 1997).

Ninety day-places per 30,000 elderly people have been recommended by the Royal College of Physicians and the Royal College of Psychiatrists (1989) in the UK. Sadly, only 63 per cent of day places are actually utilized in the UK (Department of Health, 1991).

Reasons for any non-attendance should be critically examined in any developing service to reduce wastage (Shah and Ames, 1994). Most day hospitals open on week-days during normal working hours, but models of day hospitals opening during the weekend have been developed with evidence of effectiveness (Tym, 1991; Rosenvinge et al., 1994).

Transportation to the day hospital and follow-up clinics

The exact mode of transportation will be determined by local conditions. Types of transport include taxi service, traditional ambulance service, minibus operated by service staff and 'dial a ride' (available through local government in the UK). In Melbourne (Australia), there was no difference in the cost of using the taxi service and the minibus operated by staff (Shah, 1996).

The advantages of the taxi service include convenience, flexibility and fewer stigmas to the patient (Shah and Ames, 1994). The disadvantages include lack of appropriate training of taxi drivers, difficulties with arranging nurse escorts and the problems of carrying non-ambulant patients. Theoretically, the service can institute a rolling programme of basic training for their taxi drivers if they have a bulk contract with one company, although there is no evidence that any service has tried this. Also, taxi service could be used to transport two or three patients living in close proximity with a nurse escort; this method may be more cost-effective.

The advantages of the ambulance service include medical training of staff, plus collection of multiple and non-ambulant patients and nurse escorts are possible allowing assessment of the home (Shah and Ames, 1994). The disadvantages include inconvenience of longer trips to pick up other patients and inflexibility of the timing of travel.

Social services

Management of patients at home requires availability of social support (Reddy and Pitt, 1993). Many aspects of such support are provided informally by relatives, friends and neighbours (Victor, 1991). Formal supports include availability of social workers, domiciliary services for shopping, housework and personal care, meals on wheels, day centres and befriending schemes (Victor, 1991). Ideally, these services need to work closely with the core old age psychiatry service (Wasylenki et al., 1984). Some of these services are also beginning to emerge in developing countries (Iorgulescu and Sullivan, 1995).

Inpatient

There are three types of admissions: assessment and treatment; respite; and continuing care (long-term admission). This chapter is only concerned with the first two. Indications for an admission for assessment and treatment cannot be specified in unequivocal terms. However, some broad rules can be applied. These include severity of illness, severity of the sequelae of the illness (e.g. risk of suicide or self neglect), severe distress, poor availability of satisfactory social and community support at home, need for further assessment, monitoring of side-effects and administration of certain treatment like electroconvulsive therapy (Shah and Ames, 1994; Casten and Rovner, 2000). Inpatients units should have multidisciplinary staffing similar to that described for community teams.

There is a debate about nursing 'organically' and 'functionally' ill patients together (Tym, 1991) because the clinical features, disabilities, needs and management strategies may be different for the two groups. Staff and patient satisfaction was better in units where these two groups were nursed on separate wards (Craig *et al.*, 2000). If both groups of patients are nursed on the same ward then consideration should be given to avoid mixing them in the same room (Craig *et al.*, 2000). Legislation requires British hospitals to either have single sex wards or clearly designated areas for both sexes on the ward. The size of acute wards should be small (12 to 20 beds) in order to provide a friendly home-like environment (Shah and Ames, 1994). An Israeli study surprisingly showed no difference in terms of demographic characteristics, psychiatric history and diagnosis and clinical outcome for admission between a specialist psychogeriatric unit and a general psychiatric unit (Heinik *et al.*, 1995).

The Royal College of Physicians and the Royal College of Psychiatrists (1989) recommend 45 acute admission beds per 30,000 older people in the UK. In Sydney (Australia), Snowdon (1993) has estimated similar number of required beds in one catchment area. These figures are only a guide as other factors including community resources, social service resources, day hospital places, epidemiological factors and the availability of geriatric medicine resources influence the number of required beds (Jolley and Arie, 1992).

Respite admissions are designed to give carers a break. There is paucity of methodologically sound research in this field (Brodaty and Gresham, 1992), but there is a demand for this facility. These can be on acute admission wards, continuing care wards, rehabilitation wards or as a separate 'stand alone' respite ward. The exact location will depend upon the demand, availability of community resources, and the nature of respite patients and patients on the acute, rehabilitation and continuing care wards. Only patients requiring expert psychiatry nursing and medical input (e.g. because of severe behaviour disturbance) should be admitted into inpatient respite units. Those patients needing respite, but not requiring expert psychiatric nursing or medical input, can be admitted to ordinary residential or nursing homes. It is advisable to develop locally agreed indications and operational protocols for respite admissions. There are no published norms for the required number of respite beds in a catchment area.

The role of the GP

Primary Care Physicians or GPs are pivotal in the satisfactory functioning of an old age psychiatry service. They should, if possible, be involved in the initial assessment at home. Most UK GPs consider home visits very important (Orrell *et al.*, 1998) and can formally request home visits for patients who are unable to attend hospital; there are financial incentives for the hospital specialist to visit the patient at home. Sadly, 94 per cent of such visits are made without the GP (Donaldson and Hill, 1991). In other countries including Australia and the US, due to the method of funding GPs and psychiatrists such joint visits usually do not occur (Shah and Ames, 1994; Reifler, 1997). Any developing service should seriously consider a model of assessment involving the GP. Furthermore, old age psychiatry services should take a proactive role in the training of trainee GPs and the continuing professional development of GPs (Brodaty *et al.*, 1997; Bragason, 2003). Similarly, staff of the old age psychiatry team can also learn from GPs (Orrell *et al.*, 1998).

British legislation requires GPs to offer all patients over 75 years an annual physical and mental examination (Secretaries of State Health, Wales, Northern Ireland and Scotland, 1989). This will be further supplemented by the new NSF (Department of Health, 2001) requiring individual services to develop formal referral and shared care protocols with local GPs. This has also been advocated in Australia (Brodaty *et al.*, 1994, 1997, 1998; Shah and Harris, 1997). The low cost and wide availability of GP services in developed countries suggests much could be gained by improving GPs competence in old age psychiatry assessments. This could be further facilitated by ready access to old age psychiatry services, provision of liaison service in primary care involving psychiatrists (Tyrer, 1985) and CPNs (Waterreus, 1992; Blanchard *et al.*, 1995). In India health visitors, who are an important part of the primary care system, have been trained to detect dementia in rural areas (Shaji *et al.*, 2002).

Liaison and consultation service

Liaison old age psychiatry service could be available to the following organizations:

1. Departments of geriatric medicine and the rest of general hospital (Shulman *et al.*, 1986; Anderson and Philpott, 1991; Jolley and Arie, 1992);

2. Residential facilities for the elderly (Tym, 1991; Baillon *et al.*, 1996);

3. Social services and voluntary sector day facilities (Dening, 1992);

4. Home care providers (Banerjee, 1993; Banerjee and Macdonald, 1996); and

5. Voluntary sector organisations and other local government services (Roca *et al.*, 1990; Dening, 1992).

Medically ill older inpatients in geriatric medicine units and general hospital have a high prevalence of psychiatric morbidity (Ramsey *et al.*, 1991). Psychiatric morbidity can compromise medical treatment, increase admission duration and lead to a poor prognosis (Ramsey *et al.*, 1991). Moreover, psychiatric morbidity is poorly recognized and poorly treated in medical settings (Koenig *et al.*, 1988).

Provision of a liaison service to other institutions can be valuable because there is a high prevalence of mental illness in sheltered homes (Harrison *et al.*, 1990;

Banerjee and Macdonald, 1996), hostels (Snowdon and MacIntosh, 1989), old people's homes (Ames *et al.*, 1988), special accommodation homes in Victoria (Australia) (Flicker *et al.*, 1992), nursing homes (Snowdon and Donnelly, 1986) and those receiving home care services (Banerjee and Macdonald, 1996; Nagatomo and Takigawa, 1998). Moreover, psychiatric morbidity is poorly recognized and treated in these settings (De Leo *et al.*, 1989; Ames, 1990). Furthermore, the prevalence of behavioural and psychological signs and symptoms of dementia in nursing homes is high (Shah *et al.*, 2000). Training of staff can improve the management of psychiatric morbidity in these settings (Proctor *et al.*, 1999).

A liaison old age psychiatry service may be a consultation service, a liaison service or both, and a range of multidisciplinary staff can provide this. The exact nature of the service and its staffing composition will depend on the receiving organization and the nature of advice sought. Consultation service provided by consultation/liaison and old age psychiatrists (Strain *et al.*, 1991; Cole *et al.*, 1991; Teitelbaum *et al.*, 1996; Banerjee *et al.*, 1996; Shah *et al.*, 2001), liaison nurses (Collinson and Benbow, 1998), and CPNs backed by a multidisciplinary psychogeriatric team (Blanchard *et al.*, 1995, 1999) have been formally evaluated. In Dutch nursing homes, a resident psychologist is available to fulfil this liaison role (Bleeker and Diesfeldt, 2000). Primary Care Physicians and residential home staff appreciate liaison service provided to them (Baillon *et al.*, 1996).

All recipients of the liaison service should receive information on the range of facilities provided by the local old age psychiatry service, the mechanics of making a referral, and, the types of clinical issues that require referral (Shah and Ames, 1994). The liaison service should aim to share knowledge about old age psychiatry with others to improve their ability to detect and manage mental illness. This can be done on a case-by-case basis (consultation model), by direct educational and training contribution (liaison model), and by both these means.

Carer issues

Old age psychiatry services can play an important role in carer education and this is cost-effective (Brodaty and Peters, 1991). Often the role of carer education falls on voluntary sector agencies such as the Alzheimer's Disease Society. Local partnerships between the core old age psychiatry service, social services and voluntary sector agencies can be utilized to develop a programme of carer education.

Views of carers on the quality of service provision are important. Monitoring of services by carer is feasible, allows identification of practical problems for service delivery, and allows alteration in service configuration (Meltzer *et al.*, 1996; Dening and Lawton, 1998).

Links with private sector psychiatry

As patients may move between sectors, it is useful for old age psychiatry services to develop close links with private sector psychiatry. This is important in countries where insurance schemes for mental illness are available, where central taxation (such as the Medicare levy in Australia) funds private psychiatric consultations (Flynn *et al.*, 2000), and where there is predominance of private sector psychiatry. It is less important in countries like the UK where private insurance is not available for mental illnesses (Shah, 1997b). Availability of private sector services should not be a reason for under-resourcing of public sector services (Shah and Ames, 1994).

The location of old age psychiatry services

The aim should be to provide a comprehensive service to patients close to their homes and with the philosophy of maintaining them at home as long as possible (Shah and Ames, 1994). Ideally, all components of the service should be based in a general hospital, close to geriatric medicine units, within the catchment area (Shah and Ames, 1994). This will ensure easier access to all the general hospital facilities (including facilities for medical investigations), improve communication with other specialties, reduce the stigma attached to psychiatry, reduce hardship upon relatives and allow development of a liaison service to the general hospital and GPs (Shah and Ames, 1994).

The geographical size of the catchment area, population density, the anticipated geographical distribution of psychiatric morbidity and the provision of existing services will influence the location of any newly emerging service. For inpatient units located on a different site from the general hospital, provision needs to be made for ready access to all the general hospital facilities. In countries like the UK where catchment areas are compact, the above developments are feasible. In countries with large sparsely populated rural areas such an idealistic model may not be possible. In large catchment areas there may be a case for smaller satellite units to be distributed close to population clusters (Tyrer, 1985).

Staffing levels

Multidisciplinary staffing is needed to deal with the complex medical, psychological and social factors contributing to mental illness in old age (Jolley and Arie, 1978; Shah and Ames, 1994). Staffing ought to include a consultant old age psychiatrist, psychiatric trainee and/or junior medical staff, psychiatric nurses (community, inpatient wards and day hospitals), occupational therapists, social workers, physiotherapists, speech and language therapists, chiropodists and dieticians (Jolley and Arie, 1992).

The exact CPN caseload will depend on the case-mix of patients and the specialist activity they undertake (Junaid and Bruce, 1994). An ideal caseload for CPNs is reported as 20 (Intagliata, 1982; Harris and Bergmann, 1988), but many CPNs carry a caseload of up to 35. Large caseloads can dilute their work (Waterreus, 1992). There are no clearly established norms for other disciplines. In the US, a day hospital staffing ratio of one staff member to seven patients has been suggested (Casten and Rovner, 2000).

Staffing levels for each discipline should to be based on experience, intuition and anticipated satisfactory running of the service, the exact model of service delivery, the exact nature of the work and the amount of time lost travelling (Shah and Ames, 1994). Staffing levels based on empirical grounds ought to be subject to regular audit with a view to informing modification in staffing levels as the service evolves. Regular rotation of staff through different components of the service will help improve and maintain morale, generate new ideas, and provide continuity of care across different arms of the service (Dening, 1992). Adequate structures should be in place to provide support for staff, continuing professional development, to monitor work patterns to reduce poor morale and avoid burn out (Benbow et al., 1993).

Design and equipment

Each facility should be carefully designed with the help of experienced staff (Benjamin and Spector, 1990a, b; Marshall, 1992) irrespective of it being new and purpose-built or adapted from a pre-exiting facility (Shah and Ames, 1994). Adequate space for patients and staff must be ensured and the facilities need to be secure (Casten and Rovner, 2000). For example, a secure and appropriately designed spacious facility can allow a dementia patient with wandering or pacing behaviour to be managed safely. Medical, nursing and occupational therapy equipment are required. Administrative equipment including photocopiers, fax machines, land and mobile telephones, answerphones, long-range pagers, dictaphones and computers (Jolley and Arie, 1992) should be available. Access to e-mail and the Internet has become essential (Orrell and Katona, 1998). E-mail can be used for rapid communication, including receiving referrals and forwarding reports of the assessment to the referrer and other interested parties. Access to the Internet can assist with staff education and it also allows development of web sites to share information about available services, psychiatric disorders, treatment and management issues, and relevant legal issues with any interested party. Many services use electronic methods of data collection and record keeping and this clearly needs to be encouraged and developed in new services. This will enhance clinical care and allow systematic data collection for audit to facilitate service improvements (Shah and Ames, 1994).

Administrative staff

A key component of any old age psychiatry team is the administrative assistant (Lennon and Jolley, 1991). In addition to the usual secretarial duties, they have to be able to receive referrals, facilitate access to team members and improve communication in the team. There should be satisfactory provision of secretarial time, office space and secretarial equipment (Shah and Ames, 1994). As administrative staff are often the first person the patient sees on entering a service, they need to be given basic training in dealing with distressed patients and carers.

Quality assurance and audit

The activities of the overall service and individual disciplines should be subject to internal and external audit and quality assurance monitoring (Jones, 1992a,b;

Harrison and Sheldon, 1994). Internal audit can involve peer review and the whole cycle of audit following recommendations should be completed. External audit can be organized using colleagues from another unit or by various governmental agencies. Findings of any internal or external audit should be communicated to all staff including managers and budget holders, and be closely linked to a formal mechanism for change. Provision for audit activities ought to be made as part of an ongoing professional development plan for all staff with funds identified to implement any change that result.

Education

Old Age psychiatry services should take a lead in education (Wasylenski *et al.*, 1984; Bragason, 2003; Kalasic and Javanovi, 2003). Ideally, all such services ought to be closely affiliated with an academic university department (Wattis, 1989). Training and continuing professional development need to be available to staff from all disciplines within the service and to staff working in disciplines that the service has close contact with. The latter ought to include multidisciplinary staff working in geriatric medicine, general practice, general psychiatry, residential and nursing homes and voluntary sector agencies (Saarela and Kiviharju, 1995; Weyerer and Schaufele, 2000). Ideally, all the old age psychiatry disciplines should be involved in providing education and training. Various different educational models can be used and include teaching on a case by case basis in clinical situations, by attending clinical meetings like ward rounds, and by formal lectures, seminars and workshops. Old age psychiatry teams ought to have opportunities to visit other services to learn about new innovations and also to share common problems. All the educational activity should occur on an ongoing rolling basis and staffing levels should be sufficient for time spent on education.

National educational strategies developed by governmental agencies or other national organizations are invaluable for individual services (Resnikoff, 2003; Miyoshi, 2003; Kivela, 2003). Old age psychiatry services also have a role in public education campaigns. These can be specific local campaigns on specific issues or part of national campaigns. A video on dementia in ethnic minority languages has been jointly produced by the Alzheimer's Disease Society and the authors' local service. Public education campaigns like the 'Defeat Depression' and 'Changing Minds' pursued by the Royal College of Psychiatrists in the UK can be locally implemented by the service. A similar public education role in suicide prevention campaigns has been reported in Singapore and Hong Kong.

Research

All old age psychiatry services have research potential that can be facilitated by close affiliation with academic university departments. Research activity can stimulate staff, provide diversity of work, and help reduce poor morale and burnout. However, time for research activity is a luxury that a developing service or a poorly resourced service cannot always afford. Nevertheless, research is needed for the further advancement of old age psychiatry and old age psychiatry services are instrumental in this endeavour.

Overview

Development of an efficient acute old age psychiatry core service should be underpinned by national and international guidelines, and appropriate legislation. For example, the NSF (Department of Health, 2001) in the UK is the current driving force for improving service delivery. A national strategy for dementia in Mexico will similarly encourage service delivery (Resnikoff, 2003). Consensus statements on the organization of old age psychiatry service delivery from international organizations like the World Health Organization (WHO) and the Geriatric Psychiatry Section of the World Psychiatric Association (GPWPA) also provide guidance for new services (Wertheimer, 1997; WHO and GPWPA, 1998).

The core components of an acute old age psychiatry service described in this chapter are a guide, and it is recognized that local factors will dictate the exact nature of the service.

References

Abraham, I.L., Buckwalter, K.C., Snustad, D.G., Smullen, D.E., Thompson-Heistermam, A.A., Neese, J.B., and Smith, M. (1993) Psychogeriatric outreach to rural families: the Iowa and Virginia models. *International Psychogeriatrics*, **5**, 203–11.

Ames, D. (1990) Depression among elderly residents of local authority residential homes: its nature and efficacy of intervention. *British Journal of Psychiatry*, **156**, 667–75.

Ames, D., Ashby, D., Mann, A., *et al.* (1988) Psychiatric illness in elderly residents of Part III homes in one London borough: prognosis and review. *Age and Ageing*, **17**, 249–56.

Anderson, D. and Aquilina, C. (2002) Domiciliary clinics 1: effects of non-attendance. *International Journal of Geriatric Psychiatry*, **17**, 941–4.

Anderson, D.N. and Philpott, R.M. (1991) The changing pattern of referrals for psychogeriatric consultations in the general hospital: an eight year study. *International Journal of Geriatric Psychiatry*, **6**, 801–7.

Aquilina, C. and Anderson, D. (2002) Domiciliary clinics II: a cost minimisation analysis. *International Journal of Geriatric Psychiatry*, **17**, 945–9.

Arie, T. (1970) The first year of Goodmayes psychogeriatric service for older people. *Lancet*, **ii**, 1179–82.

Arie, T. and Jolley, D. (1982) Making a service work. Organisation and style of psychogeriatric services. In R. Levy and F. Post (eds.) *The Psychiatry of Late Life*, pp 222–51. Blackwell, London.

Baillon, S., Neville, P., and Broome, C. (1996) A survey of the relationship between community mental health teams and residential homes for the elderly. *International Journal of Geriatric Psychiatry*, **11**, 807–11.

Baldwin, R. and Murray, M. (2000) Services for younger people with dementia. In J. O'Brien, D. Ames and A. Burns (eds.). *Dementia*, pp. 353–9. Arnold, London.

Ball, C., Payne, M., and Lewis, E. (1996) Doctors and nurses: referrals by general practitioners to different arms of an old age psychiatry service. *International Journal of Geriatric Psychiatry*, **11**, 995–9.

Banerjee, S. (1993) Prevalence and recognition rates of psychiatric disorder in elderly clients of a community care service. *International Journal of Geriatric Psychiatry*, **8**, 125–31.

Banerjee, S. (1998) Organisation of old age psychiatry services. *Reviews in Clinical Gerontology*, **8**, 217–25.

Banerjee, S. and Macdonald, A. (1996) Mental disorder in an elderly home care population: associations with health and social service use. *British Journal of Psychiatry*, **168**, 750–6.

Banerjee, S., Shamash, K., Macdonald, A.J.D., *et al.* (1996) Randomised controlled trial of effect of intervention by psychogeriatric team on depression in frail elderly people at home. *BMJ* **313**, 1058–61.

Benbow, S.M. (1990) The community clinic: its advantages and disadvantages. *International Journal of Geriatric Psychiatry*, **5**, 235–40.

Benbow, S.M., Jolley, D.J., and Leonard, I.J. (1993) All work? A day in the life of geriatric psychiatrists. *International Journal of Geriatric Psychiatry*, **8**, 1019–22.

Benjamin, L.C. and Spector, J. (1990a) Environments for the dementing. *International Journal of Geriatric Psychiatry*, **5**, 15–24.

Benjamin, L.C. and Spector, J. (1990b) The relationship of staff, resident and environmental characteristics to stress experienced by staff caring for the dementing. *International Journal of Geriatric Psychiatry*, **5**, 15–24.

Blanchard, M., Waterreus, A., and Mann, A. H. (1995) The effect of primary care nurse intervention upon older people screened as depressed. *International Journal of Geriatric Psychiatry*, **10**, 289–98.

Blanchard, M.R., Waterreus, A., and Mann, A.H. (1999) Can a brief intervention have a longer term benefit? The case of the research nurse and depressed older people in the community. *International Journal of Geriatric Psychiatry*, **14**, 733–8.

Bleeker, J.A.C. and Diesfeldt, H.A.F. (2000) Services for dementia. A Dutch view. In J. O'Brien, D. Ames and A. Burns (eds.) *Dementia*, pp. 300–2. Arnold, London.

Bragason, A. (2003) News from Norway: working group strives to expand presence of old age psychiatry. *IPA Bulletin*, **20** (4), 16.

Brodaty, H., Draper, B., and Lie, D. (1997) Psychogeriatrics and general practice in Australia. *International Journal of Psychiatry in Medicine*, **27**, 205–13.

Brodaty, H., Howarth, G.C., Mant, A., and Kurrle, S. (1994) General practice and dementia. A national survey of Australian GPs. *Medical Journal of Australia*, **160**, 10–14.

Brodaty, H., Clarke, J., and Ganguli, M. (1998) Screening for cognitive impairment in general practice; towards a consensus. *Alzheimer's Disease and Related Disorders*, **12**, 1–13.

Brodaty, H. and Gresham, M. (1992) Prescribing residential care for dementia- effects, side-effects, indications and dosage. *International Journal of Geriatric Psychiatry*, **7**, 357–62.

Brodaty, H. and Peters, K. (1991) Cost-effectiveness of a training programme for dementia carers. *International Psychogeriatrics*, **3**, 11–22.

Brown, M., Godber, C., and Wilkinson, D. (2000) Services for dementia: a British view. In J. O'Brien, D. Ames and A. Burns (eds.) *Dementia*, pp. 291–7. Arnold, London.

Casten, R. and Rovner, B. (2000) Services for dementia: a North American view. In J. O'Brien, D. Ames and A. Burns (eds.) *Dementia*, pp. 315–19. Arnold, London.

Challis, D., Reilly, S., Hughes, J., *et al.* (2002a) Policy, organisational and practice of specialist old age psychiatry in England. *International Journal of Geriatric Psychiatry*, **17**, 1018–26.

Challis, D., Von Abendorff, R., Brown, P., *et al.* (2002b). Care management, dementia care and specialist mental health services: an evaluation. *International Journal of Geriatric Psychiatry*, **17**, 315–25.

Clement, J. and Leger, J. (2000) Services for dementia. A French view. In J. O'Brien, D. Ames and A. Burns (eds.) *Dementia*, pp. 311–13. Arnold, London.

Cole, M.G., Fenton, F.R., Engelsmann, F., *et al.* (1991) Effectiveness of geriatric psychiatry consultation in an acute care hospital: a randomised clinical trial. *Journal of the American Geriatric Society*, **39**, 1183–8.

Cole, M.G., Rochan, D.T., Engelsmann, F., and Ducic, D. (1995) The impact of home assessment on depression in the elderly: a clinical trial. *International Journal of Geriatric Psychiatry*, **10**, 19–23.

Coles, R.J., Von-Abendorff, R., and Hertzberg, J. (1991) The impact of a new community mental health team on an inner city psychogeriatric service. *International Journal of Geriatric Psychiatry*, **33**, 57–8.

Collighan, G., MacDonald, A., Herzberg, J., *et al.* (1993) An evaluation of the multidisciplinary approach to psychiatric diagnosis in elderly people. *BMJ* **306**, 821–4.

Collinson, Y. and Benbow, S. (1998) The role of an old age psychiatry consultation liaison nurse. *International Journal of Geriatric Psychiatry*, **13**, 159–63.

Corcoran, E. and Wrigley, M. (1994) The day hospital in psychiatry of old age – what difference does it make? *Irish Journal of Psychological Medicine*, **11**, 110–15.

Craig, J., Patel, J., Lee-Jones, C., *et al.* (2000) Psychiatric assessment wards for older adults: a qualitative evaluation of two ward models. *International Journal of Geriatric Psychiatry*, **15**, 721–8.

De Leo, D., Stella, A., and Spagnoli, A. (1989) Prescription of psychotropic drugs in geriatric institutions. *International Journal of Geriatric Psychiatry*, **4**, 11–16.

Dening, T. (1992) Community psychiatry of old age: a UK perspective. *International Journal of Geriatric Psychiatry*, **7**, 757–66.

Dening, T. and Lawton, C. (1998) The role of carers in evaluating mental health services for older people. *International Journal of Geriatric Psychiatry*, **13**, 863–70.

Dennis, M., Furness, L., Lindesay, J., *et al.* (1998) Assessment of patients with memory problems using a nurse-administered instrument to detect early dementia and dementia subtypes. *International Journal of Geriatric Psychiatry*, **13**, 405–9.

Department of Health (1991) NHS day care facilities in England year ending 31 March 1990. HMSO, London.

Department of Health (2001) *National Service Framework for Older People*. Department of Health, London.

Donaldson, L.J. and Hill, P.M. (1991) The domiciliary consultation service: time to take stock. *BMJ* **302**, 449–51.

Doyle, H. and Varian, J. (1994) Crisis intervention in psychogeriatrics: a round-the -clock commitment? *International Journal of Geriatric Psychiatry*, **9**, 65–72.

Draper, B. (1990) The effectiveness of services and treatments in psychogeriatrics. *Australia and New Zealand Journal of Psychiatry*, **24**, 238–51.

Flicker, L., Keppich-Arnold, S., Chiu, E., *et al.* (1992) The prevalence of depressive symptoms and cognitive impairment in supported residential services in Victoria: a pilot study. *Australian Journal of Aging*, **11**, 16–18.

Flynn, E., Ames, D., and LoGiudice, D. (2000) Services for dementia: an Australian view. In J. O'Brien, D. Ames, and A. Burns (eds.) *Dementia*, pp. 229–333. Arnold, London.

Ginsburg, L., Hamilton, P., Madora, P. *et al.* (1998) Geriatric psychiatry outreach practices in the province of Ontario: the role of the psychiatrist. *Canadian Journal of Psychiatry*, **43**, 386–90.

Gupta, K., Coupland, L., and Fottrell, E. (1996) A two-year review of an open access multidisciplinary community psychiatric service for the elderly. *International Journal of Geriatric Psychiatry*, **11**, 795–9.

Harris, M. and Bergmann, H. C. (1988) Misconceptions about use of case management services by the chronic mentally ill: a utilisation analysis. *Hospital and Community Psychiatry*, **39**, 1276–80.

Harrison, R., Savla, N., and Kafetz, N. (1990) Dementia, depression and physical disability in a London borough: a survey of elderly people in and out of residential care and implications for future development. *Age and Ageing*, **19**, 97–103.

Harrison, S. and Sheldon, T. A. (1994) Psychiatric services for elderly people evaluating system performance. *International Journal of Geriatric Psychiatry*, **9**, 259–72.

Heinik, J., Barak, Y., Salgenik, I., and Elizur, A. (1995) Patterns of two psychogeriatric hospitalisation services in Israel: a one year study. *International Journal of Geriatric Psychiatry*, **10**, 1051–7.

Hettiaratchy, P. (1985) UK travelling day hospital. *Ageing International*, **12**, 10–12.

Howard, R. (1995) The place of day hospitals in old age psychiatry. *Current Opinions in Psychiatry*, **8**, 240–1.

Intagliata, J. (1982) Improving the quality of community care for the chronically mentally disabled: the role of case-management. *Schizophrenia Bulletin*, **8**, 655–74.

Iorgulescu, M. and Sullivan, G. (1995) The beginning of community care in Romania. *International Journal of Geriatric Psychiatry*, **10**, 623.

Jolley, D. and Arie, T. (1978) Organisation of psychogeriatric services. *British Journal of Psychiatry*, **132**, 1–11.

Jolley, D. and Arie, T. (1992) Developments in psychogeriatric services. In T. Arie (ed.) *Recent Advances in Psychogeriatrics No 2*, pp. 177–85. Churchill Livingston, London.

Jones, R. (1992a) Medical audit in geriatric psychiatry: more questions than answers. *International Journal of Geriatric Psychiatry*, **7**, 1–3.

Jones, R. (1992b) Audit for old age psychiatry. In T. Arie (ed.) *Recent Advances in Psychogeriatrics*, pp. 187–200. Churchill Livingston, London.

Junaid, O. and Bruce, J. M. (1994) Providing a community psychogeriatric service: models of community psychiatric nursing provision of a single health district. *International Journal of Geriatric Psychiatry*, **9**, 715–20.

Kalasic, A. M. and Javanovi, A. (2003) What's going on in Serbia with psychogeriatrics? *IPA Bulletin*, **20** (4), 17.

Kivela, S. (2003) Increased funding for health care in Finland. *IPA Bulletin*, **20** (4), 15.

Koenig, H. G., Meadows, K. G., Cohen, H. J., *et al.* (1988) Self-rated depression scales and screening for major depression in the elderly hospitalised patients for mental illness. *Journal of the American Geriatric Society*, **36**, 699–706.

Lennon, S. and Jolley, D. (1991) Psychiatric services for the elderly: an urban service in South Manchester. In R. Jacoby and C. Oppenheimer (eds.) *Psychiatry in the Elderly*, pp. 322–38. Oxford University Press, Oxford.

Lindesay, J., Herzberg, J., Collighan, G., *et al.* (1996) Treatment decisions following assessment by multidisciplinary psychogeriatric teams. *Psychiatric Bulletin*, **20**, 78–81.

Macdonald, A., Goddard, K., and Poynton, A. (1994) Impact of 'open access' to specialist services the case of community psychogeriatrics. *International Journal of Geriatric Psychiatry*, **9**, 709–14.

Marshall, M. (1992) Designing for confused old people. In T. Arie (ed.) *Recent Advances in Psychogeriatrics*, pp. 201–16. Churchill Livingston, London.

Meltzer, D., Bedford, S., Dening, T., *et al.* (1996) Carers and monitoring of psychogeriatric community teams. *International Journal of Geriatric Psychiatry*, **11**, 1057–61.

Miyoshi, K. (2003). Psychogeriatrics in Japan. *IPA Bulletin*, **20** (4), 14–15.

Nagatomo, I. and Takigawa, M. (1998) Mental status of the elderly receiving home health services and the associated stress of home helpers. *International Journal of Geriatric Psychiatry*, **13**, 57–63.

Neese, J.B. and Abraham, I.L. (1997) Cluster analysis of psychogeriatric characteristics and service use among rural elderly. *Issues in Mental Health Nursing*, **18**, 1–18.

Orrell, M. and Katona, C. (1998) Do consultant home visits have a future in old age psychiatry. *International Journal of Geriatric Psychiatry*, **13**, 355–7.

Orrell, M., Katona, C., Durani, S., *et al.* (1998) Do domiciliary visits in elderly people with psychiatric problems fulfil the expectations of general practitioners? *Primary Care Psychiatry*, **4**, 47–9.

Plotkin, D.A. and Wells, K.B. (1993) Partial hospitalisation (day treatment) for psychiatrically ill elderly patients. *American Journal of Psychiatry*, **150**, 266–71.

Proctor, R., Burns, A., Powell, H.S., *et al.* (1999) Behaviour management in nursing and residential homes: a randomised controlled trial. *Lancet*, **345**, 26–9.

Ramsey, R., Wright, P., Katz, A., *et al.* (1991) The detection of psychiatric morbidity and its effect on outcome in acute elderly medical admissions. *International Journal of Geriatric Psychiatry*, **6**, 861–6.

Reddy, S. and Pitt, B. (1993) What becomes of demented patients referred to a psychogeriatric unit? An approach to audit. *International Journal of Geriatric Psychiatry*, **8**, 175–80.

Reifler, B. V. (1997) The practice of geriatric psychiatry in three countries: observations of an American in the British Isles. *International Journal of Geriatric Psychiatry*, **12**, 795–807.

Resnikoff, D. (2003) Mexico develops a national plan to address dementia. *IPA Bulletin*, **20** (4), 12.

Roca, R.P., Storer, D.J., Robbins, B.M., *et al.* (1990) Psychogeriatric assessment and treatment in urban public housing. *Hospital and Community Psychiatry*, **41**, 916–20.

Rolleston, M. and Ball, C. (1994) Evaluating the effect of brief day hospital closure. *International Journal of Geriatric Psychiatry*, **9**, 51–3.

Rosenvinge, H.P., Woolford, J.E., and Martin, A. (1994) Evaluation of extension of a psychogeriatric day hospital to open Saturdays. *International Journal of Geriatric Psychiatry*, **8**, 764.

Royal College of Physicians and Royal College of Psychiatrists (1989) *Care of Elderly People with Mental Illness*. London, Royal College of Physicians.

Saarela, T. and Kiviharju, U. (1995) Evaluating the usefulness of training in psychogeriatrics. *International Journal of Geriatric Psychiatry*, **10**, 1019–22.

Secretaries of State for Health, Wales, Northern Ireland and Scotland (1989) *Working for Patients*. HMSO, London.

Seidel, G., Smith, C., Hafner, R. J., *et al.* (1992) A psychogeriatric community outreach service: description and evaluation. *International Journal of Geriatric Psychiatry*, **7**, 347–50.

Seymour, J., Saunders, P., Wattis, J., and Daly, J.P. (1994) Evaluation of early dementia by a trained nurse. *International Journal of Geriatric Psychiatry*, **9**, 37–42.

Shah, A.K. (1994) Cost comparison of psychogeriatric consultations: outpatient versus home consultations. *International Psychogeriatrics*, **6**, 179–89.

Shah, A.K. (1995) Cost comparison of hospital based and primary (general practice health centre) based psychiatric outpatient clinics. *Acta Psychiatrica Scandinavica*, **92**, 32–4.

Shah, A.K. (1996) Cost of transportation to a psychogeriatric day hospital: Taxi versus minibus. *International Journal of Geriatric Psychiatry*, **11**, 555–8.

Shah, A.K. (1997a) Cost comparison of outpatient and home geriatric psychiatry consultations in one service. *Aging and Mental Health*, **1**, 372–6.

Shah, A.K. (1997b) Private psychiatry. Can it be improved? *Journal of the Royal Society of Medicine*, **90**, 1–2.

Shah, A. and Ames, D. (1994) Planning and developing psychogeriatric services. *International Review of Psychiatry*, **6**, 15–27.

Shah, A.K., Chiu, E., Ames, D., *et al.* (2000) Aggressive behaviour in nursing homes for the elderly in Melbourne Australia. *International Psychogeriatrics*, **12**, 145–61.

Shah, A.K., Odutoye, K., and De, T. (2001). Depression in medically ill elderly inpatients: a pilot study of early identification and intervention by psychogeriatric consultation. *Journal of Affective Disorders*, **62**, 233–40.

Shah, S. and Harris, M. (1997) A survey of general practitioners' confidence in their management of elderly patients. *Australian Family Physician*, **26** (Suppl. 1), S12–17.

Shaji, K.S., Arun Kishore, M.S., Lal, K.P., *et al.* (2002) Revealing a hidden problem. An evaluation of a community dementia case finding program from the India 10/66 dementia research network. *International Journal of Geriatric Psychiatry*, **17**, 222–5.

Shulman, K.I., Silver, I.L., Hershberg, R.I., *et al.* (1986) Geriatric psychiatry in the general hospital: the integration of services and training. *General Hospital Psychiatry*, **8**, 223–8.

Snowdon, J. (1993) How many bed days for an areas psychogeriatric patients? *Australian and New Zealand Journal of Psychiatry*, **27**, 42–8.

Snowdon, J. and Donnelly, N. (1986) A study of depression in nursing homes. *Journal of Psychiatric Research*, **20**, 327–33.

Snowdon, J. and MacIntosh, S. (1989) Depression and dementia in three Sydney hostels. *Australian Journal on Ageing*, **8**, 24–8.

Strain, J.J., Lyons, J.S., Hammer, J.S., *et al.* (1991) Cost offset from a psychiatric consultation-liaison intervention with elderly hip fracture patients. *American Journal of Psychiatry*, **148**, 1044–9.

Teitelbaum, L., Cotton, D., Ginsburg, M.L., *et al.* (1996) Psychogeriatric consultation services: effect and effectiveness. *Canadian Journal of Psychiatry*, **41**, 638–44.

Tym, E. (1991) Psychiatric services for the elderly: a rural service in East Anglia. In R. Jacoby and C. Oppenheimer (eds.) *Psychiatry in the Elderly*, pp. 313–21. Oxford University Press, Oxford.

Tyrer, P. (1985) Psychiatric clinics in general practice. *British Journal of Psychiatry*, **145**, 9–14.

Victor, C.R. (1991) Who should care for the frail elderly? A survey of medical and nursing staff. *International Journal of Geriatric Psychiatry*, **6**, 743–7.

Von Abendorff, R., Challis, D., and Netten, A. (1994) Staff activity patterns in a community mental health team for older people. *International Journal of Psychiatry*, **9**, 897–906.

Wasylenki, D.A., Harrison, M.K., Britnell, J., and Hood, J. (1984) A community-based psychogeriatric service. *Journal of the American Geriatric Society*, **32**, 213–18.

Waterreus, A. (1992) Community psychiatric nursing in primary care. *International Review of Psychiatry*, **4**, 317–22.

Wattis, J.P. (1989) Old Age Psychiatry in the United Kingdom: their educational role. *International Journal of Geriatric Psychiatry*, **4**, 361–3.

Wertheimer, J. (1997) Psychiatry of the elderly: a consensus statement. *International Journal of Geriatric Psychiatry*, **12**, 430–5.

Weyerer, S. and Schaufele, M. (2000) A German view. In J. O'Brien, D. Ames and A. Burns (eds.) *Dementia*, pp. 303–5. Arnold, London.

Williams, D.D.R., Ellis, M.M., and Hardwick, F. (1997) Intensive home nursing. An innovation in old age psychiatry. *Psychiatric Bulletin*, **21**, 23–5.

World Health Organisation and GPWorldPA (1998) Organisation of care in psychiatry of the elderly – a technical consensus statement. *Aging and Mental Health*, **2**, 246–52.

Chapter 15

The role of psychogeriatric services in long-term residential care settings

John Snowdon

There are considerable differences in long-term residential care arrangements between different parts of the world, and there have been variations over time. The percentage of people who live to be old and disabled has dramatically increased, but to an extent that varies between countries. For example, the percentage of people aged over 80 years in Kenya, Egypt and the Philippines was under 0.25 per cent in 1980, but was expected to double in twenty years or so, while already in 1980 in France, the United Kingdom (UK), West Germany and Sweden about 2.5 per cent were aged over 80 years (Selby and Schechter, 1982). Some countries have devoted considerable resources to provision of long-term accommodation and services for disabled older persons, but the World Health Organization declared that *developing* countries would be unable to afford to provide institutional care and should therefore concentrate on community-based options (Kaprio, 1982). Some cultures are known for their pertinacity in supporting disabled persons at home in extended families, thus limiting the need for residential care.

To illustrate the rapidity of change, reference can be made to the provision of long-term care in England during the last sixty years (Jolley, 1992; Jolley *et al.*, 1998). In the 1940s, some former workhouses became long-term hospitals, while other older people who needed long-term care were accommodated in local authority homes. In the 1980s there was a massive increase in independent sector residential and nursing home availability in England, and many local authorities reduced or even ceased provision of residential care.

Recognizing these variations, what is said about the role of psychogeriatric services in one country or region at one point in time may not apply in other places or at other times. Historical factors, together with differences in staffing, funding, culture, ageing of the population, the size and structure of residential facilities and how they are run, the organization of health and welfare services and other factors affect whether psychogeriatric services are provided in long-term residential care settings, and if so, how.

Much of the recent literature on the provision of mental health services in nursing homes emanates from the United States (US). Many of the psychiatric and behavioural problems discussed in the literature by US clinicians are no doubt similar to those experienced in other countries, but recommendations on management may need to be adapted, depending on differences in staffing, resources, culture, etc.

This chapter will provide examples of how psychogeriatric services have been provided in aged care homes, and ways by which such services have responded to specific problems. The aim is to provoke consideration of whether and how to develop and fund (or alter) the provision of mental health services in long-term aged care facilities around the world.

The need for mental health services in long-term care facilities

Numerous surveys have revealed the high prevalence of mental disorders in nursing homes and residential care facilities. Rates vary between countries and between facilities, depending partly on admission policies, the number of long-term care places per unit of population, factors affecting quality of life and factors determining the availability of rehabilitation and treatment resources. Studies in the US have reported the prevalence of psychiatric disorders in nursing homes to be 80–91 per cent (Streim et al., 1997). Clinical studies have shown rates of dementia above 80 per cent, with 25–50 per cent of dementia patients having psychotic symptoms. Significant depressive symptoms were reported in 30–50 per cent of nursing home patients who could be assessed, and major depression was diagnosed in 6–25 per cent of residents (Rovner and Katz, 1993). Research in Australia has revealed rates of cognitive impairment, depression, anxiety disorders and behaviour disturbance in nursing homes that are comparable to those reported in the US (Snowdon, 2001). In the US, some 2.4 per cent of newly admitted residents were reported to have schizophrenia (Rovner et al., 1990). Ten per cent of US nursing home residents are said to have schizophrenia (Birkett, 2001), whereas about 5 per cent of those in Australian nursing homes have schizophrenia or a paranoid disorder (Rosewarne et al., 1997).

Studies in European nursing homes have shown similarly high prevalence rates for psychiatric conditions. For example, among residents newly admitted to ten Austrian nursing homes, 76.3 per cent had an ICD-9 psychiatric diagnosis. Some 64.9 per cent had dementia or another organic mental illness, 4.2 per cent had substance use disorders and 1.9 per cent had schizophrenia (Wancata et al., 1998).

The prevalence of mental disorders in US and Australian nursing homes appears to be increasing. As long-stay hospital wards have closed, a progressively higher proportion of patients admitted to nursing homes have been recorded as having dementia, and there has been an increase in the average severity of physical disorders among residents.

In the US in the 1980s there was mounting criticism of the care provided in nursing homes, particularly in regard to excessive use of neuroleptic and sedative medication; most prescriptions were written without any input from a mental health professional. There were continuing calls for involvement of mental health specialists in treating residents with mental disorders. The 1987 Omnibus Budget Reconciliation Act (OBRA-87) established many new rules and regulations for nursing home care. Among the Act's quality of care regulations, there are statements that residents must be 'free from unnecessary drugs', that antipsychotic drugs should not be used unless one of the allowable specific conditions is recorded as an indication in the clinical record, and that residents using antipsychotic drugs must receive 'behavioral programming', dose reductions or drug holidays in an effort at discontinuation (Ouslander *et al.*, 1991).

Surveys in some other countries at that time revealed similarly high use of psychotropic medication in nursing homes, though perhaps too little use of antidepressants (Snowdon, 1993). Subsequent reductions in sedative and neuroleptic use are largely attributable to enhanced awareness by and education of prescribers and nursing staff in those countries rather than new legislation. Increased involvement of pharmacists has certainly helped.

Since 1990, when OBRA regulations were implemented, there has been a fall in the use of antipsychotic medication in US nursing homes (34 per cent in 1976–90, 19 per cent in 2001) and of hypnotics (16 per cent to 4.2 per cent), but an increase in the use of antidepressants (13 per cent to 33.3 per cent of residents) (Ryan *et al.*, 2002).

Inadequate provision of mental health services in long-term care facilities

What is astonishing, given the OBRA-87 regulations and decades of criticism concerning the lack of appropriate psychiatric care in US nursing homes, is to read that, even now:

> Most of those residents who need mental health services do not receive them …. Nursing home administrators have estimated that two-fifths of nursing home residents need psychiatric services, yet half of nursing homes do not have access to adequate psychiatric consultation, and three-quarters are unable to obtain consultation and educational services for behavioral interventions.
>
> Bartels *et al.*, 2002

Before and at the time of OBRA implementation, few nursing home residents – 2.3 per cent in one part of the US – (Burns *et al.*, 1993) had contact with a mental health professional. Borson *et al.* (1987) commented on the lack of reliable data but suggested that less than 1 per cent of all patients with a diagnosable mental disorder received explicit mental health interventions. Conn *et al.* (1992b) found that only 46 per cent of nursing homes in Ontario had psychiatrists available to do consultations in their facilities, the percentage being lowest in rural areas.

US policies had led to a significant barrier to the recognition and treatment of mental illness in nursing homes. This arose because of concerns by designers of the federally-funded Medicaid programme in the US that States would abrogate responsibility for the costs of long-term mental health care by transferring patients from mental hospitals to nursing homes. It was decided that Medicaid funding would not be provided to long-term care facilities if more than half their patients were diagnosed as having a mental disorder; they were called 'institutions for mental disease' (IMDs). Fears of exceeding the 50 per cent threshold resulted in a disincentive to recognition or treatment of mental disorders. In order to enable Alzheimer's disease (AD) patients still to be admitted to nursing homes, AD was called a neurological rather than a psychiatric disorder. A consequence was that patients with AD were then denied State mental hospital admission even if they manifested severe behavioural problems.

OBRA-87 was intended to deal with under-servicing of those with mental disorders by arranging 'pre-admission screening and annual resident review' (PASARR). This aimed to restrict access to nursing home care for patients with mental disorders, but ensure they reached facilities where appropriate treatment was available. In some respects, this aim was successfully met. Mechanic and McAlpine (2000) quoted evidence that the prevalence of schizophrenia-related diagnoses in nursing homes declined in the decade to 1995, especially among those younger than 65 years, and Borson *et al.* (1997) agreed that the PASARR process was likely to identify most cases of schizophrenia. However, patients with physical conditions that required ongoing nursing care still needed admission to nursing homes even if they also had mental disorders; nowhere else was appropriate and available. Once admitted, care for their physical problems was funded, but the new policies did not take account of needs in such cases for assessment and treatment of their mental disorders. Drinka and Howell (1991) found it 'most ironic that those requiring basic nursing care for dementia or major medical problems who *in addition* have severe psychiatric problems will not have specific funding for an in-depth ... psychiatric evaluation'. In any case, Borson *et al.* (1997) showed that the PASARR process did *not* identify a majority of those residents who have significant depression, nor those likely to have treatable non-cognitive symptoms of dementia. OBRA-87 did not solve the problem of the unmet need for mental health services in US nursing homes (Moak and Borson, 2000). Peak bodies in the fields of geriatrics and geriatric psychiatry have stated a need for reforms that will provide incentives for improvement, so that those needing mental health services will receive them (American Geriatrics Society and American Association for Geriatric Psychiatry, 2003). They called for development of a trained workforce of mental health professionals with expertise and a commitment to practise in long-term care settings.

Some might argue that the deficiency in mental health services in US nursing homes can be blamed on the fee-for-service model, and that in countries with universal health cover arrangements it should be possible to access specialist services when needed. However, universal health coverage does not necessarily mean universal accessibility of mental health professionals to assess and advise on treatment, or to provide ongoing management recommendations. Old age psychiatry services are unavailable in some areas and under-resourced in others, even in the UK, Canada and Australia, where obtaining health care is intended to be affordable or free for all citizens. In some countries and regions, aged care teams or physicians without psychiatric training have taken responsibility (without necessarily wanting it) for providing management recommendations in relation to psychiatric problems (see Chapter 1). Some geriatricians have developed expertise in assessing and treating behavioural problems in cases of dementia. However, even when specialist help is available, doctors and facility staff may not recognize or even consider the potential benefits of referral. This could be because they have not observed such benefits in previous cases (perhaps due to unavailability of such services), or because adequate education concerning effective psychiatric treatments has not been provided. It could also be because they have ageist and negative attitudes about treating old age mental disorders. For these reasons it is important to show evidence of the benefits and to consider the most cost-effective ways of providing old age mental health services in long-term care facilities.

Models of mental health services in residential care facilities

Psychiatric services in US nursing homes, when available, are most commonly provided by a consultant psychiatrist who works alone, comes only when called to see a specific patient, and does not provide subsequent care unless called back to review the case (Bartels *et al.*, 2002). Opinions expressed by specialists from around the world suggest that this is the most common model in other countries too, though reports in the literature seem to concentrate more on multidisciplinary models. Streim *et al.* (1997) outlined the spectrum of potential roles that could be fulfilled by psychiatrists in nursing homes. Because of their specialized training in assessment, diagnosis and treatment of mental disorders, they are well placed to advise on the interactions between psychiatric disorders, comorbid medical conditions, medication, psychosocial and environmental variables, and associated behavioural disturbances. They are well equipped to address family systems issues. They can advise on medico-legal issues and may be asked to evaluate residents' decision-making capacities. If service arrangements allow, their roles may expand to be more like those of traditional consultation-liaison psychiatrists in general hospitals.

Hanchuk (1996) stated:

> Within a nursing home, a consulting psychiatrist will function as a consulting mental disorder diagnostician, as a consulting psychopharmacologist, and as a psychotherapist. The role of geriatric psychiatrist is also to be an integral and active participant of an evaluating and treating team of health care providers ... Treatment will often include education of the staff and family, therapy recommendations for the patient and caregivers, behavioral modifications to be carried out, and pharmacological interventions.

How well does this model (the visiting psychiatrist) work? Reichman *et al.* (1998) in the US found that staff of 899 nursing homes in six states were satisfied with psychiatrist input in relation to diagnosis and recommendations concerning medication, but a majority regarded other aspects of the perceived roles of psychiatrists (provision of recommendations concerning non-drug treatments, resolution of resident family problems, education of staff and management of staff stress) as inadequate.

Various authors have stressed that the role of psychiatrists should extend beyond providing a consultative service for referred patients (Bienenfeld and Wheeler, 1989;

Sakauye and Camp, 1992; Lantz and Kennedy, 1995; Gupta and Goldstein, 1999). *Liaison* as well as referral-dependent consultations results in increased awareness of, and attention to, mental health problems of unreferred residents. Liaison with staff in the form of case conferences and other educational activities has been recommended (Joseph *et al.*, 1995). Sakauye and Camp (1992) referred to six guiding principles that need emphasis in order to guide staff to think more about behavioural management options. These involve looking for depression or psychosis as a source of problems, reducing multiple medications, assuming that no behaviour is random, making the patient 'human' to staff, creating a home-like environment, providing appropriate activities, and agreeing that individuals in advanced stages of dementia may still be capable of learning new information or responding to reinforcement. Bienenfeld and Wheeler (1989) declared that the core element of their liaison service was the case conference that followed an evaluation. The importance of establishing relationships to nurses and other staff has been emphasized by Hanchuk (1996), who described liaison as teaching psychiatric and interpersonal skills to non-psychiatrists. A team approach necessitates clear communication between members, and it is best if members of the team can be present or easily available when psychiatrists talk with patients. Designation of one nurse in a facility to receive and coordinate referrals of residents for psychiatric evaluation (Bienenfeld and Wheeler, 1989) may be crucial to the flow and monitoring of mental health care (Hanchuk, 1996). As the nurse's experience with psychiatric treatments and evaluations improves, so does the level of care within the facility.

When psychiatrists and facility staff are willing and able to adopt the liaison philosophy, facilities can adopt a *multidisciplinary team approach* without having to depend on a *visiting* team of multidisciplinary staff. The visiting psychiatrist works with a team formed from staff of the nursing home. The difference between this and the criticized consultation model is that the psychiatrist and staff work together in carrying out assessments, and planning and reviewing interventions. One major limitation to this approach is if staff cannot get away from other duties to join in team discussions. To make this modification of the visiting psychiatrist model feasible, funds need to be expended to allow *time* for involvement.

Joseph *et al.* (1995) described a Mental Health Consultation Team (MHCT) established in a 120-bed Veterans' Nursing Home Care Unit. The team consisted of an interdisciplinary team of primary care providers working in the nursing home, including nurse practitioners and social workers. A visiting geropsychiatrist and mental health clinical nurse specialist each joined the MHCT for two hours per week, and the nursing home supplied four hours per week of nursing time to provide a 'unit expert' to liaise between the MHCT and the nursing staff. Referrals were discussed at triage meetings. The unit expert often performed a preliminary assessment, helped in implementation of individual treatment plans, served as a role model and facilitated communication of 'recommendations, knowledge and skills from the MHCT to bedside nurses'. The visiting clinical nurse specialist provided support to Nursing Home Care Unit nursing staff.

The authors admitted it was likely that more staff resources were available in Veterans' facilities than would be the case in other nursing homes, emphasized the need for administrative support of dedicated time for the unit expert, and stated that 8 to 12 hours would be a more appropriate time allocation if the role was to be fulfilled adequately in that setting.

Multidisciplinary teams are said to be the preferred model for mental health service provision in nursing homes (Bartels *et al.*, 2002). It is stated that research supports the belief of skilled clinicians that a multi-tiered, interdisciplinary approach is required in order to achieve an acceptable standard of care (Moak and Borson, 2000). At the same time, there has been a call for research to answer fundamental questions about optimal organization and delivery of services (Moak and Borson, 2000). Bartels *et al.* (2002) commented that studies had not assessed the cost-effectiveness of the team approach.

The usual understanding of the multidisciplinary team model is that team members come from outside the facility, and may include psychiatric nurse specialists, psychologists and/or social workers, each with their special expertise. Teams include a psychiatrist with one to four other health professionals, and vary in the roles and responsibilities they undertake (Bartels *et al.*, 2002). A team in Seattle (psychiatrist, psychiatric nurse and 'geriatric mental health specialists') provided on-site consultations and direct care psychiatric services to a number of nursing homes on a contractual basis (Loebel *et al.*, 1991). Most reports referred to consultations with individual residents, but emphasized the complementary contributions of different disciplines. The clinical nurse specialist may be more effective in developing treatment plans with facility nursing staff, while the psychiatrist may have most effect in relating to doctors, recording diagnoses and recommending medications. Psychologists have expertise in behavioural programming and neuropsychological assessment, and 'social workers may have superior skills in addressing family and social support concerns'.

Old age psychiatry services have evolved in a number of countries. Multidisciplinary teams have commonly taken responsibility for provision of mental health services for residential care facilities in their catchment areas. Arrangements vary. In the author's Central Sydney service, the psychiatrists conduct initial assessments, but may call on other members of the team (a psychologist, social worker or nurse) as appropriate. Budgetary constraints have led to under-resourcing and consequent under-availability of team members to provide follow-up review and support to facility staff. The team is indeed multidisciplinary, but when kept under-resourced it becomes in effect a psychiatrist service that liaises and works with facility staff. There is now Health Department support for pharmacists to visit and advise aged care facilities in Australia, and some nursing homes find funds to bring in psychologists and others (including herbalists) to provide treatments, but they are independent of catchment area teams.

Seidel *et al.* (1992) presented data from Adelaide concerning 100 consecutive referrals to a multidisciplinary old age psychiatry service that included four community psychiatric nurses. Seventy-three of the 100 referred persons were living in residential care.

Initially, 50 of them were rated as very or fairly disruptive, but after three months the number had fallen to 19. It was not clear from the report what role each team member played in the intervention process.

Fairbairn (2002) reported that in Britain there had been 'poor liaison between specialist teams catering for the mental health of older people and independent-sector residential/nursing homes', though Challis *et al.* (2002) found that over half of the old age psychiatry services in England had links with residential and nursing homes. Comparable attitudes have been observed in Australia among health administrators who believe that non-government facilities receive government subsidies, which should be adequate to allow payment for extrinsic mental health services. In Britain the Faculty for the Psychiatry of Old Age has contributed to guidelines on good practices, which recognize the expertise of members of community multidisciplinary teams and suggest that they can contribute to training of care staff in residential or nursing homes.

Some of the research reports reveal examples of how multidisciplinary teams may function. Brodaty *et al.* (2003) described an intervention study aimed at treating residents with dementia complicated by depression or psychosis. Treatments were supervised by geriatric psychiatrists and administered by a multidisciplinary team, including a psychologist and nurse who were experienced in aged care. Comparison groups did not receive comparably intensive interventions, but there was improvement over 12 weeks of follow-up in all groups despite depressive and psychotic symptoms reported to have been present for an average of over three years. The 'study's model of specialist mental health care provided directly or through consultative advice had no appreciable benefit over that evident in a control group'. However, all patients had been assessed for at least half a day and this included discussions with the patient's family and nursing home staff. Residents rather than homes were randomized, so that intervention directed to one group may also have affected control subjects. In addition, the presence of a psychogeriatric team, as well as focused attention resulting from participation in a research study (the Hawthorne effect), appears to have been therapeutic.

Another research report described a consultancy team (psychiatrist, psychologist and nurses) who devised strategies to reduce severe behaviour disturbance among nursing home residents with advanced dementia (Opie *et al.*, 2002).

Variations in the visiting team model have been described. Jackson and Lyons (1996) described a 'roving' clinic, whereby a psychiatrist visited residential homes for elderly people on a rotational basis, referrals being arranged in advance by care staff in consultation with residents' general practitioners. This led to a reduced need for inpatient care. A majority of referrals were of people with dementia.

Llewellyn-Jones *et al.* (1999) evaluated the effectiveness of a shared care intervention aimed at reducing late life depression in residential care facilities. The intervention was primarily delivered by general practitioners (GPs) and residential care staff, supported by a GP education programme and a health education and health promotion programme for all residents (some being in sheltered housing, some in residential homes, but none in nursing homes). Specialist consultations and advice were available if needed. The intervention was modestly effective in reducing depression levels in this population.

Some teams limit their interventions to cases of disturbed behaviour. For example, an English study in nursing and residential homes (Proctor *et al.*, 1999) relied on seven hour-long seminars by a hospital outreach team to train staff in management of dementia, agitation and screaming, and to educate them about old age psychiatric disorders and treatments. A psychiatric nurse then visited each home weekly to provide support and advice.

Behaviour Support Units have been developed in Australia to provide specialist assessment, advice, training and funding support to aged care facilities to deal with dementia complicated by 'challenging behaviours'. The federal government has funded one such unit for each State, though each has developed a different model. Generally they are staffed by registered nurses with varying contributions from allied health, geriatricians and psychiatrists.

Another innovative approach used by Tang *et al.* (2001) was the use of *telepsychiatry* to link a psychiatrist and colleagues from a hospital in Hong Kong to a 'care and attention home'. This was used to provide monthly assessments of patients who had been seen initially in an outpatient clinic.

As well as the psychiatrist-centred and multidisciplinary team models of mental health service delivery in nursing homes, Bartels *et al.* (2002) identified a *nurse-centred* model. They gave the example of a geropsychiatric nurse specialist who coordinates the services provided by other extrinsic mental health clinicians, while training facility staff to develop skills and abilities. Santmyer and Roca (1991) described such a service, where clinical supervision was provided by a geropsychiatrist during weekly two-hour visits, but referrals were made directly to the nurse – most frequently by doctors and registered nurses. The nursing home was part of a larger medical complex, of which the nurse was an employee. She was available for emergency contact five days a week, and spent two days per week in the nursing home. Apparent depression was the most common reason for referral, followed by behavioural complications of dementia. About one half of the problems prompting referral were within the expertise of the nurse specialist and did not require the psychiatrist's direct involvement. This was especially true of behaviour problems complicating nursing care, problems in adjusting to the nursing home environment, and problems in relationships with staff and other residents.

Another example of the nurse-centred approach was reported by Ballard *et al.* (2002). Problems were discussed by a team (so some might call the service multidisciplinary) but the work and liaison were conducted by an individual nurse in six facilities in Newcastle (UK), two being nursing homes and four residential homes. The nurse, who had a psychiatric qualification and a diploma in cognitive therapy, visited each facility weekly. An old age psychiatrist and a clinical psychologist, who were available for the equivalent of one day and half a day weekly respectively, gave supervision. The service aimed to improve the way medication and health service resources were used in treating people with dementia. Interventions were based on detailed evaluation of behaviours, antecedents and consequences, in order to develop individual ('tailored') management plans. 'Psychological interventions were the first line approach.'

There have been few well-designed controlled intervention studies to examine the outcomes of providing mental health services to residential facilities (Bartels *et al.*, 2002), though uncontrolled observational studies suggest that such services result in improved clinical outcomes and less use of acute services. Four of these studies reported improvement in symptoms and functioning ranging from 51–78 per cent of cases where residents received services. Bartels *et al.* (2002) referred to the randomized controlled study by Ames (1990) in residential care homes, which reported no difference in outcome between those who received psychogeriatric consultation services and those who received usual care. Brodaty *et al.*'s (2003) randomized controlled trial of different models of mental health service in nursing homes showed that residents with depression or psychosis improved significantly with time, regardless of type of service, though there were trends toward greater improvement in behavioural disturbance in the case management group. Snowden *et al.* (2003) reviewed literature concerning the benefits of various types of intervention in treating dementia-related behavioural symptoms, and concluded that, in general, there was insufficient evidence to prioritize a non-pharmacological versus a pharmacological approach. This chapter is focused on the effects of services rather than on whether particular medications or treatments have demonstrated efficacy, but the importance of environment, the design of buildings and the understanding of mental health issues by facility staff, in determining responses to mental health services or treatment needs emphasis. Special care units (SCUs) have been developed in order to provide specialist treatment for persons with continuing behavioural symptoms, and a randomized trial showed modest but significant effects on engagement, sociability and positive affect (Lawton *et al.*, 1998). However, positive behavioural outcomes can also be achieved in traditional units (Rovner *et al.*, 1996).

Several studies have suggested that targeted *educational interventions* may be successful in changing clinicians' treatment practices (Bartels *et al.*, 2002). Chartock *et al.* (1988) commented on the unpreparedness of facility staff to deal with mental health issues, and described a multidisciplinary programme that was effective in building knowledge and improving job-skills for all levels and types of staff. Studies of nurse aide training interventions had negative or mixed results (Snowden *et al.*, 2003).

Specialist mental health residential care facilities

The move towards community care for older people with mental illnesses led to reductions in long-term bed numbers in a number of countries. Psychiatric units were opened in general hospitals, but these were for acute care. Mental hospitals closed. Deinstitutionalization was meant to lead to case management in the community for those who still had psychiatric problems. Primary care practitioners were to provide treatment, but in cooperation with community mental health staff and psychiatrists. It was intended that the latter would continue their clinical review and management roles for a substantial proportion of the patients who formerly would have been in long-term hospital wards.

The new arrangements may have worked well for middle-aged people with schizophrenia. For a large proportion of the older patients, however, the change was in effect transinstitutionalization rather than deinstitutionalization, so that observers in the US commented that nursing homes had become the equivalent of long-term mental hospital wards (Schmidt *et al.*, 1977). To an extent that varied between countries, long-term beds for older people with disturbed behaviour remained available in hospitals for longer than did those for younger people. In Britain, the move out of geriatric and mental hospitals of mentally disturbed older people who needed constant supervised care was slower to occur than in the US, but now, in various countries, including the UK, US, Australia and Canada, comparatively few long-term beds remain available in the hospital system. Because accommodation for such people is now mainly in non-government facilities, psychiatrists no longer manage the beds. Their advice may be welcome but they no longer control or can insist on appropriate psychiatric care.

A majority of mentally ill younger and older persons do not need frequent review and management by mental health professionals, but some do. Mainstream residential care facilities cannot provide such specialized care. Facilities that employ no staff who have had psychiatric training should not be looking after patients who have severe mental disorders. Mental health clinicians need to be able to admit such patients to units where trained psychiatric staff can coordinate appropriate treatments and programmes. Such units are likely to be few and far between, and comparatively expensive. Experience suggests that persistently severe behavioural disturbance settles within a few months of admission to these specialized facilities in most cases. Resolution of behavioural problems is commonly attributable (at least in part) to progression of a brain disorder or the development of other debilitating or disabling physical illnesses. When patients no longer need to be in units designed and staffed to manage severe behavioural disturbance, many believe it appropriate for them to move to more peaceful surroundings, rather than for the units to be their 'homes for life'. The move (which, in large, comprehensive facilities, may be to a different unit within the same complex) is also financially appropriate, since special care units are more expensive. Their admission and discharge arrangements need to be efficient and well regulated. It will probably be best if each area has an agreed number of such beds, with access controlled by the catchment area old age psychiatry team – if there is one.

The State of Victoria in Australia has used funds from the closure of a geriatric hospital to develop a number of 30-bedded 'psychogeriatric nursing homes'.

The Australian Government subsidizes these facilities just as it funds mainstream nursing homes, but the Victorian State Department of Health arranges 'top-up' funding to pay for psychiatrically trained personnel to be on the staff, and for catchment area old age psychiatrists and their teams to coordinate psychiatric management. Admission contracts make clear to patients and their families that these facilities provide *interim care* during the time that a person is ambulant and too disturbed to be in a mainstream aged care facility.

In Sydney, Australia, it is intended to close the remaining long-term beds for older people in a psychiatric hospital, with the patients being transferred to a psychogeriatric nursing home run by a non-government organization. It will be vital to put in place a management protocol that enables the area old age psychiatry team to make clinical decisions regarding discharge, in order to admit others who need such special care. Without it, the acute hospital psychogeriatric unit will soon be over-filled as a result of nursing homes ejecting residents perceived as too mentally disturbed for them to continue living there.

These 'psychogeriatric nursing homes' need to form part of a coordinated area old age psychiatry service, and are the equivalent of small hospitals, but built to be home-like and to 'normalize' behaviour as much as possible. If all parts of the system work well, the number of beds needed in these special care facilities per elderly persons in the catchment area could be 0.5 per 1000. Also in Victoria and Sydney there are a small number of 'psychogeriatric hostels', which are 'low care' facilities that provide long-term supervision for older people who are ambulant but have schizophrenia or other mentally disabling condition. They do not have severe physical problems, and do not require intensive nursing or to be in a locked facility, but would be unable to live independently due to impaired social or daily living skills. Facility staff can ensure compliance with treatment requirements.

Other examples of units that provide special care for older people manifesting disturbed behaviour can be seen in various countries. Several studies of SCUs (including an evaluation of ten Italian facilities by Bellelli *et al.* (1998)) have shown decreases in behaviour disturbance and improved function, the improvements being attributed to staff training, care arrangements and environmental features of the units. Sloane *et al.* (1991) reported that specialized dementia units were successful in reducing the use of physical but not pharmacologic restraints. Lindesay *et al.* (1995) compared a 'domus', the 'only long-stay psychogeriatric facility for a population of 18,000 elderly people in part of one London health district', with two typical psychogeriatric long-stay wards serving another area. Twenty-four of the 27 residents had dementia. The domus is agreed to be the residents' home for life. (Note that the ratio of beds per 1000 elderly in the population was three times greater than that recommended in areas where residents move elsewhere once their behaviour has adequately settled.) A GP provides primary medical care, and residents have access to a community psychogeriatric team for assessment and advice. The authors noted markedly greater levels of activity and staff–resident interaction in the domus and thought them 'strongly indicative of a better quality of life in this setting'.

Various nursing homes have developed special units for the care of populations with particular needs (other than the management of disturbed behaviour). These include AIDS-designated centres, units for ventilator-dependent residents and palliative care units. Psychiatrists may well be needed to contribute to ongoing care (Lantz and Kennedy, 1995).

Depla *et al.* (2003) described how innovators in the Netherlands have been 'experimenting with the integration of mental health care into residential homes for the elderly'. Unlike in nursing homes, residents of these facilities live in self-contained apartments. Most of the target group had schizophrenia, recurrent depression or serious personality disorders. The researchers reviewed six programmes and concluded that residents' mental health care can be best safeguarded by having a mental health institution assign mental health professionals to take on psychiatric care duties in these residential homes.

Comparisons between outcomes for residents in the various SCUs and other innovative facilities for older persons with disturbed behaviour, and the psychogeriatric nursing homes, are inappropriate because of differences in the populations admitted and policies regarding how long they may stay. Certainly, however, those providing mental health services to long-term residential care facilities need to be able to refer, or themselves be able to take ongoing clinical care of, that minority of residents who need care in a specialized mental health care facility because of persistent and severely disturbed behaviour. If referral is impossible, the alternative is usually unacceptable chemical restraint. Alternatives *must* be found!

Who pays?

In countries such as the UK, Canada and Australia, mental health services for residents in long-term care facilities are provided at little or no cost to patients or the facilities. Mental health services are funded to assess and review residents referred from within their area. It sounds better than the US system, but a drawback is the under-resourcing and therefore relative under-availability of health professionals to provide such services. GPs may also refer their patients to doctors in private practice, who can claim payment from their country's health cover system (in Australia, Medicare).

In the US, two models for nursing home consultation reimbursement are in use (Gupta and Goldstein, 1999). One model is fee-for-service, the consultant seeking reimbursement from Medicare, Medigap and Medicaid. Careful documentation of the complexity of the case is required to justify the billing code. Residents too rich for Medicaid have to pay for themselves. There is no Medicare provision for reimbursements for time spent in consultation with nursing staff or telephone consultations. Camp *et al.* (2002) pointed out inconsistencies and difficulties in arranging reimbursement.

Medicare covers only 50 per cent of approved psychiatric and psychological services, compared with 80 per cent of approved medical services. In many States, Medicaid does not cover a 50 per cent co-payment, and payments vary by region because fiscal intermediaries have different interpretations of regulations. Further, reviews by the Office of the Inspector-General have suggested that a quarter to one third of nursing home mental health services billed to Medicare, particularly psychological testing, were unnecessary (Streim *et al.*, 2002). The other model is where a nursing home agrees to an hourly rate for the visiting mental health clinician's time, and then may bill the patient or third party-payer for services (Gupta and Goldstein, 1999). Moak and Borson (2000) called for changes to reimbursement and regulation, including creation of mechanisms for expanding the role of consultant pharmacists. They commented that then-current cost-containment strategies for long-term care were exerting counter-pressures against expansion of services to nursing homes despite a clear need.

The range of referrals and recommendations for treatment

Long-term care facilities differ considerably in many ways. Some are described as 'high care' (nursing homes, usually requiring 24-hour nursing care), others as 'low care' (staffed, but without necessarily having trained nursing staff, and commonly unlocked). They vary in their ability and willingness to provide care to patients with psychotic problems, severe dementia, particular behavioural manifestations (such as wandering or aggression), particular physical disabilities, and so on. Much depends on the structure of buildings and the expertise and attitudes of staff. Some facilities specialize in management of particular problems.

Loebel *et al.* (1991) described reasons for referral to their psychiatric service from six nursing homes over a two-year period. Nearly half of the 197 referred patients had a previous psychiatric history, with 19 per cent of the referrals being for follow-up of an established mental disorder after transfer from another clinician's care. Ninety-six residents (49 per cent) were referred because of behavioural problems, 35 per cent for mood-related reasons and 16 per cent because of psychotic features. Cognitive impairment, functional disability and adjustment problems were each cited as reasons for referral in less than 10 per cent of cases. Some patients were referred for more than one reason.

The authors commented that the problems for which psychiatric consultations were sought were similar across diagnostic categories. For example, the 96 patients referred because of behavioural problems were diagnosed as having dementia (45), affective or anxiety disorders (13), adjustment disorder (13), schizophrenia or paranoid disorder (11) or 'other' (14). Problems were thought to 'arise from the interaction of a broad range of emotional, cognitive, behavioral and illness-related factors in the context of caregiving relationships'.

The range of mental health problems on which advice may be sought is illustrated by the titles of chapters in books on psychiatric care in nursing homes (Conn *et al.*, 1992a;

Reichman and Katz, 1996; Birkett, 2001). The medical interface, death and dying, sexuality and sleep disorders are considered, along with delirium, personality disorders and the diagnoses mentioned by Loebel *et al.* (1991). There are also chapters on cognitive and behavioural therapy, psychotherapy, helping the family, and medico-legal and ethical issues. This emphasizes the breadth of the roles of mental health clinicians in residential care situations.

Much has been written concerning treatment of agitation in nursing homes, particularly in relation to use of neuroleptic medication. Herrmann and Lanctôt (1997) attempted to provide a rationale for why pharmacological treatments may be effective in cases of behavioural disturbance. Clinicians specializing in long-term residential care psychiatry must have extensive knowledge concerning geriatric psychopharmacology and medication trial reports in order to advise on management, and will know whether non-pharmacological treatments may be feasible and appropriate, sometimes *with* medication, in a particular setting. Camp *et al.* (2002) have reviewed the effectiveness of such interventions for a variety of behavioural problems, while Cody *et al.* (2002) discussed barriers to their more widespread use. The first step in treatment must be to try to understand reasons for the behaviour. The hypothesized explanation may lead to suggestions on how best to treat it. Cohen-Mansfield *et al.* (1990) and Cariaga *et al.* (1991) described situations where residents screamed, and commented that it may be a response to social isolation. Behavioural treatments work in some cases, but others appear resistant – most often when there is no obvious reason for the behaviour.

The various forms of depression, including demoralization, will also be a frequent focus of attention for the residential care psychiatrist, and aspects of treatment have been considered extensively (Rubinstein and Lawton, 1997). Katz *et al.* (1989) wrote that in long-term care facilities 'essentially all depressions can be considered secondary disorders, arising in the context of medical illness, neurological disease, or irreversible dementia'. They went on to say that the high prevalence of dysphoria and depression demands that psychotherapeutic services be made available in long term care. Rosen *et al.* (1997) reported that psychosocial interventions that restored a sense of choice and control to nursing home residents resulted in improvement in mood, whether or not they were taking antidepressants, and whether or not they fulfilled criteria for major depression.

Katz *et al.* (1990) and others have demonstrated that depression in residential care settings (most often comorbid with dementia) may well respond to antidepressants, though there is evidence that in this situation placebo treatments are nearly as effective. This points to the importance of psychosocial factors in relation to maintenance and outcome of such depressions. Grief-work, environmental adjustments, helping people to adjust to situations, and positive action in relation to disabilities and pain may be as important as pharmacology, or more so, if mood change is to be achieved and distress relieved.

Referrals to mental health clinicians will only be made if primary care doctors or facility staff recognize that there is a problem to be addressed or a disorder to be treated. To help alert staff and doctors that a resident may be depressed, it is appropriate to use screening instruments such as the Geriatric Depression Scale (Yesavage *et al.*, 1983) or the Cornell Scale for Depression in Dementia (Alexopoulos *et al.*, 1988). Most important of all is for staff to be alert to what residents say, to have time to discuss what they are feeling, and to document and report aspects that might suggest that a resident is worried, anxious, deluded or in any way distressed. The doctors need to work with facility staff as a team. It certainly helps restore optimal mental health to residents if staff have acquired expertise in recognizing mental disorders and in knowing whom to refer.

The future

Governments around the world have expressed concerns about the financial consequences of ageing of their populations. The mean age of people living in nursing homes is about 85 years. The proportion of the populations of various countries who are aged over 80 years will double within a generation, with obvious implications regarding needs for long-term care. About 20 per cent of those aged over 80 years have dementia. At least half of these will have moderate or severe dementia, and if current practices continue, a majority of such persons in the US, UK and countries with comparable long-term care arrangements, will be admitted to nursing homes. Governments will be looking to limit expenditure on such care. Alternative funding possibilities will be examined. There may well be expectations that people will provide for their own retirement needs, including the possibility of needing nursing home care. Some countries already rely on extended family arrangements in relation to care of persons with severe dementia, and many do not have accessible mental health services to advise and help with disturbed behaviour among this group. Long-term care provision in such countries has been insufficiently discussed in old age psychiatry journals. Even in some developed parts of the world there has been a move to separate dementia services (including care for people in nursing homes) from mental health services, with the result that behavioural disturbance and psychiatric problems comorbid with dementia do not receive attention from staff with psychiatric training. This concern may be somewhat diminished if psychologists are employed as part of the 'dementia service'.

The future requires attention now. A major problem in the long-term care residential sector in many places is a form of demoralization, with staff feeling under-appreciated, under-paid, and insufficiently supported, and a sense that no one is doing anything about it. Self-esteem of those who work in residential care facilities is not helped by the low status attached to such employment, and criticisms of the care provided there. What is needed, and soon, in countries such as the US, UK, Australia and Canada, is advocacy by government representatives and deliberate positive discrimination to ensure improved pay and morale, adequate staffing and an emphasis on restorative treatments.

As part of this process, there needs to be proper funding and support for mental health services. This includes education, but also, aged care facilities should be integrated as components of a local health service.

One initiative that received support twenty years ago was the concept of the *teaching nursing home* (Schneider, 1983; Libow, 1984). Inclusion of long-term care facilities as venues where academics could enable students (medical, nursing, etc.) to acquire knowledge about mental disorders, palliative care, treatment of pain, rehabilitation and long-term consequences of illnesses is desirable for many reasons. Those who have relatives in such institutions would surely welcome a new positive and inclusive approach. The risk is that governments will concentrate on the costs rather than the benefits of such initiatives, and long-term care facilities (which many populations will demand remain available) will be left to continue in a state of demoralization.

A description of long-term residential care facilities that foster optimal interventions and management for those with mental disorders, and optimal settings for preventing development of such disorders, would provide a satisfying conclusion to this chapter. However, what is ideal and possible in one situation (for example, central London) may not be in another (such as rural Texas or downtown Bangkok). Philosophies, cultures and funding possibilities differ. Ideally, residents of such facilities in any country will retain self-esteem through having as many opportunities for choice and control over their lives as their cognitive and physical function will allow. The setting will be home-like and the staff will respect and support residents, facilitating anything that contributes to positive self-regard. Caregiving will be person-centred, with recognition of 'the individuality, complexity and diversity of the dementia experience' (Sixsmith *et al.*, 1993). Staff will have adequate time to provide emotional as well as physical care, will enjoy their work and will be appropriately remunerated. Ongoing education will ensure that they recognize mental health problems and draw them to the attention of other team members. Residents' doctors will be knowledgeable and positive about the complex health needs of older people, and mental health professionals will be available as team members when needed to coordinate or conduct interventions in cases of psychiatric or behavioural disturbance. The concept of 'team approach' is important, though models will vary. The ideal outcome is for residents to be content and well settled, visitors to be confident that the residents are in appropriate surroundings, and for staff and visiting team members to know that optimal health care is being provided.

Leaders in the residential care field can of course have profound effects on morale. Where there are medical directors, it is important that they ensure high standards of medical care (including mental health services), and work with managers and directors of nursing to create positive attitudes among residents, relatives and staff. Good care includes an emphasis on identifying and treating reversible mental disorders, removing (as far as possible) reasons for demoralization, and maintaining or restoring self-esteem. Ideally, facility residents and their carers should be proud of what they are doing, and should say so.

References

Alexopoulos, G.S., Abrams, R.C., Young, R.C., and Shamoian, C.A. (1988) Cornell Scale for depression in dementia. *Biological Psychiatry*, **23**, 271–84.

American Geriatrics Society and American Association for Geriatric Psychiatry (2003) The American Geriatrics Society and American Association for Geriatric Psychiatry recommendations for policies in support of quality mental health care in US nursing homes. *Journal of the American Geriatrics Society*, **51**, 1299–304.

Ames, D. (1990) Depression among elderly residents of local-authority residential homes: its nature and the efficacy of intervention. *British Journal of Psychiatry*, **156**, 667–75.

Ballard, C., Powell, I., James, I., *et al.* (2002) Can psychiatric liaison reduce neuroleptic use and reduce health service utilization for dementia patients residing in care facilities? *International Journal of Geriatric Psychiatry*, **17**, 140–5.

Bartels, S.J., Moak, G.S., and Dums, A.R. (2002) Models of mental health services in nursing homes: a review of the literature. *Psychiatric Services*, **53**, 1390–6.

Bellelli, G., Frisoni, G.B., Bianchetti, A., *et al.* (1998) Special care units for demented patients: a multicenter study. *Gerontologist*, **38**, 456–62.

Bienenfeld, D. and Wheeler, B.G. (1989) Psychiatric services to nursing homes: a liaison model. *Hospital and Community Psychiatry*, **40**, 793–4.

Birkett, D.P. (2001) *Psychiatry in the Nursing Home*, 2nd edn. Haworth, New York.

Borson, S., Liptzin, B., Nininger, J., and Rabins, P. (1987) Psychiatry and the nursing home. *American Journal of Psychiatry*, **144**, 1412–18.

Borson, S., Loebel, J.P., Kitchell, M., Domoto, S., and Hyde, T. (1997) Psychiatric assessments of nursing home residents under OBRA-87: should PASARR be reformed? *Journal of the American Geriatrics Society*, **45**, 1173–81.

Brodaty, H., Draper, B.M., Millar, J., *et al.* (2003) Randomized controlled trial of different models of care for nursing home residents with dementia complicated by depression or psychosis. *Journal of Clinical Psychiatry*, **64**, 63–72.

Burns, B.J., Wagner, R., Taube, J.E., Magaziner, J., Permutt, T., and Landerman, L.R. (1993) Mental health service use by the elderly in nursing homes. *American Journal of Public Health*, **83**, 331–7.

Camp, C.J., Cohen-Mansfield, J., and Capezuti, E.A. (2002) Use of nonpharmacologic interventions among nursing home residents with dementia. *Psychiatric Services*, **53**, 1397–401.

Cariaga, J., Burgio, L., Flynn, W., and Martin, D. (1991) A controlled study of disruptive vocalizations among geriatric residents in nursing homes. *Journal of the American Geriatrics Society*, **39**, 501–7.

Challis, D., Reilly, S., Hughes, J., Burns, A., Gilchrist, H., and Wilson, K. (2002) Policy, organisation and practice of specialist old age psychiatry in England. *International Journal of Geriatric Psychiatry*, **17**, 1018–26.

Chartock, P., Nevins, A., Rzetelny, H., and Gilberto, P. (1988) A mental health training program in nursing homes. *Gerontologist*, **28**, 503–7.

Cody, M., Beck, C., and Svarstad, B.L. (2002) Challenges to the use of nonpharmacologic interventions in nursing homes. *Psychiatric Services*, **53**, 1402–6.

Cohen-Mansfield, J., Werner, P., and Marx, M.S. (1990) Screaming in nursing home residents. *Journal of the American Geriatrics Society*, **38**, 785–92.

Conn, D.K., Hermann, N., Kaye, A., Rewilak, D., Robinson, A., and Schogt, B. (eds.) (1992a) *Practical Psychiatry in the Nursing Home. A Handbook for Staff.* Hogrefe and Huber, Seattle.

Conn, D.K., Lee, V., Steingart, A., and Silberfeld, M. (1992b) Psychiatric services: a survey of nursing homes and homes for the aged in Ontario. *Canadian Journal of Psychiatry*, **37**, 525–30.

Depla, M.F.I.A., Pols, J., de Lange, J., Smits, C.H.M., de Graaf, R., and Heeren, T.J. (2003) Integrating mental health care into residential homes for the elderly: an analysis of six Dutch programs for older people with severe and persistent mental illness. *Journal of the American Geriatrics Society*, **51**, 1275–9.

Drinka, P.J. and Howell, T. (1991) The burden of mental disorders in the nursing home. *Journal of the American Geriatrics Society*, **39**, 730–3.

Fairbairn, A.F. (2002) Principles of service provision in old age psychiatry. In R. Jacoby and C. Oppenheimer (eds.) *Psychiatry in the Elderly*, 3rd edn. Oxford University Press, Oxford.

Gupta, S. and Goldstein, M.Z. (1999) Psychiatric consultation to nursing homes. *Psychiatric Services*, **50**, 1547–50.

Hanchuk, H.T. (1996) Psychiatric consultation and liaison. In W. E. Reichman and P. R. Katz (eds.) *Psychiatric Care in the Nursing Home*. Oxford University Press, New York.

Hermann, N. and Lanctôt, K.L. (1997) From transmitters to treatment: the pharmacotherapy of behavioural disturbances in dementia. *Canadian Journal of Psychiatry*, **42** (Suppl. 1), 51S–64S.

Jackson, G. and Lyons, D. (1996) Psychiatric clinics in residential homes for the elderly. *Psychiatric Bulletin*, **20**, 516–18.

Jolley, D. (1992) Nursing homes: the end of a great British tradition? *International Journal of Geriatric Psychiatry*, **7**, 71–3.

Jolley, D., Dixey, S., and Read, K. (1998) Residential and nursing homes. In R. Butler and B. Pitt (eds.) *Seminars in Old Age Psychiatry*. Gaskell, London.

Joseph, C., Goldsmith, S., Rooney, A., McWhorter, K., and Ganzini, L. (1995) An interdisciplinary mental health consultation team in a nursing home. *Gerontologist*, **35**, 836–9.

Kaprio, L.A. (1982) A statement from WHO. In P. Selby and M. Schechter (eds.) *Aging 2000: A Challenge for Society*. MTP Press, Lancaster.

Katz, I.R., Lesher, E., Kleban, M., Jethanandani, V., and Parmelee, P. (1989) Clinical features of depression in the nursing home. *International Psychogeriatrics*, **1**, 5–15.

Katz, I.R., Simpson, G.M., Curlik, S.M., Parmelee, P.A., and Muhly, C. (1990) Pharmacologic treatment of major depression for elderly patients in residential care settings. *Journal of Clinical Psychiatry*, **51** (Suppl. 7), 41–7.

Lantz, M.S. and Kennedy, G.J. (1995) The psychiatrist in the nursing home, part I: collaborative roles. *Psychiatric Services*, **46**, 15–16.

Lawton, M.P., Van Haitsma, K., Klapper, J., Kleban, M.H., Katz, I.R., and Corn, J. (1998) A stimulation-retreat special care unit for elders with dementing illness. *International Psychogeriatrics*, **10**, 379–95.

Libow, L.S. (1984) The teaching nursing home: past, present and future. *Journal of the American Geriatrics Society*, **32**, 598–603.

Lindesay, J., Briggs, K., Lawes, M., Macdonald, A., and Herzberg, J. (1995) The domus philosophy: a comparative evaluation of residential care for the demented elderly. In E. Murphy and G. Alexopoulos (eds.) *Geriatric Psychiatry. Key Research Topics for Clinicians*. Wiley, Chichester.

Llewellyn-Jones, R.H., Baikie, K.A., Smithers, H., *et al.* (1999) Multifaceted shared care intervention for late life depression in residential care: randomised controlled trial. *British Medical Journal*, **319**, 676–82.

Loebel, J.P., Borson, S., Hyde, T., *et al.* (1991) Relationships between requests for psychiatric consultations and psychiatric diagnoses in long-term-care facilities. *American Journal of Psychiatry*, **148**, 898–903.

Mechanic, D. and McAlpine, D.D. (2000) Use of nursing homes in the care of persons with severe mental illness: 1985–1995. *Psychiatric Services*, **51**, 354–8.

Moak, G. and Borson, S. (2000) Mental health services in long-term care. Still an unmet need. *American Journal of Geriatric Psychiatry*, **8**, 96–100.

Opie, J., Doyle, C., and O'Connor, D.W. (2002) Challenging behaviours in nursing home residents with dementia: a randomised controlled trial of multidisciplinary interventions. *International Journal of Geriatric Psychiatry*, **17**, 6–13.

Ouslander, J.G., Osterweil, D., and Morley, J. (1991) *Medical Care in the Nursing Home*. McGraw-Hill, New York.

Proctor, R., Burns, A., Powell, H.S., *et al.* (1999) Behavioural management in nursing and residential homes: a randomised controlled trial. *Lancet*, **354**, 26–9.

Reichman, W.E., Coyne, A.C., Borson, S., *et al.* (1998) Psychiatric consultation in the nursing home. A survey of six states. *American Journal of Geriatric Psychiatry*, **6**, 320–7.

Reichman, W.E. and Katz, P.R. (eds.) (1996) *Psychiatric Care in the Nursing Home*. Oxford University Press, New York.

Rosen, J., Rogers, J.C., Marin, R.S., Mulsant, B.H., Shahar, A., and Reynolds, C.F. (1997) Control-relevant intervention in the treatment of minor and major depression in a long-term care facility. *American Journal of Geriatric Psychiatry*, **5**, 247–57.

Rosewarne, R., Opie, J., Bruce, A., Ward, S., and Doyle, C. (1997) *Care Needs of People with Dementia and Challenging Behaviour Living in Residential Facilities. Resident Profile Survey*. Commonwealth of Australia, Canberra.

Rovner, B.W., German, P.S., Broadhead, J., *et al.* (1990) The prevalence and management of dementia and other psychiatric disorders in nursing homes. *International Psychogeriatrics*, **2**, 13–24.

Rovner, B.W. and Katz, I.R. (1993) Psychiatric disorders in the nursing home: a selective review of studies related to clinical care. *International Journal of Geriatric Psychiatry*, **8**, 75–87.

Rovner, B.W., Steele, C.D., Shmuely, Y., and Folstein, M.F. (1996) A randomized trial of dementia care in nursing homes. *Journal of the American Geriatrics Society*, **44**, 7–13.

Rubinstein, R.L. and Lawton, M.P. (eds.) (1997) *Depression in Long-term and Residential Care. Advances in research and treatment*. Springer, New York.

Ryan, J.M., Kidder, S.W., Daiello, L.A., and Tariot, P.N. (2002) Psychopharmacologic interventions in nursing homes: what do we know and where should we go? *Psychiatric Services*, **53**, 1407–13.

Sakauye, K.M. and Camp, C.J. (1992) Introducing psychiatric care into nursing homes. *Gerontologist*, **32**, 849–52.

Santmyer, K.S. and Roca, R.P. (1991) Geropsychiatry in long-term care: a nurse-centered approach. *Journal of the American Geriatrics Society*, **39**, 156–9.

Schmidt, L.J., Reinhardt, A.M., Kane, R.L., and Olsen, D.M. (1977) The mentally ill in nursing homes. New back wards in the community. *Archives of General Psychiatry*, **34**, 687–91.

Schneider, E.L. (1983) Teaching nursing homes. *New England Journal of Medicine*, **308**, 336.

Seidel, G., Smith, C., Hafner, R.J., and Holme, G. (1992) A psychogeriatric community outreach service: description and evaluation. *International Journal of Geriatric Psychiatry*, **7**, 347–50.

Selby, P. and Schechter, M. (1982) *Aging 2000: A Challenge for Society*. MTP Press, Lancaster.

Sixsmith, A., Stilwell, J., and Copeland, J. (1993) 'Rementia': challenging the limits of dementia care. *International Journal of Geriatric Psychiatry*, **8**, 993–1000.

Sloane, P.D., Mathew, L. J., Scarborough, M., Desai, J.R., Koch, G.G., and Tangen, C. (1991) Physical and pharmacologic restraint of nursing home patients with dementia. Impact of specialized units. *Journal of the American Medical Association*, **265**, 1278–82.

Snowden, M., Sato, K., and Roy-Byrne, P. (2003) Assessment and treatment of nursing home residents with depression or behavioural symptoms associated with dementia: a review of the literature. *Journal of the American Geriatrics Society,* **51**, 1305–17.

Snowdon, J. (1993) Mental health in nursing homes. Perspectives on the use of medication. *Drugs and Aging,* **3**, 122–30.

Snowdon, J. (2001) Psychiatric care in nursing homes: more must be done. *Australasian Psychiatry,* **9**, 108–12.

Streim, J.E., Oslin, D., Katz, I.R., and Parmelee, P.A. (1997) Lessons from geriatric psychiatry in the long term care setting. *Psychiatric Quarterly,* **68**, 281–307.

Streim, J.E., Beckwith, E.W., Arapakos, D., Banta, P., Dunn, R., and Hoyer, T. (2002) Regulatory oversight, payment policy, and quality improvement in mental health care in nursing homes. *Psychiatric Services,* **53**, 1414–18.

Tang, W.K., Chiu, H., Woo, J., Hjelm, M., and Hui, E. (2001) Telepsychiatry in a psychogeriatric service: a pilot study. *International Journal of Geriatric Psychiatry,* **16**, 88–93.

Wancata, J., Benda, N., Hajji, M., Lesch, O., and Müller, C. (1998) Prevalence and course of psychiatric disorders among nursing home admissions. *Social Psychiatry and Psychiatric Epidemiology,* **33**, 74–9.

Yesavage, J.A., Brink, T.L., Rose, T.L., *et al.* (1983) Development and validation of a geriatric depression screening scale: a preliminary report. *Journal of Psychiatric Research,* **17**, 37–49.

Chapter 16

Specialized service components

David K. Conn

The purpose of this chapter is to describe a number of specialized psychogeriatric services including the day hospital, memory clinic, consultation-liaison service, respite service and services for younger individuals suffering from dementia. These services are ideally components of a larger comprehensive psychogeriatric programme, which would also include inpatient and community outreach services (Sadavoy and Conn, 1994). In addition some special issues relevant to academic psychogeriatric services will be addressed.

Good quality of care for older people with mental health problems should be comprehensive, accessible, responsive, individualized, transdisciplinary, accountable and systematic as described in the Consensus Statement issued by the World Health Organization and World Psychiatric Association (Graham *et al.*, 1998). This Consensus Statement also outlines the full range of psychogeriatric services that would be provided in an ideal system. Unfortunately, an international survey found that only three countries (the Netherlands, UK and Switzerland) consistently provided a full range of long-term, hospital-based and community-based geriatric programmes (Reifler and Cohen, 1998). A comprehensive review of the effectiveness of old age psychiatry services (Draper, 2000) reported a growing increase in service evaluation data, although much of it had been generated from uncontrolled audits. Fortunately, the number of controlled trials demonstrating the efficacy of service provision was noted to be increasing.

Day hospitals

Craft defined a day hospital as 'one where full hospital treatment is given under medical supervision to patients who return to their homes each night' (Craft, 1959). The American Association for Partial Hospitalization set out the following definition in 1980:

> Partial hospitalization is an ambulatory treatment program that includes the major diagnostic, medical, psychiatric, psychosocial and prevocational treatment modalities for serious mental disorders which require coordinated, intensive, comprehensive and multidisciplinary treatment not provided in an outpatient clinic setting. It allows for a more flexible and less restrictive treatment program by offering an alternative to inpatient treatment.
>
> Casarino *et al.*, 1982

It has been suggested that older patients are more likely to be treated in a day programme in the United Kingdom as compared to the United States (Tourigny-Rivard and Potoczny, 1996). Indeed, geriatric psychiatry day hospitals are a mandated component of the British health care system, where established guidelines recommend two to three geriatric psychiatry day hospital places per 1,000 older people (Peace, 1982). Studies from the UK have shown higher numbers of patients with dementia than with functional psychiatric disorders in geriatric psychiatry day hospital programmes. In North America, some of these individuals may be treated in day care rather than day hospital programmes.

Wagner (1991) has described seven guiding principles in specialized partial hospitalization for older people:

1. Services that meet a continuum of needs of older adults;

2. Services that are cost-effective and economically viable;

3. Services that are accessible and acceptable;

4. Programmes that provide an interdisciplinary orientation;

5. Individualized assessment and treatment planning;

6. Enhancement of family and community supports; and

7. Restitution of capacity.

It has been suggested that in order to fulfill these guidelines, the geriatric psychiatry day hospital should ideally be staffed by a multidisciplinary team. Some key issues in the organization of geriatric day hospitals include the large variations in diagnostic groups, potential dependency on the programme, discharge planning with the goal of short-term admissions and the practical aspects of transportation to and from the day hospital. Because of the potentially therapeutic value of time spent travelling with other patients, the term 'transport therapy' has been used, although others have used the term pejoratively.

There has been significant debate regarding the effectiveness of geriatric day hospitals. Draper (2000), in his review of the effectiveness of old age psychiatry services notes that the role of day hospitals in acute care, remains unresolved and rated the level of evidence for effectiveness to be low. He noted that there is some evidence that day hospitals may diminish the need for inpatient admissions, but this evidence is unconvincing.

Several uncontrolled studies have demonstrated that patients treated in day hospitals improve over time (Steingart, 1992; Conn et al., 2000; Plotkin and Wells, 1993). In one study better outcomes were associated with mood disorders, initial functional status, greater social support, a low level of stress and longer duration of treatment (Plotkin and Wells, 1993). Fasey (1994) and Howard (1994) debated the case for and against geriatric day hospitals. Murphy (1994), in an accompanying editorial, noted that day hospitals are not homogeneous institutions. She noted that many day hospitals in the UK provide daily respite care relief for relatives of people with dementia and suggested that this type of respite does not need to be provided in a hospital, or necessarily staffed by health care professionals. On the other hand, some day hospitals focus on the care of older people with functional psychiatric illness where attendance is time limited, focused on specific treatment regimens and where patients will benefit from specialist care. Unfortunately, some patients with depressive illnesses are not willing to attend a day hospital and, as a result, these services are not always effective alternatives to admission for the patient who needs close supervision. Fasey (1994), arguing against day hospitals, suggested that they are usually staffed by expensive health service professionals, but provide very little in the way of specific care or treatment. Fasey also suggested that day hospitals probably do not prevent admission to acute or continuing care facilities. He argued that day hospitals may actually increase family burden and workload rather than diminish it because attending a day programme disrupts familiar routines. He noted that further research was required to compare psychiatric treatment in different settings. Howard (1994) on the other hand, emphasized the effectiveness of day hospitals as alternatives to inpatient admission and noted that discharge from inpatient wards can be made earlier using the day hospital as a halfway house, while the patient gains confidence and competence at home and a social network is re-established. He also noted that the day hospital may provide a convenient venue for a full assessment that requires complex investigations. He argued that in some cases day hospitals do provide important relief for burdened caregivers. He also emphasized the difference between day hospitals and day-care centres. He stressed that levels of staff satisfaction are very high in day hospitals and that day hospitals have an important role in the maintenance of morale on geriatric psychiatry services. He reiterated the proposal of Donaldson et al. (1986), suggesting a research strategy with data to be collected in four main areas:

1. Comparisons of outcomes for subgroups of day hospital patients with similar subgroups utilizing alternative models of care;

2. Costing of each patient's consumption of care within treatment and subsequent service use, over a determined time period;

3. Standardized collection of clinical, social and psychological outcome data and measures of dependency at the beginning, during and at the end of the study period; and

4. Some measure of patient and caregiver satisfaction with the treatment received.

Memory clinics

Memory clinics were first established in North America in the 1970s and, subsequently, in the United Kingdom in the following decade (Phipps and O'Brien, 2002). Wright and Lindesay surveyed British memory clinics in 1995. Twenty memory clinics were identified and in most cases the profile of the memory clinic was as a specialized multidisciplinary hospital-based assessment service linked to a programme focusing most commonly on anti-dementia drug trials. The overall goal of memory clinics is to improve dementia care, with the clinic as one part of the pathway towards high quality of care. A repeat survey of British memory clinics (Lindesay et al., 2002) reported an increased number of clinics to at least 58. The authors reported the development of a broader range of service models from traditional academic research clinics to newer clinics funded by the National Health Service, which tend to be smaller and to concentrate more on service provision than research or education. The core functions were described by the authors as specialist assessment; information and advice to patients, caregivers and doctors; initiation and monitoring of treatment; and education and training. Phipps and O'Brien (2002) offer a generic specification for memory clinic development with a focus on mild cognitive impairment, as an illustration of the standards of quality that might be achieved. The authors offer a series of useful recommendations, for example, 'the extent to which diagnostic information is discussed with patients should be negotiated individually and sensitively with them in response to their wishes'. The authors also note that management plans should be formulated to include pharmacological and non-pharmacological aspects of care.

Lindesay et al. (2002), in their recent extensive survey of memory clinics in the British Isles, noted that the substantial growth in number of clinics has been stimulated by the licensing of cholinesterase inhibitor drugs for Alzheimer's disease and the development of services for early-onset dementia. They reported that most of the new memory clinics had been set up within old age psychiatry programmes. The lead clinician in 66 per cent of responders was a geriatric psychiatrist. A wide range of professionals work in these clinics, including psychiatrists (79 per cent of clinics), nurses (71 per cent), psychologists (60 per cent), physicians/geriatricians (28 per cent), occupational therapists (16 per cent), speech therapists (10 per cent) and neurologists (21 per cent). Of interest was the fact that only 33 per cent of the clinics routinely follow-up all of their patients. Other clinics follow up diagnostically uncertain cases and/or selected diagnostic groups only. The number of patients per clinic receiving cholinesterase inhibitors varied considerably, ranging from six to 400. Other commonly used treatments and interventions included aspirin, vitamin E, ginkgo biloba, anxiety management and memory training. The authors note that there have been few outcome studies of memory clinics, although one study suggested that the provision of education, counselling and onward referral to support services can improve the quality of life of caregivers (LoGiudice et al., 1999). Although there was significant improvement in psychosocial health related quality of life among caregivers in this study, there was no significant difference in caregiver psychological morbidity, caregiver burden or caregiver knowledge of dementia.

Much of the literature on memory clinics focuses on the issue of the detection of potentially reversible cognitive impairment. It has been reported that the rate of both potential and actual reversibility of dementia is low in memory clinic patients.

Patients whose condition improves with intervention are more likely to have early and milder cognitive deficits (Freter *et al.*, 1998). It has also been suggested that a routine battery of laboratory investigations should be replaced with selected investigations based on clinical indicators (Burke *et al.*, 2000). An interesting study from Melbourne comparing non-English-speaking patients to English-speaking patients found that non-English-speaking patients with dementia presented at a later stage of their disease and that non-English-speaking patients were more likely to present with a functional psychiatric disorder (particularly depression) or normal cognition (LoGiudice *et al.*, 2001). A study by van Hout (2001) evaluated the opinions of memory clinic users. It was reported that patients, caregivers and general practitioners had positive opinions about the diagnostic value of the memory clinic. The author suggested that quality improvement could focus on clarity of the diagnostic information for patients and on better advice to relatives.

Flynn *et al.* (2000) described the development of 14 regional cognitive, dementia and memory services (CDMS) across the state of Victoria in Australia. The aim is to provide integrated dementia services at all levels of the health care system. A number of clinical indicators have been developed to evaluate services, including prompt response to assessment of referrals, adequate counselling of caregivers and development of linkages with GPs and other care services. It is also noted that patients should have the option of being assessed at home where possible.

As more advances are made in the treatment of Alzheimer's disease and other forms of dementia, it is likely that the development of memory clinics around the world will continue. These clinics are most likely to succeed when they are multidisciplinary and when they are fully integrated with the rest of the health care system. Studies focusing on the cost-effectiveness of memory clinics would be most helpful. Some critics note that these clinics are generally expensive, labour intensive and inefficient – often adopting a standardized battery of assessments and investigations. Another criticism is that the 'clinic' approach often provides medication but limited psychosocial interventions. Nevertheless memory clinics do generally provide comprehensive assessments, good training and opportunities for research.

Consultation-liaison services

As early as 1983 Lipowski underlined the need to integrate consultation-liaison psychiatry and psychiatry of old age. There is considerable overlap between the two sub-specialties because approximately 30–40 per cent of patients admitted to general hospitals are aged 65 years or older and the actual number of bed days for seniors is more than 50 per cent of the total. In addition, approximately 30 per cent of psychiatric consultations in general hospitals are for elderly patients. Rabins *et al.* (1983) compared psychiatric consultations of elderly patients with those of a younger group of patients. Despite the fact that 28.5 per cent of the hospital beds were occupied by patients over the age of 60, only 21 per cent of all consultations were carried out on these patients. The authors suggested several reasons for the fewer than expected geriatric consultations, including decreased severity of illness, lack of recognition by referring physicians, atypical disorders and ageism. The most common diagnoses among the elderly who received consultations were cognitive disorders (54 per cent) and depression (27 per cent). Popkin *et al.* (1984) reported 1,072 consultations of patients. Organic mental disorders were the most common (46 per cent) for the elderly, 23 per cent of whom suffered from affective disorders. The authors noted that patients aged 60 or older were referred less often than younger patients, with requests for referral coming later during the hospitalization, and suggested a number of explanations for the lower than expected geriatric referral rate. They suggested that referring physicians may be too tolerant of cognitive dysfunction and behavioural abnormalities, that organic mental disorders may be under diagnosed and that treatment of these patients may be carried out by the attending physician or referred to other specialties such as neurology. Ruskin (1985) described 67 geriatric consultations on patients 60 years of age and older. These consultations represented 16.5 per cent of the total number of patients referred for consultations. The most common reasons for referral were: requests for competency evaluations; help in diagnosing and treating specific symptoms; and assistance with psychotropic use. Fifty-four per cent of the patients were suspected of having an underlying organic component in their psychiatric presentation.

Small and Fawzy (1988) proposed a collaborative model of care for the geriatric patient in the general hospital, making elderly patients the central focus of four existing services, i.e. general medicine, consultation-liaison psychiatry, geriatric medicine and geriatric psychiatry. The authors reported on 160 psychiatric consultations performed by the consultation-liaison service of UCLA and described differences between a younger group of patients and an older group (over the age of 60). Referring physicians asked for evaluations of depression and mental status examinations more often for older than for younger patients. Older patients required longer consultation notes and tended to have more family members involved during the hospitalization. Treatment recommendations differed between groups, with older patients receiving antidepressants and psychostimulants more often, as well as more laboratory investigations, such as thyroid function tests and CT scans.

A number of studies have compared the liaison approach to a more traditional consultation approach in the care of the hospitalized elderly. Reported benefits from a liaison approach have included higher referral rates, more referrals for depression, a higher degree of diagnostic accuracy by referring doctors, more reviews by the psychiatric consultant and increased compliance with psychotropic recommendations (Draper, 2000). Scott *et al.* (1988) described referrals to a psychogeriatric consultation-liaison service in Newcastle. They describe 217 patients who had been referred over a three-year period with a median age of 79.5 years. The most prevalent psychiatric diagnoses were dementia, delirium and depression. Interestingly, the pattern of referrals changed significantly following the introduction of a liaison service to the hospital's geriatric unit. The number of referrals increased by over 100 per cent and there was a significant increase in the recognition and referral of functional psychiatric disorders, especially depression. DeLeo *et al.* (1989) described a six-year experience of psychiatric consultation in a geriatric hospital in Italy. The most common referrals were for patients with cardiovascular and gastrointestinal problems and the most frequent reasons for referral were mood disorders, anxiety disorders and organic mental disorders. Interestingly the most common final diagnoses were dysthymic disorder, anxiety disorders and adjustment disorder. The study confirmed the high prevalence of minor affective disorders among the hospitalized elderly. During the study, a new psychogeriatric unit was established and the services offered by the team subsequently underwent considerable innovation. There was a higher availability of psychiatrists, which resulted in improved interpersonal relationships. There also appeared to be a marked reduction in the length of hospital stays.

Draper (2000) noted that there have been few controlled trials of C-L services for the elderly and the overall results in terms of psychiatric outcome have been modest, with two studies demonstrating only non-significant trends towards improvement on measures of depression and cognitive function (Cole *et al.*, 1991; Strain *et al.*, 1991). Nevertheless, the study by Strain *et al.* did show impressive cost reductions and reductions in length of stay when elderly patients with hip fractures received a psychiatric C-L intervention. In addition, Levitan and Kornfeld (1981) reported that elderly patients with hip fracture who received psychiatric consultation spent 12 fewer days in hospital and were discharged home more often, when compared with the patients who did not receive a consultation.

Unützer and Small (1996) offer some practical advice with regard to the practice of geriatric consultation-liaison psychiatry. They focus on the need to work with the medical team by establishing a working relationship, the importance of defining the question asked by the consultee, bearing in mind that consultation requests often contain stated and unstated questions. They also describe an optimal approach for providing recommendations, which should be concise and easily understood by non-psychiatric colleagues. They also make reference to some of Pasnau's 'Ten Commandments of Medical Etiquette for Psychiatrists', which urged a consultant to communicate in person with the clinician who requested advice, to respect them as fellow physicians and colleagues, to be available and prompt, to give concrete suggestions, to follow up and 'not to preach' (Pasnau, 1985).

Respite care

Respite care can be defined as a caregiving service that provides a planned, temporary, break from the ongoing responsibility of caring for a dependent person who is living at home (Flint, 1995). Five major categories of respite care were described by Hegeman (1989):

1. in home

2. in the community

3. in institutions caring for elderly individuals

4. in hospitals

5. combination models.

Caregivers of individuals with dementia living in the community often experience extreme levels of stress and caregiver burden has been associated with significant emotional, physical, social and financial costs (Morris *et al.*, 1988). The potential goals of respite care include providing caregivers with a rest, reducing caregiver burden and stress and postponing, or avoiding, nursing home placement.

In their 1991 review Zarit and Teri reported that the first generation studies of interventions and services for caregivers had demonstrated 'an expectedly modest amount of improvement, given the complexity of caregivers' lives and the relatively limited magnitude of the interventions'. In their review of residential respite care, Brodaty and Gresham (1992) concluded that there was little empirical evidence for the efficacy of this intervention despite it being the most popularly requested help by caregivers. In one study (Mohide *et al.*, 1990), there was evidence of a clinically significant improvement in the quality of life of caregivers. Burdz *et al.* (1988) found that patients' problematic behaviour improved with institutional respite care, but, unfortunately, caregivers reported a significant worsening of the relationship following respite.

Flint (1995) carried out a systematic review of respite care studies. Ultimately, only four studies met the inclusion and validity criteria. The types of respite care included in these studies were institutional, in home and day care. The duration of respite care varied from ten weeks to 12 months. Flint concluded there was little evidence that formal respite care has a significant effect on caregivers' burden, psychiatric status or physical health, or on patients' cognition, function, physical health or rate of institutionalization. Nevertheless, the author cautions that given the small number of controlled studies and their methodological and conceptual limitations, the data should be interpreted with caution. Gräsel (1997) focused on temporary institutional respite (TIR) or residential respite care. Although there appeared to be evidence of only a slight reduction of subjective burden for caregivers, Gräsel points out that there is a clear need for respite services because many caregivers are at high risk themselves of physical or mental illness. Studies have shown that TIR is utilized primarily by adult child caregivers (daughters and daughters-in-law) who are affected by a high subjective burden.

A report from Canada (Canadian Study of Health and Aging, 1994) suggests that TIR is not commonly utilized by caregivers of non-institutionalized clients. Only 3.1 per cent of dementia patients utilized temporary institutional respite within a one-year period. Brodaty and Gresham (1992) described a number of barriers that limit caregiver's utilization of respite care. These include barriers that may derive from the caregivers themselves: caregiver guilt, financial reasons, cultural attitudes and lack of information. Structural barriers include: unavailability, lack of publicity, long waiting lists and lack of identification of at-risk caregivers. Barriers that may derive from the patients include: severe problem behaviours, immobility, incontinence, wandering and inability to communicate. They recommended that respite care needs to be 'prescribed' with the same rigour as for medications, with indications, contraindications and possible adverse reactions (e.g. increased behavioural disturbance on return home). In addition, caregivers should be educated in the best way to use respite care. Both Flint and Gräsel suggest that improved methodology is required in future studies of respite care.

Services for younger people with dementia

The prevalence of Alzheimer's disease for individuals aged 45–64 has been estimated to be 34.6 per 100,000 (Newens et al., 1993). In addition, the rates for pre-senile vascular dementia were 11.7 per 100,000, and 27 per 100,000 for other types of pre-senile dementia. It has been estimated that there are approximately 17,000 younger people with dementia in Britain (Baldwin and Murray, 2000). Difficulties obtaining a diagnosis of dementia in younger patients have been frequently cited (Ferran et al., 1996).

The Alzheimer's Association of Australia commissioned a survey because of concern about lack of information regarding younger people with dementia and their caregivers, and relative neglect in service planning for this group (Luscombe et al., 1998). One hundred and two responses were analysed representing caregivers of 49 individuals with Alzheimer's disease, 24 with Huntington's disease and 29 with other dementias. The average age of these individuals at the time of the survey was 53.3. Diagnostic problems were reported by 71 per cent of the caregivers. The mean time until diagnosis had been 3.4 years. Fifty-nine per cent of working caregivers reduced their hours or stopped working after the diagnosis and 89 per cent of all caregivers had experienced financial problems subsequent to the diagnosis. Caregivers who were considered to be most vulnerable to psychological distress were younger females caring for males with pre-senile dementia and children caring for parents. The authors suggested that services needed to be aware of the special issues facing younger people with dementia and hoped that greater community awareness of dementia in this age group would encourage earlier presentation, reduce denial and inspire community initiatives to help. Because of unmet needs, a declaration of rights for younger people with dementia was developed in 1991 by the Mersey Regional Health Authority, UK (Baldwin and Murray, 2000). These rights include full medical assessments, recognition of the need for specialist services, access to day care services, appropriate residential care, case management and welfare benefits and retrospective reinstatement of rights and benefits.

One study compared the diagnostic practices of two teaching hospital departments (neurology and geriatric psychiatry) in the investigation of younger people with cognitive problems (Allen and Baldwin, 1995). Individuals assessed in the neurology department were more likely to receive a comprehensive medical assessment and neuropsychological testing as well as brain imaging. Given the difficulty making the diagnosis and the frequent overlap between mood disorders and cognitive disorders in this age group, Baldwin and Murray suggest that the optimum model is for a neurologist and a psychiatrist to work together.

It has been suggested that younger people with dementia may have a more rapid downhill course, but Newens *et al.* reported that the mean survival time from onset to death was over nine years. Baldwin (1994) found greater morbidity from behavioural and other non-cognitive symptoms than from cognitive impairment in a study of 44 patients with early-onset dementia.

The Faculty of Old Age Psychiatry of the Royal College of Psychiatrists (UK) has proposed guidelines for the development of services for younger people with dementia (Baldwin and Murray, 2000). It is recommended that a small, dedicated multidisciplinary team should be developed in each area with a population base of 500,000. In smaller communities it is suggested that a designated community nurse be made available for this population. Initial service development should focus on diagnostic and community services, whereas a comprehensive service comprises additional day programmes, respite care and specific long-stay care programmes. Baldwin and Murray (2000) provide practical advice regarding the planning of services for younger people with dementia and also described samples of successful services that have been developed in Manchester, Merseyside and Newcastle (UK).

Academic psychogeriatric services

Academic psychogeriatric services face the difficult challenge of integrating comprehensive clinical care with teaching and training, while at the same time developing an adequate infrastructure for research. The challenges associated with running a combined clinical and academic programme include recruitment of staff with a keen interest in academics, obtaining adequate funding to support teaching and research, and ensuring that staff dedicate adequate time to patient care. The benefits include the creation of a highly stimulating work environment, the extra care provided by trainees, opportunities for patients to participate in research studies of newly available therapies and increased opportunities for collaboration with colleagues in other regions or countries.

An international survey of 55 countries found that in most nations training programmes in geriatric psychiatry are in relatively early stages of development (Reifler and Cohen, 1998). Only five countries achieved a mean score of 2.5 out of 4 on a scale that focused on the development of training programmes and subspecialization (the UK, US, Finland, Canada and Sweden). Within medical schools there is a vital need to develop first-rate training programmes for postgraduate trainees and advanced training for those wishing to specialize. It is also critically important that exposure to psychogeriatrics be available for undergraduate students in medicine and other disciplines.

Halpain and colleagues (1999) have described training needs and strategies in geriatric mental health in the US. They reported that the American Association for Geriatric Psychiatry had approximately 1500 members, and 2300 psychiatrists had passed the American Board of Psychiatry and Neurology examination for added qualifications in Geriatric Psychiatry. Nevertheless, the authors note that the number of geriatric and gerontologic specialists in mental health available across disciplines is exceptionally small given the need, and emphasize that the supply of both specialists and resources cannot meet current or future demands. On the positive side, the existing cadre of academics, although small in number, are highly devoted to the field, as clinicians, teachers, and researchers, despite limited recognition during an era of limited support. Among the specific recommendations described were: a need to expand the core curriculum on aging and late life mental disorders in professional programmes; a need to increase incentives for individuals who seek specialty training in geriatric mental health and; a need to diversity the range of advanced training opportunities available.

Lieff *et al.* (2003a) recently examined the effect of training and other influences on the development of career interests in geriatric psychiatry. The timing of individualized teaching exposure as well as lectures in geriatric psychiatry was associated with the development of first interest in the field. The most important influences on the development of interest included specific teacher attributes, training experiences, personal experiences with seniors, and characteristics cited as unique to geriatric psychiatry, such as the medical, neuropsychiatric and multifactorial nature of the field. The authors emphasize that it behooves geriatric psychiatry programmes to create exemplary educators and commit them to teaching in the early years of general psychiatry programmes as well as in medical school. Lieff and Clarke (2002) recently reported that the nature of the educational experience during a psychiatry residency had a significant influence on whether graduates would see older patients in their practices.

Geriatric educational requirements in postgraduate training programmes for psychiatrists vary considerably from country to country. For example, in the United States, residents have been required to complete one month of training in geriatric psychiatry since 2001. In Canada, training guidelines guidelines were developed in 1989 by the section on geriatric psychiatry of the Canadian Psychiatric Association (Thorpe *et al.*, 1993). A survey conducted in the fall of 1991 found that more than 80 per cent of Canadian training centres required residents to have a formal rotation in geriatric psychiatry, which was generally three months in length. Shulman *et al.* (1986) described the early development of geriatric psychiatry services in a university general hospital, noting that an integrative model enhanced the quality of health care delivery to the elderly, while at the same time improving training and recruitment. Lieff *et al.* (2003b) recently surveyed 62 geriatric psychiatry fellowship programmes in the United States, reporting that the number of programmes had slowly increased over the previous seven years. Although training directors reported that the application rates for fellowship positions were stable during the academic years 1999–2002, the fill-rate for first year fellowship positions dropped from 84 per cent in 1999/2000 to 61 per cent in 2001/2002. The authors concluded that recruiting high quality graduates into geriatric psychiatry fellowship programmes remains a challenge. They also suggested that specific strategies are required to stimulate undergraduate and graduate interest in careers in clinical and academic geriatric psychiatry.

There has been rapid growth in the development of psychogeriatric research programmes in recent years, primarily in academic centres. For example a recent review of research into depressive disorder in late life found a total of 1002 publications between the years of 1998 and 2001 (Baldwin, 2002). However, less than 10 per cent represented randomized control studies, and there were comparatively few studies of psychological and psychosocial interventions. Two-thirds of all publications originated in north America or northern Europe. The need for special attention to neglected late life mental disorders such as schizophrenia, anxiety disorders, alcohol dependence, and personality disorders has been emphasized (Kennedy, 2002). Rabins (1999) notes that the research agenda in geriatric mental health has been broad, focusing on psychosocial, behavioural, and biological aspects. He noted that federal funds in the US through The National Institute of Mental Health and The National Institute on Aging have been complimented by private foundations. Advances range from molecular biological studies of normal and pathological aging, through neuroimaging studies of common late life disorders, to health services research, descriptive clinical studies, and demonstration of the benefit of psychopharmacological and psychotherapeutic interventions. Rabins also notes that in the future, primary and secondary prevention will become increasingly important and hopefully will add to the quality of life of older citizens.

Challenges for geriatric researchers include the unique ethical issues related to conducting research with elderly subjects. Jeste *et al.* (2003) described an approach for empirical research with the goal of assessing and possibly improving decisional capacity in older people with severe mental illness. Cherniack (2002) notes that alterations in methods of obtaining consent may help individuals to be more informed and even enable subjects, who lack the capacity to consent, to participate in research.

Shulman (1994) provided suggestions for consideration, which would ensure a strong future for geriatric psychiatry. He emphasized the need for collaborative research with a focus on improved diagnostic discrimination and outcome studies. He noted the need for better integration with geriatric medicine and gerontology and the need to maintain a focus and priority on service delivery and health care systems. In particular, he underlined the need for the development of an academic base and academic credibility, which will ensure the advancement of the field, while attracting the brightest of young psychiatrists. Shulman also noted the need for charismatic and credible leadership, and individuals with the qualities of social consciousness, clinical astuteness and academic inquisitiveness. Although these comments were made almost a decade ago, they remain equally relevant and particularity important for those organizing academic psychogeriatric services.

References

Allen, H. and Baldwin, B. (1995) The referral, investigation and diagnosis of presenile dementia: two services compared. *International Journal of Geriatric Psychiatry*, **10**, 185–90.

Baldwin, R.C. (1994) Acquired cognitive impairment in the presenium. *Psychiatric Bulletin*, **18**, 463–5.

Baldwin, R.C. (2002) Research into depressive disorder in later life: who is doing what? A literature search from 1998–2001. *International Psychogeriatrics*, **38**, 335–46.

Baldwin, R. and Murray, M. (2000) Services for younger people with dementia. In J. O'Brien, D. Ames and L. Flicker (eds.) *Dementia*, 2nd edn, pp. 353–9. Arnold, London.

Brodaty, H. and Gresham, M. (1992) Prescribing residential respite care for dementia: effects, side-effects, indications and dosage. *International Journal of Geriatric Psychiatry*, **7**, 357–62.

Burdz, M.P., Eaton, W.O. and Bond, J.B. Jr (1988) Effect of respite care on dementia and non-dementia patients and their caregivers. *Psychology and Aging*, **3**, 38–42.

Burke, D., Sengoz, A., and Schwartz, R. (2000) Potentially reversible cognitive impairment in patients presenting to a memory disorders clinic. *Journal of Clinical Neurosciences*, **7**, 120–3.

Canadian Study of Health and Aging (1994) Patterns of caring for people with dementia in Canada. *Canadian Journal on Aging*, **13**, 470–87.

Casarino, J.P., Wilner, M., and Maxey, J.T. (1982) American Association for Partial Hospitalization (AAPH) standards and guidelines for partial hospitalization. *International Journal of Partial Hospitalization*, **1**, 5–21.

Cherniack, E.P. (2002) Informed consent for medical research by the elderly. *Experimental Aging Research*, **28**, 183–98.

Cole, M.G., Fenton, F.R., Engelsmann, F., and Mansouri, I. (1991) Effectiveness of geriatric psychiatry consultation in an acute care hospital: a randomized clinical trial. *Journal of the American Geriatrics Society*, **39**, 1183–8.

Conn, D.K., Clarke, D., and Van Reekum, R. (2000) Depression in holocaust survivors: profile and treatment outcome in a geriatric day hospital program. *International Journal of Geriatric Psychiatry*, **15**, 331–7.

Craft, M. (1959) Psychiatric day hospitals. *American Journal of Psychiatry*, **116**, 251–4.

DeLeo, D., Baiocchi, A., Cipollone, B., Pavan, L., and Beltrame, P. (1989) Psychogeriatric consultation within a geriatric hospital: a six-year experience. *International Journal of Geriatric Psychiatry*, **4**, 135–41.

Donaldson, C., Wright, K., and Maynard, A. (1986) Determining value for money in day hospital care for the elderly. *Age and Aging*, **15**, 1–7.

Draper, B. (2000) The effectiveness of old age psychiatry services. *International Journal of Geriatric Psychiatry*, **15**, 687–703.

Fasey, C. (1994) The day hospital in old age psychiatry. *International Journal of Geriatric Psychiatry*, **9**, 519–23.

Ferran, J., Wilson, K.C.M., and Doran, M. (1996) The early onset dementias: a study of clinical characteristics and service use. *International Journal of Geriatric Psychiatry*, **11**, 863–9.

Flint, A.J. (1995) Effects of respite care on patients with dementia and their caregivers. *International Psychogeriatrics*, **7**, 505–17.

Flynn, E., Ames, D., and LoGiudice, D. (2000) Services for dementia: an Australian view. In J. O'Brien, D. Ames and L. Flicker (eds.) *Dementia*, 2nd edn, pp. 329–333. Arnold, London.

Freter, S., Bergman, H., Gold, S., Chertkow, H., and Clarfield, A.M. (1998) Prevalence of potentially reversible dementias and actual reversibility in a memory clinic cohort. *Canadian Medical Association Journal*, **159**, 657–62.

Graham, N., Diener, O., Dyfey, A.-F., *et al.* (1998) Organization of care in psychiatry of the elderly – a technical consensus statement. *Aging and Mental Health*, **2**, 246–52.

Gräsel, E. (1997) Temporary institutional respite in dementia cases: who utilizes this form of respite care and what effect does it have? *International Psychogeriatrics*, **9**, 437–48.

Halpain, M.C., Harris, M.J., McClure, F.S., and Jeste, D.V. (1999) Training in geriatric mental health: needs and strategies. *Psychiatric Services*, **50**, 1205–8.

Hegeman, C.R. (1989) *Geriatric Respite Care: Expanding and Improving Practice*. Foundation for Long-Term Care. Albany, New York.

Howard, R. (1994) Day hospitals: the case in favour. *International Journal of Geriatric Psychiatry*, **9**, 525–9.

Jeste, D.V., Dunn, L.V., Palmer, B.W., *et al.* (2003) A collaborative model for research on decisional capacity and informed consent in older patients with schizophrenia: Bioethics unit of a geriatric psychiatry intervention research center. *Psychopharmacology (Berlin)*. May 27. [Epub ahead of print].

Kennedy, G.J. (2002) *Testimony: President's New Freedom Commission on Mental Health*. http://www.aagponline.org/advocacy/testimony.asp?viewfull=11

Levitan, S. and Kornfeld, D. (1981) Clinical and cost benefits of liaison psychiatry. *American Journal of Psychiatry*, **138**, 790–3.

Lieff, S.J., Tolomiczenko, G.S., and Dunn, L.B. (2003a) Effect of training and other influences on the development of career interest in geriatric psychiatry. *American Journal of Geriatric Psychiatry*, **11**, 300–8.

Lieff, S.J., Warshaw, G.A., Bragg, E.J., Shaull, R.W., Lindsell, C.J., and Goldenhar, L.M. (2003b) Geriatric psychiatry fellowship programs in the United States: findings from the association of directors of geriatric academic programs' longitudinal study of training and practice. *American Journal of Geriatric Psychiatry*, **11**, 291–9.

Lieff, S. and Clarke, D. (2002) Canadian geriatric psychiatrists: why do they do it? A Delphi study. *Canadian Journal of Psychiatry*, **47**, 250–6.

Lindesay, J., Marudkar, M., van Diepen, E., and Wilcock, G. (2002) The second Leicester survey of memory clinics in the British Isles. *International Journal of Geriatric Psychiatry*, **17**, 41–7.

Lipowski, Z.J. (1983) The need to integrate liaison psychiatry and geropsychiatry. *American Journal of Psychiatry*, **140**, 103–5.

LoGuidice, D., Waltrowicz, W., Brown, K., Burrows, C., Ames, D., and Flicker, L. (1999) Do memory clinics improve the quality of life of carers? A randomized trial. *International Journal of Geriatric Psychiatry*, **14**, 626–32.

LoGuidice, D., Hassett, A., Cook, R., Flicker, L., and Ames, D. (2001) Equity of access to a memory clinic in Melbourne ? Non-English speaking background of attenders are more severly demented and have increased rate of psychiatric disorders. *International Journal of Geriatric Psychiatry*, **16**, 327–34.

Luscombe, G., Brodaty, H., and Freeth, S. (1998) Younger people with dementia: diagnostic issues, effects on careers and use of services. *International Journal of Geriatric Psychiatry*, **13**, 323–30.

Mohide, E.A., Pringle, D.M., Streiner, D.L., Gilbert, J.R., Muir, G., *et al.* (1990) A randomized trial of family caregiver support in the home management of dementia. *Journal of the American Geriatrics Society*, **38**, 446–54.

Morris, R.G., Morris, L.W., and Britton, P.G. (1988) Factors affecting the emotional wellbeing of the caregivers of dementia sufferers. *British Journal of Psychiatry*, **153**, 147–56.

Murphy, E. (1994) The day hospital debate. *International Journal of Geriatric Psychiatry*, **9**, 517–18.

Newens, A.J., Forster, D.P., Kay, D.W., Kirkup, W., Bates, D., and Edwardson, J. (1993) Clinically diagnosed presenile dementia of the Alzheimer type in the Northern Health Region: ascertainment, prevalence, incidence and survival. *Psychological Medicine*, **23**, 631–44.

Pasnau, R.O. (1985) Ten commandments of medical etiquette for psychiatrists. *Psychosomatics*, **26**, 128–32.

Peace, S.M. (1982) Review of day-hospital provision in psychogeriatrics. *Health Trends*, **14**, 92–5.

Phipps, A.J. and O'Brien, J.T. (2002) Memory clinics and clinical governance – a UK perspective. *International Journal of Geriatric Psychiatry*, **17**, 1128–32.

Plotkin, D.A. and Wells, K.B. (1993) Partial hospitalization (day treatment) for psychiatrically ill elderly patients. *American Journal of Psychiatry*, **150**, 266–71.

Popkin, M.K., Mackenzie, T.B., and Callies, A.L. (1984) Psychiatric consultation to geriatric medically ill in-patients in a university hospital. *Archives of General Psychiatry*, **41**, 703–7.

Rabins, P.V. (1999) The history of psychogeriatrics in the United States. *International Psychogeriatrics*, **11**, 371–3.

Rabins, P., Lucas, M.J., Teitelbaum, M., Mark, S.R., and Folstein, M. (1983) Utilization of psychiatric consultation for elderly patients. *J Am Geriatr Soc*, **31**, 581–5.

Reifler, B.V. and Cohen, W. (1998) Practice of geriatric psychiatry and mental health services for the elderly: results of an international survey. *International Psychogeriatrics*, **10**, 351–7.

Ruskin, P.E. (1985) Geropsychiatric consultation in a university hospital: a report on 67 referrals. *American Journal of Psychiatry*, **142**, 333–5.

Sadavoy, J. and Conn, D. (1994) A comprehensive geriatric psychiatry program in Canada. *Hospital and Community Psychiatry*, **45**, 329–30.

Scott, J., Fairbairn, A., and Woodhouse, K. (1988) Referrals to a psychogeriatric consultation-liaison service. *International Journal of Geriatric Psychiatry*, **3**, 131–5.

Shulman, K.I. (1994) The future of geriatric psychiatry. *Canadian Journal of Psychiatry*, **39**, S4–8.

Shulman, K.I., Silver, I.L., Hershberg, R.I., and Fisher, R.H. (1986) Geriatric psychiatry in the general hospital: the integration of services and training. *General Hospital Psychiatry*, **8**, 223–8.

Small, G.W. and Fawzy, F.I. (1988) Psychiatric consultation for the medically ill elderly in the general hospital: need for a collaborative model of care. *Psychosomatics*, **29**, 94–103.

Steingart, A.B. (1992) Geriatric psychiatry day hospital: a treatment program for depressed older adults. In M. E. Bergener (ed.) *Aging and Mental Disorders*, pp. 338–55. Springer, New York.

Strain, J.J., Lyons, J.S., Hammer, J.S., *et al.* (1991) Cost offset from a psychiatric consultation-liaison intervention with elderly hip fracture patients. *American Journal of Psychiatry*, **148**, 1044–9.

Thorpe, L., Leclair, K., Donnelly, M., and MacBeath, L. (1993) Geriatric psychiatry: training guidelines and their application. Section on Geriatric Psychiatry of the Canadian Psychiatric Association. *Canadian Journal of Psychiatry*, **38**, 90–5.

Tourigny-Rivard, M.-F., and Potoczny, W.M. (1996) Acute care inpatient and day hospital treatment. In J. Sadavoy, L. W. Lazarus, L. F. Jarvik and G. T. Grossberg (eds.) *Comprehensive Review of Geriatric Psychiatry – II*, 2nd edn, pp. 973–1002. American Psychiatric Press, Washington DC.

Unützer, J. and Small, G.W. (1996) Geriatric consultation-liaison psychiatry. In J. Sadavoy, L. W. Lazarus, L. F. Jarvik and G. T. Grossberg (eds.) *Comprehensive Review of Geriatric Psychiatry – II*, 2nd edn, pp. 937–72. American Psychiatric Press, Washington DC.

van Hout, H.P., Vernooij-Dassen, M.J., Hoefnagels, W.H., and Grol, R.P. (2001) Measuring the opinions of memory clinic users: patients, relatives and general practitioners. *International Journal of Geriatric Psychiatry*, **16**, 846–51.

Wagner, B.D. (1991) Specialized partial hospitalization for older adults: a clinical description of an intermediate-term program. *The Psychiatric Hospital*, **22**, 69–76.

Wright, N. and Lindesay, J. (1995) A survey of memory clinics in the British Isles. *International Journal of Geriatric Psychiatry*, **10**, 379–85.

Zarit, S.H. and Teri, L. (1991) Interventions and services for family caregivers. *Annual Review of Gerontology and Geriatrics*, **11**, 287–310.

Chapter 17

Integrated service delivery and quality of care

Pamela Melding

The chief difficulty Alice found at first was in managing her flamingo … and when she had got its head down, and was going to begin again, it was very provoking to find that the hedgehog had unrolled itself, and was in the act of crawling away: besides all this, there was generally a ridge or furrow in the way wherever she wanted to send the hedgehog to, and, as the doubled-up soldiers were always getting up and walking off to other parts of the ground, Alice soon came to the conclusion that it was a very difficult game indeed.

The Queen's croquet-ground, Chapter 8, *Alice in Wonderland*. Lewis Carroll, 1866

In thinking about integrating services, we need to begin at the 'centre' – with the patient. Consider the following scenario. Sandy Jones, a former head teacher, is 75 years old and had a stroke yesterday. This was not the first time, or the worst, but this latest event is another huge hurdle for Sandy to overcome. Luckily, a friendly neighbour heard Sandy fall and came to investigate, as Sandy lives alone and has no immediate family. Life has not been particularly kind as Sandy, an only child brought up by overprotective, critical parents, married an alcoholic abusive partner who died some years ago, and then a drunk driver killed Sandy's only daughter at the age of twenty-six in a horrific road crash. Not surprisingly, Sandy has had several bouts of depression in the past requiring hospitalization and treatment.

Sandy could be male or female because this story is an invention. However, very few readers of this book would not be familiar with such a scenario, as such stories are an everyday reality for geriatric psychiatry services. Put yourself in Sandy's shoes and 'walk a mile' in them. If you were Sandy, what would you want from the health services you are about to confront?

You would probably want someone to organize your access to treatment. Certainly, you would want immediate assessment and stabilization of the medical condition, and rehabilitation to restore your functioning as much as possible. Having a stroke is emotionally devastating especially if support is limited and with your history of depression, you are especially vulnerable to anxiety, depression, and loneliness following a major medical trauma, so you might want someone to look after your emotional needs. You might despair of ever being able to live an independent existence again but you are determined to try, with help if that is available. If you cannot manage it, you want to have someone recognize that the struggle is too much and arrange for you to have the appropriate care or find you nice sheltered accommodation where you can see out your days. Above all, you want to be treated humanely, with respect and with care. You hope any treatment you receive has been tried and tested well before it reaches you and you can trust that the health professionals are up to date and offering you the highest quality treatment available. You do not want people experimenting on you or using you as a 'guinea pig'; at least if they do, then you want to have the opportunity to consent. Above all, you want to feel that 'someone' is looking after your interests and needs as you negotiate the medical system.

Our mythical patient, Sandy, needs a range of services in the journey through the health system. The interfaces between domains of health care for the older person are numerous and include the general practitioner, a geriatrician, a geriatric psychiatrist, clinical psychologists, nurses, occupational therapists, physiotherapists, meals on wheels, community support workers, social workers, perhaps nursing home caregivers, and possibly a consumer organization such as Age Concern, or a Stroke Foundation. What Sandy hopes for is a patient-centred needs-based service that facilitates access to all these domains and interfaces and does not allow patients to 'fall through the cracks'. Integration of elder care services has been advocated repeatedly in several countries including the UK Audit Commission Report (2000), the New Zealand Strategy for Health of Older People (2002) and the Commonwealth Department of Health and Ageing in Australia. These policies represent a sea change in health strategies from funding of programmes to funding health of populations.

Integrated services

An integrated service is one with a single point of entry providing interventions and support in multiple domains and dimensions (New Zealand Guidelines Group, 2003). A domain is a broad area of health care, such as mental health, physical functioning, safety, personal care, social functioning etc: a dimension is a subset of a domain such as depression, anxiety, cognitive impairment, elder abuse, respiratory disease. More simply, integrated services provide continuity of care.

This book cites many references on different types of geriatric psychiatry services, yet there are very few on fully integrated services. Similarly, there are many reports on the effectiveness of individual components of geriatric psychiatry services (e.g. Burns et al., 2001) but little on the effectiveness of total comprehensive services. Furthermore, there is great variation in the degree to which geriatric psychiatry services have integrated with other elder care providers (Challis et al., 2002). The Audit Commission (2000) found the range of services available in different health authorities in the UK was patchy and coordinated care between health and social services was lacking. Britain is not alone, as similar shortcomings occur in many other countries. Poorly integrated services with inadequate communication between domains and deficient information systems are a risk in themselves. Patients in such a system are in danger from polypharmacy, poor discharge planning, loss to follow-up, and insufficient carer support. Some places have embraced the 'Arie Model' (Arie, 2002) and developed comprehensive 'Departments of Health Care for the Elderly' that include geriatrics and geriatric psychiatry, with links to community services and resources; others are working towards this end. However, in reality, true integrated services, the patient-centred 'one-stop shop' for elders with multiple geriatric needs, appear to be rare. Intuitively, most people would think that an integrated continuum of care is the ideal to which we should all aspire. This begs the question, why are they not the norm today? They have had their advocates for at least twenty years. The answer is of course that integrating services into a coordinated holistic model is 'a very difficult game'. Indeed, one that requires organizational, cultural and conceptual paradigm shifts.

Few have the luxury of creating an integrated service from scratch; most have to bring together a disparate set of already established work groups or services, the minority of which are structured to be truly patient-centred. If we are really honest with ourselves, many services are set up to develop professional interests as much as patients' interests. Changing a service delivery paradigm from provider-centred to patient-centred is challenging. Carroll's story of the croquet game is a metaphor for what can go wrong when different players will not integrate into a functional team. In the story, Alice tries to play an uncoordinated game of croquet with flamingos for mallets, hedgehogs for balls and playing card soldiers for hoops, all of whom have their own independent ideas and objectives for the game. The purpose of the 'game' is lost in trying to regulate the idiosyncratic players. Most health professionals want to play the 'game' of providing a broad spectrum of care for older people, but unfortunately, like Alice, they are defeated by the many barriers that get in the way.

Barriers to integrating services – 'playing games'
Strong professional identities

Health services are fortunate that its workforce is tertiary educated, intelligent and idealistic. There are multiple professional groups and professional identities are very strong. Many pursue their highly specialized careers through several organizations and rather than identify themselves with the organization for which they work, they identify themselves with the norms and values of their professional group, which are strengthened by relationships with their professional organizations outside the immediate workplace. The more complex and specialized the work, the stronger the professional identity becomes. To complicate the issue in health systems, some professions are organized in strict hierarchies as with line management, others by expertise as with professional specialists. The different inherent values in the two systems can lead to disputes and conflict. Even if different specialist professionals successfully mix within a team or department (see below), the result can be that the team or department acquires an equally strong identity of its own. The paradox for integration is that the stronger a common identity forms *within* a team or department the more difficult it will be to integrate *between* teams or departments (Child, 1984).

Professional arrogance

Strong professional identities are useful in developing a specialized area, but total belief in the supremacy of one's own professional schemata can lead to professional arrogance. Many examples can be seen in everyday practice. Thus, we have teams refusing to delegate to other teams; primary care or geriatric physicians who refuse to have their patients assessed by psychiatric nurses; psychiatrists who do not consider geriatricians capable of doing competency assessments; health professionals who refuse to discharge patients as they do not believe that another can manage their patient successfully.

Territory

Marking one's territory seems to be an inherent feature of most life forms, but human beings are somewhat more sophisticated in their territorial marking. In the health professional sphere, territory can be physical space such as offices or wards. Territory also can be resource materials, or conceptual professional 'turf' as in areas of work, research, or special interest (Handy, 1993). Territorial disputes are common even within teams, for example, when office space is allocated on hierarchy rather than function so that who has the biggest office becomes more important than whether there is an office at all. Integrating different teams' territories has its difficulties especially if there are winners and losers, unless properly negotiated. Boundaries, in the form of rigid access policies, are often erected around team territory and the stronger the 'turf' – the firmer the boundary.

Departmental rivalries

Occasional friction is the norm as even the closest of people quarrel from time to time. However, strong professional identity, professional arrogance and firm boundaries can lead to interdepartmental rivalries. This often manifests itself as labelling and stereotyping of other teams or departments. Misinterpretation of other departments' motivations can lead to overuse of privacy and confidentiality issues so that essential information is withheld from appropriate people (Stevenson, 1999). An entrenched 'them and us' mentality is toxic and usually indicates antipathy based on misunderstanding of others' work practices, norms and objectives. Organizational expert John Child (1984) considers that these are significant barriers to integration and it is essential that such dynamics are worked through and dispelled.

Dysfunctional teams

Multidisciplinary teams are ubiquitous in geriatric health care, more so in geriatric psychiatry than in geriatrics or geriatric community care teams. They are composed of several specialist members, doctors, clinical psychologists, nurses, social workers, occupational therapists and physiotherapists. These members are disparate in educational training, status, perceived responsibility, privileges, and sophistication of knowledge, power and remuneration. They are not groups of equals. The idea that such teams are unproblematic, with the professional body engaged in skilled, comprehensive shared care with no conflicts of professional interests, is subject to increasing challenge (Opie, 1999, p. 184; Adamson *et al.*, 1995). In contrast to the ideal, teams can be playing fields for interdisciplinary contest, unequal power struggles and protection of professional 'turf'. Other professionals (Adamson *et al.*, 1995) have repeatedly challenged medical dominance of such teams. It is virtually impossible to integrate services if the individual teams are dysfunctional in the first place, as they will carry their 'baggage' with them to the new integrated service, with the interprofessional dynamics being acted out on a bigger playing field.

Empire building

When individual teams or departments have built reputations for research, develop specific areas of clinical excellence or have otherwise established a name for themselves, it is not surprising that they will resist any attempt to subsume their team or services into a greater whole. Such units, whilst no doubt serving patient interests, also serve professional interests, possibly more. Integrating 'empires' that incorporate considerable personal investments can lead to power struggles and heated discussions about which should be the 'lead' service in the group, 'lead' clinician or 'lead' administrator.

Management systems and funding

Departments established for some time will have management systems that often duplicate other departments or services and each assumes that certain tasks are the responsibility of the other services, resulting in gaps in delivery. This is indeed a very good argument for integration, but if integration reduces duplication and causes redundancies, resistance can ensue.

Funding that is 'ring fenced' or 'quarantined' i.e. for one purpose only, can also be a problem for integration. Usually, protected funding occurs because the service was initially under-resourced or had its resources diverted to other health interests, in order to stop any further plundering. Strict ring fencing, when funds are only available for a single purpose such as 'mental health', or 'geriatric' or 'disability support' assumes that patients fall neatly into categories. Problems arise when patients needs cross these silos, creating gaps in delivery.

Indicators of poor integration
Proliferation of committees and meetings

Committees are useful as an integrative tool, in that discussion of competing interests can take place and interdepartmental power balanced. Problem areas can be identified and plans made to work through them. When integration is not working, an early sign is that the work of committees starts to stall, issues become fudged, and decisions procrastinated. A sure red light sign is when other committees start to look into the work of the original committees and a proliferating hierarchy of meetings and committees ensues without any outcomes (Child, 1984).

Red tape rituals

Integration usually involves a change in some procedures or communication channels between the arms of the whole service. These may be documented in protocols, policies, guidelines or procedures. When staff fail to take these seriously and monitoring becomes meaningless rituals of red tape to keep the administrators happy, then integration is not working (Child, 1984). The current thrust towards 'single assessment processes' by many jurisdictions involved in elder care has the potential to become such a red tape ritual unless there is full support for the assessment process by all involved parties.

Overloading with administrators

Integrating services into an administrative whole usually means streamlining of management systems. However, as problems with coordination between teams are referred to management, they consume valuable time and divert managers from other tasks. Thus, if there are many problems to sort out, there is often a proliferation of coordinators, administrators, or liaison officers engaged to deal with difficulties.

Complaints by consumers

A sure sign of poor integration is patients being passed from department to department, or they are given information from one arm of the service that conflicts with another, or they have to negotiate several departments for the same problem, or they perceive indifference to their needs – 'sorry, not our department'.

Improving the game

According to Burns *et al.* (2001), in the UK 'specialist mental health services for older people have grown rapidly and successfully over the past two decades, aiming to offer services that are comprehensive, accessible, responsive, individualized, multidisciplinary, accountable, and systematic'. To meet all these objectives, components of specialist geriatric psychiatry services need to be integrated amongst themselves and with other elder care services with whom they interface on a regular basis.

Many services develop as independent pieces in the jigsaw and integration of all, from an administrative perspective, may not be possible. Often geriatric psychiatry and geriatrics are managed as completely separate divisions, and their services may not be even co-located, never mind co-joined. However, from the patient's point of view, if not administratively co-joined, they need to be *functionally* integrated and have systems that deal with problem interfaces.

Geriatric psychiatry services contact many other services and have numerous interfaces in their work. These are highlighted in Figure 17.1.

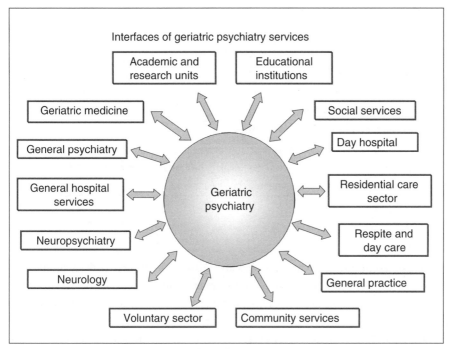

Figure 17.1 Functional relationships and interfaces in geriatric psychiatry.

The principles of integration

Arie and Jolley (1982) articulated the principles of achieving integrated comprehensive geriatric psychiatry secondary care services many years ago (see Chapters 1 and 2). These are – flexibility, responsiveness, availability, non-hierarchical use of staff, domiciliary assessment and willingness to collaborate with other services and agencies. These principles are as true today as they were then. Components of services all have a slightly different emphasis or focus. Transforming disparate teams or services each with their own identities and culture into an integrated system creates tensions. However, an integrated system needs both the concept of 'systemness' without diminishing the component part identities (Wolf *et al.*, 2004).

Vision

There needs to be an agreed common purpose or vision that all the teams and professions accept and develop, irrespective of individual team differences. A vision needs to anticipate any future developments, the ultimate goal. A detailed situational analysis of current realities, problems and issues and an assessment of anticipated future development will probably demonstrate a large disparity. This 'gap', according to Wolf *et al.* (2004), causes a tension that initiates the momentum for change towards the desired

Table 17.1 Principles of integrating services

- Common vision, values and goals shared by services
- Able leadership –transactional and transformational
- Situational analysis, external, internal and future
- Attention to potential interface problems
- Focus on teams' development
- Shared comprehensive assessment processes
- Clear administrative, clinical and funding structures
- Interdependent cooperation in education, training, professional development and research
- Good clinical governance and attention to quality

---

system and commitment to group vision and goals. A situational analysis should cover external influences such as social or environmental needs, national or organizational strategic planning and take into account government recommendations, guidelines plus economic realities. It should also cover internal processes such as practices, resources, and culture, which underpin the current services' organizational status (Outhwaite, 2003).

Leadership

Leadership can be transactional or transformational and both are crucial to integrating teams and systems. Transformational skills are essential to develop an integrated system if the challenges are to be faced and conceptual and cultural shifts made. They are needed to allow the team or teams to work together and be innovative in their approaches. Walshe (2000a) notes that 'There is a vast and daunting literature on leadership, which both attempts to describe the characteristics of effective leaders and to analyze the processes or methods which leaders use.'

These leaders exhibit what may be essential ingredients of transformational leadership. They;

- have a vision of the ultimate goal
- excel in communicating this vision and values to others
- inspire openness, trust and confidence
- help others to feel capable and to realize their own potential
- have enormous energy and drive, and are action-oriented.

Transformational skills create an environment that encourages and supports the team member's individual development and leadership skills (Corrigan and Garman, 1999). This contrasts with transactional leadership, which focuses on formal systems and processes, planning and process design, accountability and monitoring.

Detmer and Ford (2001) assert that leadership is not something separate from clinical practice:

> Leadership is a continuous and everyday activity that is an explicit part of all senior clinical roles. Many clinicians see that leadership is somebody else's business and that clinicians should not be troubled by having to manage their services. Effective clinical leaders, through their relationships and actions, make a broader contribution to patient well being well beyond their individual impact as clinicians. They show personal courage, take personal risk and accept responsibility. This form of leadership takes an intelligence, knowledge and wisdom significantly broader that that of even the most expert practitioner.

Relationships and multidisciplinary teams

Multidisciplinary or interdisciplinary teams provide most geriatric psychiatry service delivery. For such teams to be effective they need to understand each other's roles, communicate with a common language, and value each other's perspectives. The clearer team members are as to how each member contributes to the team and how the team contributes to the service, the more effective it will be. Health care research confirms that these team characteristics are prerequisite to effective patient care in a range of contexts including mental health (Millward and Jefferies, 2001).

Given the importance of the multidisciplinary team in psychiatry, it is not surprising that the 'team', 'teamship' and 'team functions' should be a focus for considerable study (Opie, 1999; Ovretveit, 1993). The literature on multidisciplinary team development cites the importance of organizational support (Ovretveit, 1993) together with a need for clarity on how decisions are made, responsibilities, supervision and support. Whilst teamwork itself can be broken down into aspects of shared attitudes, knowledge and skills, the complexity of the health care environment requires a much more sophisticated approach to team learning (Firth-Cozens, 2001). Groups of people do not become a 'team' just because someone tells them they are one. There is a growth cycle of learning and development. First, there is some exploration at an individual level; second, pooled learning and gradual sharing; third, integration of different perspectives and learning beyond usual boundaries; and fourth, collective learning, knowledge sharing and a spirit of enquiry (Dechant et al., 1993). Teams move backwards and forwards along this learning curve depending on the issue and the disciplines involved, but as 'teamship' develops and greater understanding of collective service provision arises, members move towards collective knowledge sharing and enquiry (Eve, 2004). Interestingly, as a functional team identity develops, the individual professional identities become less important (Opie, 1999) and more collaborative interdisciplinary style of functioning (King et al., 1998) emerges.

King et al. (1998) define a *multidisciplinary* team as a team of health professionals and support staff who need to meet frequently to agree and coordinate interventions. The team is typically physician-led, with most interaction being between the physician and individual team members and less lateral communication between team members (as in the interdisciplinary team). They define an *interdisciplinary* team as a team of

Example of matrix to analyse inter-team relationships

Community team					**Scoring of relationships**
	Community team				Relationships between these units are:
					1. Soundñperfect unity
Inpatient psychiatry team	2	Inpatient psychiatry team			2. Almost full unity
					3. Better than average
					4. Average
Geriatric ATR	4	4	Geriatric ATR		5. Somewhat of a breakdown
					6. Almost complete breakdown
					7. Couldn't be worse!
Community support services	3	4	2	Community support services	
Day hospital	2	2	2	2	Day hospital
Long-stay geriatric hospital	5	6	5	5	5	Long-stay geriatric hospital

Figure 17.2   Matrix of relationships between component parts of the system. Adapted from a concept in Child, J. (1984).

health professionals and support staff working collectively with group decision-making and group responsibility for developing optimal treatment and support management plans. This approach facilitates lateral communication between team members and freer exchange of ideas, with the aim of more effective problem-solving.

There are often inter-team relationship problems in integration. Potential problems can be anticipated by developing a matrix of relationships (Child, 1984) between the individual components. Relationships are scored on a Likert scale. The problem areas are quickly spotted and the barriers can be explored and resolved.

Whilst relationships between component parts of a system are important to develop, there also needs to be a major focus on individual team development. An integrated service is only as good as its weakest link (Wolf *et al.*, 2004). Consequently, successful integration depends on continuing development of its component parts. Despite the obvious importance of multi- or inter-disciplinary team functioning in providing effective health services, few teams actually have written protocols of team practice. Very few professional health personnel are given training either in their undergraduate years or subsequently on how to be a team member. What there is focuses on team dynamics and management of interpersonal relations (Opie, 1999). Functional teams are more likely to integrate, to have the qualities of flexibility, responsiveness and willingness to collaborate, highlighted by Arie and Jolley (1982) as important in achieving comprehensive integrated services.

Shared assessment processes – comprehensive geriatric assessment

Older people, their GPs or other referrers do not want to be sent from team to team until they hit the right one. Patients have to tell the same story repeatedly. Multiple assessments are not only irritating to consumers but are inefficient and a waste of scarce resources (Stevenson, 1999). Different disciplines have their own modes of assessment but despite individual difference, it is useful to have some common information for all teams and multidisciplinary groups, irrespective of who takes the main responsibility for the patient. Consequently, there has been increasing advocacy for the comprehensive geriatric assessment (CGA). The intention of a CGA is to cover the main domains and dimensions of assessment. There is a good body of evidence indicating that a CGA improves outcomes (Reuben *et al.*, 1995, 1999; Nickolaus *et al.*, 1999; Burns *et al.*, 2000; Morris *et al.*, 1997). Whilst CGAs have an important role, they do require personnel to work across professional and agency barriers (Stevenson, 1999). Nevertheless, as Stevenson asks, 'Surely this is in the interests of all people concerned including consumers?'

Yet CGAs are by no means universal, or have been incorporated voluntarily in many places. Recently, (April 2004) the UK Department of Health required local authorities to implement a *single* assessment process (SAP) into each health district. The chosen SAP is to be audited (DOH, 2004). It is left up to the local authorities whether they design their own assessment or use an 'off the shelf' tool. Similar moves are being made by the New Zealand and Australian health departments, indicating the importance being placed on patient centred single assessment processes by these governments. Table 17.2 gives a list of some of the tools suggested for use in a single assessment process.

Table 17.2 Some comprehensive assessment tools suggested as useful for a single or comprehensive geriatric assessment process

- Camberwell Assessment of Needs of the Elderly - CANE[1]
- EASY-Care 2002–2005[2]
- Functional Assessment of the Care Environment FACE[3]
- Minimum Data Set for Home Care MDS-HC[4]
- Minimum Data Set –Residential Assessment Instrument MDS-RAI[5]
- The Long Term Care resident assessment instrument Inter-RAI[6]

[1] Reynolds et al. (2000)
[2] EASY-Care http://www.shef.ac.uk/sisa/easycare/ accessed May 28 2004
[3] FACE recording and measuring systems http://www.facecode.com/ accessed May 28 2004
[4] InterRAI home care http://www.interrai.org/instruments/home_care.php accessed May 28, 2004
[5] InterRAI residential care http://www.interrai.org/instruments/nursing_facility.php accessed May 28 2004
[6] InterRAI residential care http://www.interrai.org/instruments/nursing_facility.php accessed May 28 2004

Table 17.3 Criteria for assessment tools

- ◆ Capable of detecting risk factors, impaired health or function
- ◆ Have good validity
- ◆ Have good sensitivity
- ◆ Have good inter-rater reliability
- ◆ Be standardized
- ◆ Be acceptable to different ethnic groups
- ◆ Have provision for open ended comment
- ◆ Be practical to administer
- ◆ Be compatible with or supportive of carer needs assessment
- ◆ Be supported by and able to contribute data to a database to allow for ongoing monitoring and evaluation

---

Adapted from New Zealand Guidelines Group, Assessment Processes for Older People. Adapted and reproduced with kind permission

The work involved in services joining forces to agree on a CGA or SAP mirrors the importance of shared collaboration in integrating services. It is important that all disciplines contribute to ensure that all the important domains and dimensions are covered, as successful implementation depends upon this process. What might work in one area might be problematic in another. Some countries or areas may have special legislation that covers certain areas of health e.g. an accident compensation health scheme, or ethnic groups, for which current 'off the shelf' tools are inappropriate. Assessors also need training in tools and processes. Of course, a SAP or CGA can vary in its comprehensiveness of covering the relevant domains and dimensions. They can be aimed at different levels, e.g. screening, proactive assessment or when a person presents to primary care, or on entering secondary care services.

The advantages of a single comprehensive geriatric assessment are several. First, their design can ensure that the patient is a partner in the assessment. Second, they can include multiple domains so that important dimensions of health e.g. depression in Parkinson's disease or the possibility of elder abuse is not missed. Third, they can be standardized, thus allowing for data analysis across time, national, and international locations. This has obvious benefits for trends analysis, planning of future services and research (Morris, *et al.*, 1997; Wasson, *et al.*, 1999). Fourth, staff ownership of the process and willingness to work with each other across team boundaries in developing a common assessment procedure for a particular area will assist greatly with functional integration of the services.

The mere act of doing a CGA will not improve outcomes (Reuben *et al.*, 1995, Nickolaus *et al.*, 1999). The assessment, which should include the patient views, needs to

Table 17.4 Domains and dimensions

DOMAINS AND DIMENSIONS OF ASSESSMENT FOR A COMPREHENSIVE GERIATRIC ASSESSMENT

Areas of need of most importance to older people

- Personal care
- Social participation
- Control over daily life
- Nutrition
- Safety

Domains and dimensions

These are areas in which impairment can be detected at an early stage.

Domains	Key dimensions
Physical health and functioning	Chronic illness, continence, nutrition, gait, mobility, cardiac conditions, gastrointestinal conditions, pulmonary conditions, cerebrovascular conditions, co-morbidities, ADLs and IADLs (including self-care and domestic abilities), iatrogenic disease (specifically due to polypharmacy), sexual functioning, speech and language impairment, dental/oral health, vision and hearing, safety
Mental health and functioning	Anxiety, depression, other mental illness, cognitive functioning, dementia, substance abuse, iatrogenic disease due to polypharmacy, emotional well-being
Social functioning	Financial status and management, housing, family support/contact, social networks, social activities and support

Presence and roles of carers, especially informal carers

- Carer stress
- Need for respite
- Relationships with care recipient

Risk factors

- Aged 75 years or older
- Socially isolated and/or living alone
- Divorced/separated, never married, single or widowed
- Recently bereaved
- Has no children
- Has poor or limited economic resources
- Recently discharged from hospital
- Presenting at an emergency department
- Recent change in health status with an impact on capacity for independent living
- Has multiple disorders or illness

Continued

Table 17.4 Domains and dimensions—Cont'd

Also consider:

- Alcohol, tobacco and/or substance use
- Abuse of the person by another
- Cognitively impaired
- Poor self-perceived health
- High or low body mass index
- At the lower extreme of functional impairment
- Low physical activily
- Taking 3 or more prescription/nonprescription medications
- Impairment in sight or hearing
- Carer showing signs of stress/change of carer
- Carer requests an assessment for the older person

Adapted from the New Zealand Guidelines Group, Assessment Process for Older People, 2003, with kind permission

produce recommendations for interventions for any domains and dimensions highlighted as problematic. Failure to follow-up can lead to adverse outcomes (Reuben *et al.*, 1995, Martin *et al.*, 1999; Nickolaus *et al.*, 1999; Aminzadeh and Dalziel, 2002). In our perfect integrated system, these recommendations will be promptly acted upon by the clinicians committed to the concept of patient-centered care, at all levels of the system, both primary and secondary care. Unfortunately, non-adherence by clinicians to the recommendations of a single comprehensive assessment process is a major threat to integration. CGAs have potential to become red tape rituals.

Non-adherence to recommendations generated by an assessment process occurs at all levels of the system, including primary care and secondary care (Aminzadeh, 2000; Reuben *et al.*, 1999). Comprehensive Geriatric Assessments are sometimes seen as undermining the expertise of the specialist. Aminzadeh (2000) reviewed the literature on adherence to comprehensive geriatric assessments and found that physician adherence varies from 49–79 per cent. Adherence is better if:

- There are good communications between physicians in primary and secondary care
- Recommendations are prioritized and limited
- Physicians are satisfied with the shared assessment programme
- Physician has had less years in practice
- The physician is female
- Illness is severe
- Non-adherence has legal liability.

Patients may also not adhere to treatment recommendations (Anderson *et al.*, 2000). Patient adherence to plans is similar to that of doctors at 46–76 per cent (Aminzadeh, 2000). Non-adherence is also a major problem for mental health services (Maidment *et al.*, 2002). The barriers to adherence of treatment recommendations (Anderson *et al.*, 2000; Aminzadeh, 2000) are:

- Poor health status, changing health status and complex disease states
- Cognitive impairment
- Challenging behaviours
- Changing addictive behaviours or lifestyle
- Poor social support
- Polypharmacy
- Clinician ageism or nihilism
- Patient beliefs.

On the other hand, there are some strategies to support adherence (Aminzadeh, 2000).

- Identify barriers and work though potential problems
- Good communication between clinician and patient
- Gaining rapport
- Understanding patient goals and beliefs (Glazier *et al.*, 2004)
- Giving written information as well as verbal
- Jargon-free treatment plans given to patient
- Involvement of family and usual carers (Glazier *et al.*, 2004)
- Close follow-up, community services and teams in conjunction with GP.

Administrative structures and funding streams

Integrating services with multiple interfaces usually requires some system reconfiguration, setting up new administrative structures and funding streams. Arie and Jolley (1982) described the Nottingham comprehensive service with co-located but separate geriatric medicine and geriatric psychiatry under the administrative structure of 'health care of older people'. This is still considered the ideal by many professionals, both clinicians and administrators (Shah and Ames, 1994). Services need to have clearly defined roles, responsibilities, and processes for collaboration set out in protocols. Such a configuration allows for the development of distinct therapeutic environments for the physically ill and for those with psychiatric conditions. Services can work in unison, enabling cross-fertilization of ideas and approaches to joint care. Consultation and liaison between services can assist in joint approaches to older people with complex needs. Funding streams also need to be simplified. Information systems, particularly patient management systems, need designing, developing and implementing to support the team's work (Weiner *et al.*, 2003).

Interdependent cooperation in education, training, professional development and research

Clinical services have important roles in teaching training ongoing professional development and in clinical, evaluation and systems research. These can also be important means of cross-fertilization, the dissemination of ideas between related services and teams. Joint meetings may be preferred by some, others will prefer to invite presenters from other related services to join in a predominately psychiatric or geriatric continuing education programme. Involvement of several disciplines in undergraduate or postgraduate teaching programmes can be useful for disseminating a broader perspective to prospective health professionals intending to work with older people. Ageing interest groups that include primary and secondary care and cross disciplines are also useful. Collaboration in research projects is another area that can support integration.

The importance of functional integration with primary care

Integrated services that are patient-centred must include primary care. Older people mostly live in their own homes, with usually less than 10 per cent living in institutions. In addition, the majority of mental health problems are treated in primary care and not by specialist services (Lyness *et al.*, 1999). Several studies have looked at mental health of older people in primary care and note that many problems go undetected and undertreated. Mere cooperation between mental health services and primary care is insufficient to improve outcomes. Both Arthur *et al.* (2002) and Unützer *et al.* (2001) found, in randomized controlled trials, that collaborative-shared care between primary care and secondary care specialists, treating older people with depression had only modest effects. *Mental health enhanced primary care* might be more successful. Sayers *et al.* (2002) demonstrated that education of primary care nurses in recognition of mental disorders and use of screening instruments can improve identification. Training practice nurses in brief assessment scales such as the Geriatric Depression Scale may also be useful to improve detection in primary care (Arthur *et al.*, 1999). Powell and Peile (2000) report a British initiative aimed at keeping older people out of hospital with improved home support involving four primary care practices, a health authority, a community trust and social services department, including the appointment of a nurse coordinator and six support workers offering a 24-hour service. The scheme reduced hospital admissions and lengths of stay. What seems to have promise is the idea of 'embedding' nurses into primary care practices who have the skills necessary to identify health problems and coordinate care for older people. One such scheme, currently being evaluated, operates in Canterbury, New Zealand – The Coordinators of Services for the Elderly (COSE) scheme. The COSE nurses work within a primary care practice to coordinate across health, mental health, community and the accident services.

The primary care physician is crucial to patient care from start to finish, not only in identifying people who are at risk but also for any post hospital discharge care. Even if patients or their caregivers can self-refer to secondary services, it is important not to bypass the GP. The key to successful cooperation between primary and secondary services is communication (Bull and Roberts, 2001). Simple things can enhance the interface between primary care and secondary services such as geriatric mental health personnel being readily available for telephone advice or consultation. Ideally, primary care physicians, patients and caregivers should be able to contact a district central agency, a 'one-stop shop', to which enquiries and referrals to older peoples' services are directed. When community mental health staff are treating a patient in the community, a clear management plan, which includes primary care and gives direct feedback from community mental health nurses to the GP after a visit to their patient, is courteous and prevents misunderstandings.

Mentally ill patients, sick enough to be referred to secondary services, usually have complex needs and vary in functional capacity. Some are incapable of returning to their previous living situation but many others can be supported in the community after discharge with additional help. Supports may include functional aides, community physiotherapy, meals on wheels, home help, caregiver support, community mental health team support and primary care supervision. The roles and expectations of the various personnel working with an individual need to be clarified and understood by all, including the patient and caregivers.

There is great potential for improved cooperation between primary care and secondary geriatric psychiatry services. Examples include understanding the epidemiology of mental health in primary care (Gallo *et al.*, 1997), education and training of primary care practitioners in screening and identification of mental health problems (Sayers *et al.*, 2002). Other initiatives include involvement of mental health professionals in continuing medical education courses for GPs, and in having health practitioners with specialized skills in assessment, psychotherapy and coordination of elder care within primary care practices (Gilbody *et al.*, 2003).

Hospital to home interface

Specialist care services successfully integrated at the secondary care level can fall down if the secondary to primary care interface is not adequate. Mentally ill older patients discharged from medical, surgical or other wards are often poorly managed. For example, Druss and colleagues (2001) analysed over 88,000 records of patients hospitalized for myocardial infarction and found that the presence of a mental disorder was associated with a 19 per cent increase in one-year mortality and with a much poorer quality of aftercare. After controlling for all variables, the data suggested that the increased mortality in the mentally ill group was due to the lower level of care. Several studies, evaluating the types of medication prescribed by physicians, found that there was a lower quality of care for older individuals with mental disorders (Bartels, 2002). Many other studies indicate similar findings. These are major concerns and require early identification of older people with mental disorders who are at risk, well before they leave the hospital. There is a place for geriatric psychiatry consultation and liaison in the medical and surgical wards in shortening lengths of stay and improving function (Slaets *et al.*, 1997; Draper, 2001) but a key element appears to be the aged care community team's collaboration with the staff on the acute ward in discharge planning (Robinson and Street, 2004).

For inpatients, discharge planning should begin as soon as a patient is admitted to inpatient secondary services (Bull and Roberts, 2001) and include the GP. Discharge summaries are an area of discontent and poor communication between secondary geriatric services, including psychiatry, and primary care. Surveys of discharge arrangements sent to the GP showed that these vary in their receipt, from a few days to two months (Bull and Roberts, 2001). Meara *et al.* (1992) reported in one study that no communication from the hospital was received for 33 per cent of the discharges. It is extremely unlikely that these problems are confined to the areas surveyed and the problem of poor discharge communication is probably ubiquitous. Whilst often regarded as a chore by junior medical staff, detailed discharge summaries to GPs are essential communications about subsequent patient care in the community.

Clinical governance and quality – winning the game

Quality

There is an enormous body of literature covering 'quality' and this chapter can only briefly overview the subject. Nevertheless, 'quality' is fundamental to integrated services and it is important to address key concepts, albeit superficially. There is considerable evidence that points to poor quality in service delivery for geriatric and geriatric psychiatry patients (Martin *et al.*, 1999; Wenger *et al.*, 2003; Higashi *et al.*, 2004). Inadequate services, lack of services and poorly integrated services all lead to poor quality care and adverse events. Particular problem areas are in care for people with dementia, either home dwelling or in nursing homes, overuse of psychotropic drugs, and poor access for mentally ill older people to health services.

We live in an era of accounting and accountability. Funding has not kept up with expansion in the health sector and services need to demonstrate continually that they are giving maximum value for money spent. Staff are bombarded by an array of terms regarding quality, with segments of services or even whole departments in a health organization devoted to quality. The concept 'quality' (from old Latin *qualitas* – 'of which kind') literally means an inherent, essential, distinguishing characteristic of something. It implies superiority. The concept of quality can also be a means of 'gluing' a service matrix together. Commitment to quality service delivery, acceptable to the consumer, is key to the cultural change required for integrated services to be patient-centred.

Quality is broadly defined in health services as *meeting and exceeding the needs of the consumers.* If so, then the views of consumers are integral to 'quality' processes. Wensing (2003) states:

> Efforts to improve health care will be wasted unless they reflect what patients want from the service. But to be sure those surveys of patient's views are valid and have an effect, they must be evaluated rigorously.

Data from patients can be collected from a qualitative and quantitative perspective. *Preferences* are ideas about what should occur in health care systems. They refer to individual patient's views about their clinical treatment. Focus groups of several patients can help them to distinguish between preferences and experiences (Wensing, 2003). Several models have been developed to collect and analyse preference data, including the expectancy-value model, the Quality Adjusted Life Year (QALY) model and conjoint analysis models or discrete choice experiments (Froberg and Kane, 1989; Ryan, 2004). The choice of methods will influence the results. *Priorities* describe the preferences of a population. *Evaluations* are patients' reactions to their experience of health care, for example, whether the process or outcome of their care was good or bad. Evaluations can be used to change interventions that can form testable hypotheses. *Reports* represent objective, quantitative observations of organization or process of care by patients, regardless of their preferences or evaluations. For instance, patients can register how long they had to wait in the waiting room for an appointment, or whether they were given their rights or sufficient information.

Wensing (2003) asserts that the important factors to think about in designing instruments to collect patient relevant data are:

- Use of qualitative and quantitative data
- Responsiveness, discrimination, good test–retest validity
- Internal consistency
- Attention to sampling bias
- Mindful of respondent shielding. Non-responders to surveys are likely to be sicker, less satisfied, or making less use of health care
- Design chooses processes and outcomes that are relevant to patient views
- Awareness of any adverse effects e.g. unrealistic expectations of health care; defensive behaviour of care providers, resulting in higher numbers of unnecessary clinical procedures; undermining of professional morale and increased costs.

Quality of Care

Quality of care is the provision of an acceptable standard of service delivery. If we define quality as meeting the needs of the consumer, then the arbiter or an acceptable quality of care should also be the consumer. However, professional attempts to incorporate patient views in attempts to define quality of care are rare (Reuben *et al.*, 2003). Such research is essentially qualitative, time-consuming and often difficult, so it is perhaps unsurprising that health services seek alternative ways of determining quality. Nevertheless, although a challenge, research can look at several aspects of patient care from a consumer point of view. Sixma and colleagues (2000) used focus groups and a standardized instrument, the QUOTE-Elderly (Quality of care through the patient's eyes), to determine elderly person's appraisal of services. Access, attention to accessibility (for the disabled), being treated respectfully and communication about risks received the highest ratings.

In the absence of a literature on how patients define quality of care, what mostly defines it is a proliferation of protocols, clinical pathways, evidenced-based reports and clinical guidelines, written by expert panels. Several authors, including Reuben and colleagues (2003), consider that some of these approaches limited in elder care because they neither consider the question of interest nor comorbidities that can sometimes render guideline recommendations inappropriate.

Quality of care should be progressive and advances in knowledge redefine it continuously. Reversals of former recommendations can change guidelines rapidly, outdating them sometimes within two or three years (Shekelle *et al.*, 2001). Well-known examples of reversals of recommendations include hormone replacement therapy, originally thought to be protective of heart disease and dementia, now thought to increase these problems. Another example is the new atypical antipsychotics, originally heralded as an advance in the treatment of behavioural signs and symptoms of dementia (BPSD) but recently the subjects of warnings that they may increase the incidence of adverse cerebrovascular events in patients with pre-existing risk factors. If guidelines are to be useful tools, they must be revised and updated, regularly (Reuben *et al.*, 2003; Shekelle *et al.*, 2001).

To be effective in defining and raising quality of care, clinical practice guidelines should not stay on bookshelves but be implemented. To do so requires adequate personnel, resources and support. As the evidence base for most protocols and practice guidelines comes from research settings, usually with focused problems, under ideal conditions, their generalizability to complex clinical situations in geriatrics and geriatric psychiatry is unclear. In underprivileged areas or poorly resourced services, staff struggling to provide the best quality of care they can, find the standards in guidelines sometimes demoralizingly impossible to achieve in their 'real world' conditions. Despite these issues, practice guidelines are achieving importance in medico-legal circumstances and in clinical governance as definers of quality of care.

Whilst medical personnel have an important leadership role in quality of care, they have not been enthusiastic implementers of clinical practice guidelines. Some of the factors cited earlier as contributing to non-adherence to treatment recommendations from comprehensive geriatric assessment are similar to those leading to inertia in the use of guidelines. Cabana *et al.* (1999) reviewed 76 studies looking at use of practice guidelines by doctors. The most common reasons cited were lack of awareness or familiarity with the guidelines or consensus statements, disagreement with specific guidelines or guidelines in general, poor outcome expectancy and disbelief that adherence to guideline-specified care processes would lead to the desired outcomes. In addition, lack of self-efficacy to perform the required care process and inability to overcome existing practice habits were common barriers. Even when a national institute is set up to provide guidance on clinical practice interventions, as with the UK's National Institute for Clinical Excellence (NICE), there is sparse data on the effectiveness of their guidance in changing clinical practice (Dent and Sadler, 2002). It would seem we have considerable research yet to do in the usefulness and impact of clinical practice guidelines in defining quality of care in geriatric psychiatry.

Quality assurance

Quality assurance is the process by which quality of care is evaluated. It meets the need to continually update, maintain and raise standards. The first person to bring quality assurance into healthcare was Florence Nightingale, who in the 1850s attempted to standardize nursing throughout Great Britain. Later the theories of W. T. Deming (Walton, 1986) on quality control and Donabedian (1980) on quality assurance attracted the attention of health care organizations. These theorists also held that the focus should be on consumer outcomes and that quality of health care was dependent upon structure, process and outcome. Structure refers to the availability of facilities, equipment and drugs; process refers to the care delivered to patients and outcomes refer to the results of treatment. As a measure of quality, outcome is difficult to assess, as there is not a linear relationship between quality of care and outcome. Superb quality of care sometimes leads to poor outcome and appalling quality can produce a good outcome. For some conditions, the outcome may only be realized years after the health care has been delivered. Thus, quality assurance in many health care organizations has relied on structure and process measures as proxies for quality of care. The problem with this is that they are not a causal chain and outcome may have very little to do with either structure or process. Their relevance to mental health is also questionable (for more detailed discussion, see Chapter 20). What they really measure is performance.

Quality assurance activities vary considerably depending on the type of practitioner and the type of setting, including geographical area. Activities may include adherence to standards of practice protocols, checklists of guideline recommendations, feedback of clinical work, peer review, accreditation, credentialing, reports on practice activities and audit. The main goal of quality assurance activities is to ensure that health care is delivered in a consistent manner of high quality across all members of a professional group. However, for staff working in mental health services many quality assurance activities, particularly if externally imposed, seem to be time-consuming red tape rituals, extraneous to what should be the main focus of quality, the patient–health professional interface. Valenstein *et al.* (2004) surveyed 654 mental health providers on their attitudes to quality monitoring activities. The majority expressed ambivalence to many monitoring activities with similar barriers to those described above. The most acceptable quality activities were patient satisfaction surveys or other patient indicators, as the staff considered these more relevant to their work. Unfortunately, satisfaction surveys tend to be denigrated as unscientific and over favourable.

The concept of 'quality assurance' has been partly derailed by it appearing to be an ideological management device to get more for less, burdens of a seemingly endless stream of paper work, and demands to meet ever changing goalposts.

As Baroness Onora O'Neill (2002) puts it:

> Professionals have to work to ever more exacting – if changing – standards of good practice and due process, to meet relentless demands to record and report, and they are subject to regular ranking and restructuring. I think that many public sector professionals find that the new demands damage their real work.

For older person's services, the problem is often that the 'real work' is in the patient–health professional interaction, and this is not the focus of the usual activities of quality assurance, which are more applicable to the curative specialties.

Cure versus caring

Francis Peabody in 1927 said: 'The secret of the "care" of the patient is in the caring for the patient.' In 1930, he considered that 'The physician who attempts the care of the patients while neglecting the emotional life is as unscientific as the investigator who neglects to control all the conditions that may affect his experiment.'

This is no secret to geriatric psychiatry personnel, but it does seem to have been overlooked by many health care organizations' quality programmes. Health care systems can get excellent ratings for 'quality of care,' despite gross violations of human caring (Feinstein, 2002). For geriatric psychiatry services, much of the work involves interpersonal relationships between patient and health professional – 'the caring'.

There are barriers to the measurement of 'caring'. Many quality programmes are very focused on cure rather than care (Feinstein, 2002). Disease management is prominent and interpersonal targets are neglected. Reimbursement policies are focused on outputs, with technical procedures reimbursed more than communication specialties. Minimum conversation targets e.g. screening or surveys are popular, which might suit surgeons. There is inadequate data on clinician patient interactions; whilst the technical is assessed easily, the interpersonal is assessed only with great difficulty and recognition of suffering is overlooked (Cassell, 1999). In geriatric psychiatry, whilst we do spend time on 'cure' we spend far more on the hard to measure 'caring' activities with those who can't be cured, promoting health, preventing injury and further breakdown of health, hopefully avoiding premature death and relieving suffering of both patients and caregivers. Many clinicians consider these to be the real work and where the real quality is manifest. Feinstein (2002) challenges us:

> If the process of caring is to be emphasized and appraised appropriately, new methods will be required. They can be developed to identify specific activities in caring and perhaps to include evaluations of accomplishment for what patients say they want done.

'Quality' does needs to be something more than a red tape ritual and is fundamental to the common vision, goals and objectives of an integrated service. Just as it is vital for teams working in integrated services to develop and share a common vision, goals and objectives, similar principles need to be applied to quality activities. The bulk of data on the effectiveness of quality assurance activities suggests that involvement of staff in the development of the activity, be they patient focus groups, grounded theory research, guidelines, algorithms, standards, or formal quality assurance programmes, is crucial to the acceptance, implementation and ultimate success of the activity. Clinicians need to have investment in such activities. They also need commitment and support from management systems of health care organizations. Recently, the focus has moved away from quality being the sole responsibility of clinicians towards system-wide clinical governance.

Total Quality Improvement (TQI)/Management (TQM) and Clinical Governance

Total Quality Improvement (or Management) is a management philosophy aiming to improve the level of performance of key processes in the health care organization. The idea was to make quality everyone's business, including management and not just the clinical workforce. However, the concept of TQM was recently reincarnated as *clinical governance*. The World Health Organization first described the model in 1983 but it only gained traction in the late 1990s. The major motivations for its rise to prominence were multiple enquiries into adverse events due to failure of care (of which a large number were mental health) despite quality activities such as clinical audit being in place, together with increasing liability of health care organizations for damages awarded by the courts to victims of medical error. Poor quality care is an expensive liability! Other drivers of clinical governance were the rare but highly publicized cases of 'bad apple' providers and a culture of blame that prevented open enquiry into system failures. In addition, the introduction of 'best practice' guidelines and protocols has had the effect of identifying significant access problems and wider systems issues. So, is clinical governance the answer?

Clinical governance – partnership in maintaining quality

Lugon and Secker-Walker (1999) define clinical governance as:

> The action, the system or the manner of governing clinical affairs. This requires two main components; an explicit means of setting clinical policy and an equally explicit means of monitoring compliance with such policy.

Clinical governance is about creating an open quality culture involving everyone in the organization. The World Health Organization report on Quality Assurance (1983) considered clinical governance as having four key elements:

1. Professional performance

2. Efficiency of resource use

3. Management of risk of injury or illness associated with the service provided

4. Patient satisfaction with the service provided.

To these, Walshe (2000a) added professional education and development, clinical effectiveness and knowledge management to aid professional performance, an ongoing quality programme and whole systems responsibility for quality management.

Clinical and corporate governance are together responsible for clinical quality. Both must consider the impact of their actions on clinical quality. Management's task is to provide a solid foundation of workforce planning and continuous professional development, ensuring there is enough resources and the workforce are properly trained to do their tasks. There needs to be a comprehensive programme of quality improvement systems. These can include any of the quality assurance activities described above, be externally mandated process measures or patient-relevant research e.g. looking at outcomes from the patients' as well the clinicians' points of view. Knowledge management and effectiveness includes the use of evidence-based practice clinical guidelines. A further requirement is for integrated procedures for all professional groups to identify and remedy poor performance, that move away from a blaming the individual culture to addressing one of system failure. There needs to be a whole system's approach to risk management; systems for risk accountability, for risk identification, for risk analysis, and risk reduction.

Blumenthal and Kilo (1998) and Walshe (2000a,b) note some lessons for clinical governance from a whole systems approach. It is essential that clinicians are committed, involved and provide leadership. An initial focus on clinical issues or priorities where quick and visible gains can be made for both patients and staff encourages clinicians' participation and support. Time needs to be allocated – clinicians should not be expected to undertake this work in their lunch break or 'after hours'. Terminology should incorporate all disciplines and avoid jargon. General training and awareness-raising programmes are a waste of time. They have little long-term impact and can breed cynicism. Training needs to identify skill and knowledge deficits. Senior management needs to own clinical governance, be involved and value it.

Clinical governance as a means of ensuring quality in health systems and reducing risk is relatively new and its effectiveness largely unevaluated. Notwithstanding, the concept has captured the imagination of many health care organizations in many countries. How successful this will be will depend on whether it is seen as a good idea by clinicians or just another means of workforce control or a red-tape ritual. There are differences in approach. The UK has adopted clinical governance as a 'top-down' government policy, whereas Australia and New Zealand are committed to a 'bottom-up' culture change. The history of previous quality initiatives needs to be remembered. Unless the process is owned and developed by the workforce it will not be accepted. Indeed, Wallace and Stoten (1999) and Walshe *et al.* (2000) found that the implementation of clinical governance in 47 hospitals and trusts in the West Midlands was undermined by the failure:

to take a systematic approach to the design and implementation of organizational interventions that could impact on the culture change goals of clinical governance .... It seems that the key goal of clinical governance, building a shared culture, has been left to chance.

Clinical governance requires very similar characteristics to those needed for successful integration of services, such as the important role of clinical leadership, the need for everyone to develop and be committed to the programme, emphasis on professional development and clear processes for administration and accountability.

Geriatric psychiatry is already familiar with working in multi- or inter-disciplinary teams and collaborating with others. In clinical governance, with its emphasis on clinical leadership and development of clinician-led quality programmes, there could be an opportunity to develop new and more pertinent quality initiatives in conjunction with patients that overcome some of the barriers experienced with previous quality activities. To quote Baroness Onora O'Neill (2002) again:

Serious and effective accountability, I believe, needs to concentrate on good governance, on obligations to tell the truth and needs to seek intelligent accountability. I think it has to fantasize much less about Herculean micro-management by means of performance indicators or total transparency. If we want a culture of public service, professionals and public servants must in the end be free to serve the public rather than their paymasters.

Quality of care and caring has to be a major focus for integrated services in serving the public. It needs to be part of the common vision for all participants. The keys to success in developing high quality integrated services lies in three dimensions – they are *patient-centred*; there is *partnership* with patients, health professional colleagues and administrators to develop good clinical governance, and staff all exhibit a high degree of *professionalism.*

Brennan (2002) highlights professionalism as having:

- Commitment to professional competence
- Commitment to honesty with patients
- Commitment to patient confidentiality
- Commitment to maintain appropriate relations with patients
- Commitment to improving quality of care
- Commitment to improving access of care
- Commitment to just distribution of finite resources
- Commitment to scientific knowledge
- Commitment to maintain trust by managing conflict of interest.

The real effectiveness of services depends upon the ability of health personnel to collaborate together, to facilitate the quality of the everyday interactions between clinicians so that patients are enabled to increase their participation in life's activities and enjoy a better quality of life. The challenge is to demonstrate this, so that patients such as 'Sandy' have the very best possible care from their encounters with geriatric psychiatry services.

References

Adamson, B., Kenny, D., and Wilson-Barnett, J. (1995) The impact of perceived medical dominance on the workplace satisfaction of Australian and British nurses. *Journal of Advanced Nursing*, **21** (1), 172–83.

Aminzadeh, F. (2000) Adherence to recommendations of community-based comprehensive geriatric assessment programmes. *Age and Ageing*, **29** (5), 401–7.

Aminzadeh, F. and Dalziel, W.B. (2002) Older adults in the emergency department: a systematic review of patterns of use, adverse outcomes, and effectiveness of interventions. *Annals of Emergency Medicine*, **29** (2), 254–64.

Anderson, R., Ory, M., Cohen, S., and McBride, J.S. (2000) Issues of Aging and adherence to health interventions. *Controlled Clinical Trials*, **21**, 171S–183S.

Arie, T. (2002) The development in Britain. In J. R. M. Copeland, M. T. Abou-Saleh, and D. G. Blazer (eds.) *Principles and Practice of Geriatric Psychiatry*, 2nd edition. Wiley, London.

Arie, T. and Jolley, D. (1982). Making services work: organisation and style of psychogeriatric services. In R. Levy and F. Post (eds.) *The Psychiatry of Late Life*. Blackwell, Oxford.

Arthur, A., Jagger, C., Lindesay, J., Graham, C., and Clarke, M. (1999) Using an annual over-75 health check to screen for depression: validation of the short Geriatric Depression Scale (GDS15) within general practice. *International Journal of Geriatric Psychiatry*, **14** (6), 431–9.

Arthur, A.J., Jagger, C., Lindesay, J., and Matthews, R.J. (2002). Evaluating a mental health assessment for older people with depressive symptoms in general practice: a randomised controlled trial. *British Journal of General Practice*, **52**, 202–7.

Audit Commission (2000) *Forget Me Not: Mental Health Services for Older People*. Audit Commission, London.

Bartels, S. (2002) Quality, costs, and effectiveness of services for older adults with mental disorders: a selective overview of recent advances in geriatric mental health services research. *Current Opinion in Psychiatry*, **15** (4), 411–16.

Blumenthal, D. and Kilo, C. (1998) A report on continuous quality improvement. *Millbank Quarterly*, **76** (4), 625–48.

Brennan, T. (2002) Renewing professionalism in medicine: the physician charter. *Spine*, **27** (19), 2087.

Bull, M. and Roberts, J. (2001) Components of a proper hospital discharge for elders. *Journal of Advanced Nursing*, **35** (4), 571–81.

Burns, A., Dening, T., and Baldwin, R. (2001) Mental health problems. *BMJ*, **322** (7289), 789–91.

Burns, R., Nichols, L., Martindale-Adams, J., and Graney, M. (2000) Interdisciplinary geriatric primary care evaluation and management: to-year outcomes. *Journal of the American Geriatrics Society*, **48**, 8–13.

Cabana, M.D., Rand, C.S., Powe, N.R., Wu, A.W., Wilson, M.H., Abboud, P.A., and Rubin, H.R. (1999) Why don't physicians follow clinical practice guidelines? A framework for improvement. *Journal of American Medical Association*, **282** (15), 1458–65.

Cassell, E. (1999) Diagnosing suffering: a perspective. *Annals of Internal Medicine*, **131** (7), 531–4.

Challis, D., Reilly, S., Hughes, J., Burns, A., Gilchrist, H., and Wilson, K. (2002) Policy, organisation and practice of specialist old age psychiatry in England. *International Journal of Geriatric Psychiatry*, **17** (11), 1018–26.

Child, J. (1984). *Organization. A Guide to Problems and Practice*, 2nd edn. Paul Chapman Publishing: London.

Corrigan, P. and Garman, A. (1999) Transformational and transactional leadership skills for mental health teams. *Community Mental Health Journal*, **35**(4), 301–12.

Dechant, K., Marsick, V., and Kasl, E. (1993) Towards a model of team learning. *Studies in Continuing Education*, **15**, 1–14.

Dent, T.H.S. and Sadler, M. (2002) From guidance to practice: Why NICE is not enough. *BMJ*, **324** (7341), 842–5.

Department Of Health (2004) *Single Assessment Process For Older People. Audit of Progress up to 1 April 2004 and Further Developments During 2004/05*. Department of Health, London.

Detmer, D. and Ford, J. (2001) Educating leaders for healthcare. *Clinicians in Management*, **10**, 3–5.

Donabedian, A. (1980) *The Definition of Quality and Approaches to Its Assessment: Exploring in Quality Assessment and Monitoring*. Health Administration Press, Ann Arbor, MI.

Draper, B. (2001) Consultation liaison geriatric psychiatry. In P. Melding and B. Draper (eds.) *Geriatric Consultation Liaison Psychiatry*, pp. 3–34. Oxford University Press, Oxford, New York.

Druss, B.G., Bradford, W.D., Rosenheck, R.A., Radford, M.J., and Krumholz, H.M. (2001) Quality of medical care and excess mortality in older patients with mental disorders. *Archives of General Psychiatry*, **58** (6), 565–72.

EASY-Care http://www.shef.ac.uk/sisa/easycare/ accessed 28 May 2004.

Eve, J.D. (2004) Sustainable practice: how practice development frameworks can influence team work, team culture and philosophy of practice. *Journal of Nursing Management*, **12** (2), 124–30.

FACE recording and measuring systems http://www.facecode.com/accessed 28 May 2004.

Feinstein, A.R. (2002) Is 'Quality of Care' being mislabeled or mismeasured? *The American Journal of Medicine*, **112** (6), 472–8.

Firth-Cozens, J. (2001) Cultures for improving patient safety through learning: the role of teamwork. *Quality in Healthcare*, **10** (Suppl. II), 26.

Froberg, D.G. and Kane, R.L. (1989) Methodology for measuring health-state preferences. 1. Measurement strategies. *Journal of Clinical Epidemiology*, **42**, 345–54.

Gallo, J.J., Rabins, P.V., and Iliffe, S. (1997) The 'research magnificent' in late life: psychiatric epidemiology and the primary health care of older adults. *International Journal of Psychiatry in Medicine*, **27** (3), 185–204.

Gilbody, S., Whitty, P., Grimshaw, J., and Thomas, R. (2003) Educational and organizational interventions to improve the management of depression in primary care: a systematic review. *Journal of American Medical Association*, **289** (23), 3145–51.

Glazier, S.R., Schuman, J., Keltz, E., Vally, A., and Glazier, R.H. (2004) Taking the next steps in goal ascertainment: a prospective study of patient, team, and family perspectives using a comprehensive standardized menu in a geriatric assessment and treatment unit. *Journal of the American Geriatrics Society*, **52** (2), 284–9.

Handy, C. (1993) *Understanding Organizations*. Oxford University Press, New York, Oxford.

Higashi, T., Shekelle, P.G., Solomon, D.H., Knight, E.L., Roth, C., Chang, J.T., Kamberg, C.J., MacLean, C.H., Young, R.T., Adams, J., Reuben, D.B., Avorn, J., and Wenger, N.S. (2004). The quality of pharmacologic care for vulnerable older patients. *Annals of Internal Medicine*, **140** (9), 714–20.

InterRAI home care http://www.interrai.org/instruments/home_care.php accessed 28 May 2004.

InterRAI residential care http://www.interrai.org/instruments/nursing_facility.php accessed 28 May 2004.

King, J.C., Nelson, R., Heye, M.L. Turturro, T.C., and Titus, M.N. (1998) Prescriptions, referrals, order writing and the rehabilitation team function. In J. A. DeLisa, B. M. Gans, W. L. Bockenek, D. M. Currie, S. R. Geiringer, L. H. Gerber, J. A. Leonard, M. C. McPhee, W. S. Pease, and N. E. Walsh (eds.) *Rehabilitation Medicine: Principles and Practice*, 3rd edn, pp. 269–85. J. B. Lippincott, Philadelphia.

Lugon, M. and Secker-Walker, J. (1999) *Clinical Governance: Making it Happen.* Royal Society of Medicine Press, London.

Lyness, J.M., Caine, E.D., King, D.A., Cox, C., and Yoediono Z. (1999) Psychiatric disorders in older primary care patients. *Journal of General Internal Medicine.* **14** (4), 249–54.

Maidment, R., Livingston, G., and Katona, C. (2002) Just keep taking the tablets: adherence to antidepressant treatment in older people in primary care. *International Journal of Geriatric Psychiatry,* **17** (8), 752–7.

Martin, M.A., Pehrson, J., and Orrell, M. (1999) A survey of social services needs assessments for elderly mentally ill people in England and Wales. *Age and Ageing,* **26** (6), 575–8.

Meara, J.R., Wood, J.L., Wilson, M.A., and Hart, M.C. (1992) Home from hospital: a survey of hospital discharge arrangements in Northamptonshire. *Journal of Public Health Medicine,* **14**, 145–50.

Millward, L. and Jefferies, N. (2001) The team survey: a tool for health care team development. *Journal of Advanced Nursing,* **35** (2), 276–87.

Morris, J., Fries, B.E., Steel, K., Ikegami, N., Bernabei, R., Carpenter, G.I., Gigen, R., Hirdes, J. P., and Topinkova, E. (1997). Comprehensive clinical assessment in community settings: applicability of the MDS-HC. *Journal of the American Geriatrics Society,* **45**, 1017–24.

New Zealand Guidelines Group (2003) *Assessment Processes for Older People.* Government Press: Wellington.

New Zealand Strategy for Health of Older People (2002) Ministry of Health; Government Press: Wellington

Nickolaus, T., Specht-Leibel, N., Bach, M., Oster, P., and Schlierf, G. (1999) A randomized trial of comprehensive geriatric assessment and home intervention in the care of hospitalized patients. *Age and Ageing,* **28** (6), 543–50.

O'Neill, O. (2002) *Called to Account.* The Reith Lectures No. 3. http://www.bbc.co.uk/radio4/reith2002/

Opie, A. (1999) In P. Davis and K. Dew (eds.) *Health and Society in Aoteraroa New Zealand,* pp. 181–98. Oxford University Press, Melbourne.

Outhwaite, S. (2003) The importance of leadership in the development of an integrated team. *Journal of Nursing Management,* **11** (6), 371–6.

Ovretveit, J. (1993) *Coordinating Community Care: Multidisciplinary Teams and Case Management.* Open University Press: Buckingham and Philadelphia.

Peabody, F.W. (1930) Doctor and Patient. Macmillan, New York.

Peabody, F.W. (1927) The care of the patient. *Journal of the American Medical Association,* **88**, 877–82.

Powell, D. and Peile, E. (2000) Joint working. It's a stitch-up. *Health Service Journal,* **110** (5702), 24–5.

Reuben, D.B., Frank, J.C., Hirsch, S.H., McGuigan, K.A., and Maly, R.C. (1999) A randomized clinical trial of outpatient comprehensive geriatric assessment coupled with an intervention to increase adherence to recommendations. *Journal of American Geriatrics Society,* **47** (3), 269–76.

Reuben, D.B., Borok, G., Wolde-Tsadik, G., Ersoff, D., Fishman, L., Ambrosini, V., Yunbao, L., Rubenstein, L., and Beck, J. (1995) A randomized controlled trial of comprehensive geriatric assessment in the care of hospitalized patients. *New England Journal of Medicine,* **332** (20), 1345–40.

Reuben, D.B., Shekelle, P.G., and Wenger, N.S. (2003) Quality of care for older persons at the dawn of the third millennium. *Journal of American Geriatrics Society,* **51** (Suppl. 7), S346–50.

Reynolds, T., Thornicroft, G., Abas, M., Woods, B., Hoe, J., Leese, M., and Orrell, M. (2000) The Camberwell Assessment of Need for the Elderly (CANE) development, validity, and reliability. *British Journal of Psychiatry*, **176**, 444–52.

Robinson, A. and Street, A. (2004) Improving networks between acute care nurses and an aged care assessment team. *Journal of Clinical Nursing*, **13** (4), 486–96.

Ryan, M. (2004), Discrete choice experiments in health care. *BMJ*, **328** (7436), 360–1.

Sayers, J., Watts, S., and Bhutani, G. (2002) Early detection of mental health problems in older people. *British Journal of Nursing*, **11** (18), 1198–203.

Shah, A.K. and Ames, D. (1994). Planning and developing psychogeriatric services. *International Review of Psychiatry*, **6**, 15–27.

Shekelle, P.G., Ortiz, E., Rhodes, S. *et al.* (2001) Validity of the agency for healthcare research and quality clinical practice guidelines: how quickly do guidelines become outdated? *Journal of the American Medical Association*, **286**, 1461–7.

Sixma, H.J., Crétien van Campen, J.J., and Kerssens, L.P. (2000). Quality of care from the point of view of elderly persons: the QUOTE-elderly instrument. *Age and Ageing*, **29**, 173–8.

Slaets, J.P.J., Kauffmann, R.H., Duivenvoorden, H.J., Pelemans, W., and Schudel, W.J. (1997) A randomized trial of geriatric liaison intervention in elderly medical inpatients. *Psychosomatic Medicine*, **59**, 585–91.

Stevenson, J. (1999) *Comprehensive Assessment of Older People: Kings Fund Rehabilitation Programme. Developing rehabilitation opportunities for older people.* Kings Fund; London.

Unutzer, J., Katon, W., Williams, J.W. Jr., Callahan, C.M., Harpole, L., Hunkeler, E.M., and Hoffing, M. (2001) Improving primary care for depression in late life: the design of a multicenter randomized trial. *Medical Care*, **39**, 785–99.

Valenstein, M., Mitchinson, A., Ronis, D., Alexander, J., Duffy, S.A., Craig, T.J., and Barry, K.L. (2004) Quality indicators and monitoring of mental health services: what do frontline providers think? *American Journal of Psychiatry*, **161** (1), 146–53.

Wallace, L. and Stoten, B. (1999) Clinical governance in the late show. *Health Service Journal*, **109** (5644), 24–5.

Walshe, K., Freeman, T., Latham, L., Spurgeon, P., and Wallace, L. (2000) Clinical governance. Scope to improve. *Health Service Journal*, **110** (5728), 30–2.

Walshe, K. (2000a) Systems for clinical governance: evidence of effectiveness. *Journal of Clinical Governance*, **8**, 174–80.

Walshe, K. (2000b) *Clinical Governance: A Review of the Evidence.* Health Services Management Centre, University of Birmingham, Birmingham.

Walton, M. (1986) *The Deming Management Method.* Putnam: New York.

Wasson, J., Stuckel, T., Weiss, J., Hays, R., Jette, A., and Nelson, E. (1999). A randomized trial of the use of patient self-assessment data to improve community practices. *Effective Clinical Practice*, **2** (1), 1–10.

Weiner, M., Callahan, C., Tierney, W.M., Overhage, J.M., Mamlin, B., Dexter, P.R., and McDonald, C.J. (2003) Using information technology to improve the health care of older adults: determinants of successful aging: developing an integrated research agenda for the 21st century. *Annals of Internal Medicine*, **139** (5, Part 2, Suppl. 2), 430–6.

Wenger, N.S., Solomon, D.H., Roth, C.P., MacLean, C.H., Saliba, D., Kamberg, C.J., Rubenstein, L.Z., Young, R.T., Sloss, E.M., Louie, R., Adams, J., Chang, J.T., Venus, P.J., Schnelle, J.F., and Shekelle, P.G. (2003) The quality of medical care provided to vulnerable community-dwelling older patients. *Annals of Internal Medicine*, **139** (9), 740–7.

Wensing, M.E. (2003). Methods for incorporating patients' views in health care (Education and debate: improving the quality of health care). *BMJ*, **326** (7394), 877–9.

Wolf, GA., Hayden, M., and Bradle, J.A. (2004) The transformational model for professional practice: a system integration focus. *Journal of Nursing Administration*, **34** (4), 180–7.

WHO (World Health Organization) (1983) *The Principles of Quality Assurance. Report on a WHO Meeting.* World Health Organization, Copenhagen.

Chapter 18

Rural service delivery

Jane B. Neese

To provide a thorough examination of psychogeriatric service delivery, this chapter presents a review of rural mental health, barriers and service delivery issues related to the older adult population. This chapter focuses on the United States and many of the issues identified are relevant to rural areas in other countries, but there are also likely to be differences. The term 'rural' carries many definitions depending upon the academic institution, politicians and country. According to Coward and colleagues (1994), an acceptable definition of rural has been elusive. Most traditional methods of identifying rural areas are based on population size, sparseness of towns, remoteness or distance to urban resources, degree of economic activity and commuting pattern (Magilvy *et al.*, 1994). In health services research, rural areas are designated based on the population size living in a particular geographic area, the distance from a large metropolitan area and the density of the population.

Rural areas, residents and health and mental health services are not homogeneous in any country. While rural older adults are diverse in terms of where they live, their economic base and their cultural group, they do have common stressors. The term 'farm stress' was developed in the 1980s to describe the emotional and physical stress experienced by United States farmers in the Midwest due to the slumping agricultural industry. The term now is used to imply declining employment opportunities, agricultural viability, or loss of the major employer of the area (Elkind *et al.*, 1998). Symptoms of farm stress include difficulty sleeping, depression, alcohol and drug abuse, spousal and child abuse, an increase in accidents and physiological symptoms such as headaches and chest and abdominal pains. Farm stress continues to be a major concern, especially with the current weakened United States economy and soaring fuel and energy costs (Letvak, 2002).

Defining rural

The US Census Bureau (2000) defines rural as consisting of all territory, population and housing units outside of an urbanized area or urban cluster (defined as population density of 1,000 people per square mile and overall density of 500 people per square mile) and having less than 2,500 residents. The US Census Bureau bases their definition on a combination of population density, relationship to cities and population size while Office of Management and Budget (OMB), an office that dispenses financial resources to areas, defines rural in population size and degree of integration with larger cities. These slight differences in definition become apparent in comparing the Census Bureau classification of 61.7 million (25 per cent) of the US population is rural versus the OMB classification of 55.9 million (23 per cent) of the US population as rural (Letvak, 2002). Although the definitions differ slightly, the financial resources, which translate into both health and social services, can greatly affect the rural area and its population.

Rural demographics

Within the United States, 25 per cent of the population lives within rural-designated areas. Of those rural residents, 12.8 per cent are individuals who are 65 years and over (US Census Bureau, 2000). Similar to national statistics, the majority of rural older adults are women (54.7 per cent) compared to men (45.3 per cent) and women comprise 67.4 per cent of the 85 and older age group. Women also tend to live alone and be more impoverished than their male rural counterparts (Coward et al., 1994). Rural residents as a whole tend to be more impoverished (15.9 per cent compared to 13.2 per cent in urban areas), have less access to mental health professionals, and 41 per cent of rural women are depressed or anxious as compared to 13–20 per cent prevalence rates in urban women (Mulder et al., 2001). Rural areas have a slightly greater number of elders who are 75 years and older than urban areas. Approximately 656,000 minority older adults live in non-metropolitan areas as compared to 2.7 million minority elders residing in metropolitan areas. Within the rural population, 525,000 (10.7 per cent) are African American elders compared to a higher proportion (25 per cent) of the US white elders (US Census Bureau, 1992; Harper and Alexander, 1990).

Those with mental illness who reside in rural communities are at a greater disadvantage because of limited access to health care, a scarcity of resources and traditional cultural belief systems (Coburn and Bolda, 1999; Letvak, 2002). Economic decline from changes in economy and job opportunities has led to the emigration of the young adult population from the rural US, resulting in a rapidly ageing rural population. With the rural population becoming more elderly, a higher prevalence of chronic health problems has resulted in a concomitant need for more health care services (Ermann, 1990). Rural elders report more chronic illnesses, physical impairments, chronic activity limitation and more days limited to bed than those residing in urban areas (Wagenfeld, 1990). Rural farm elders have 25 per cent more acute conditions, more days of restricted activity and more days confined to bed than the average older adult (Palmore, 1983–1984). Chronic illnesses among rural elders have been estimated as high as 87 per cent with 36 per cent more bed disability days than urban elders (US Congress, 1973). Nyman and colleagues (1991) found that rural elders needed more assistance with instrumental activities of daily living (IADLs) such as yard work, shopping, minor repairs, handling money and transportation. Rural elders also were more likely to be impaired in their hearing and vision (Nyman *et al.*, 1991).

The prevalence of psychiatric disorders has been estimated as high as 25 per cent among rural elders (Rosen *et al.*, 1981). In the Epidemiologic Catchment Area Study, cognitive impairment was found to be more prevalent among rural elders than among urban elders, even though depression rates were similar (Blazer *et al.*, 1985). Nyman and colleagues (1991) found that the rural elders were more likely to experience symptoms of depression and loneliness. In rural areas, alcohol dependence/abuse has been found to be more prevalent than in urban areas, with the incidence of alcohol dependence higher among black rural elders (Blazer *et al.*, 1985, 1987).

Robbins and Regier (1994) found that 23 per cent to 56 per cent of individuals with a diagnosed DSM–III Axis I psychiatric disorder are more likely to have a coexisting chemical dependency disorder. Among mental health professionals, these coexisting psychiatric and substance abuse disorders are referred to as 'dual diagnoses' because both the 'primary' psychiatric disorder and the chemical dependency disorder, whether alcohol or substance, are both listed on Axis I of the multi-axial assessment categories of the *Diagnostic and Statistical Manual of Mental Disorders – TR* (DSM-IV-TR) (APA, 2000). Although some studies suggest that the prevalence of alcohol and substance abuse and dependence disorders are not higher in rural areas than urban areas, there are towns and regions where a specific drug, such as methamphetamine, is a problem, (National Rural Health Association, 1999).

Murray and Lopez (1996) report that mental disorders collectively account for 15 per cent of the overall burden of disease in the US, which is more than the burden associated with all forms of cancer. It is estimated that up to 20 per cent of all people diagnosed with a medical diagnosis have some type of mental health illness. Roberts *et al.* (1999) found that 13–19 per cent of rural residents experience significant psychiatric impairment. According to Bushy (2000), rural residents experience a higher degree of depression, alcohol abuse, domestic violence, incest and child abuse than their urban counterparts. Views of mental illness within the rural community are generally more negative and stigma attached to mental illness is often more magnified, which prevents people from seeking health care at all (Letvak, 2002). Despite these marked health needs, rural elderly receive less health and mental health care than their urban counterparts. As Palmore (1983–1984, p. 40) noted, 'Fewer farm elders get hospitalized; fewer rural elders get surgical treatment; and rural elders have fewer physician and dental visits than the average elder.'

While rural areas are not homogeneous, but diverse in population size, age groups, geographic terrain, structure, and distance to dense populations, there are several common trends in examining health and service delivery in rural areas among older adults. Rural areas tend to be medically underserved both in quantity and range of available services and in number of health care providers as compared to metropolitan areas. According to Weinert and Burman (1996), rural health care varies and has fewer resources available to deliver basic as well as specialty services. As much as 80 per cent of care to rural elders is provided through informal human and fiscal resources (Havens and Kyle, 1993). The low ratio of primary care physicians to community population can affect an older adult's ability to obtain timely acute care and preventive services (Auchincloss *et al.*, 2001). Beidler and Bourdonniere (1999) discovered that

> Care services for the aging rural population suffer from uneven development. Lower availability of providers in rural areas results in lower utilization of health services by older people in rural areas. The implications are that many older rural residents receive no care at all.
>
> Beidelr and Bourdonniere, 1999, p. 34

Even though the need for services is high among rural elders, service utilization rates are low. Only between 1 per cent (Scheidt and Windley, 1982) and 7 per cent (Kermis, 1987) of rural elderly use mental health services. Stefl and Prosperi (1985) reported that only 8.9 per cent of rural elders diagnosed with mental health problems used the available mental health services and only 5 per cent of rural residents used the available substance abuse services (US Congress, 1990). Stigma attached to psychiatric and mental health services can deter rural elders from using these services (Stefl and Prosperi, 1985); however, service utilization for physical illnesses also is lower among rural elders than their urban counterparts (Coward and Lee, 1985).

In the last two decades, scholars have determined several barriers in delivery of health and mental health care in rural areas. A direct relationship exists between barriers and the health care needs: as the need for services increases, so do the barriers to meeting those needs. Reduced availability (awareness and location of services), compromised accessibility (ease of getting to services), acceptability (stigma and perception) and affordability (costs) are the greatest barriers (Stefl and Prosperi, 1985; US Congress, 1990). These barriers continue to be relevant today and leave rural elderly particularly at risk for premature institutionalization and hospitalization.

Affordability of rural mental health services

For impoverished rural residents, payment of mental health services is a complex array of entities. In the US, methods for health care payment are in a constant flux with changing funding streams from federally-funded Medicare and state-funded Medicaid to privately paid health insurance. In order to pay for health and mental health care, many older persons have multiple sources of health insurance coverage (Cohen *et al.*, 1997). US citizens 65 and older are eligible for basic hospital costs and related post-hospital services via Medicare Part A, a federally funded insurance (Office of the Federal Register, 1998). In addition, all US citizens 65 and older may purchase Medicare Part B, which adds physician and surgeon services and a variety of hospital and ambulatory services. Those older adults ineligible for Medicare Part B may purchase Medicare Part B (Auchincloss *et al.*, 2001). For many older adults, the combination of Medicare Part A and B will not cover all health, mental health, or medication expenses.

In the US poverty, income, and insurance coverage have a direct effect on utilization of services. Poverty has been linked with poor health status, which influences use of health care services. Rural elder residents are more likely to have lower incomes than urban elders. In 1987, elders typically spent 15 per cent of their income on health care, an average of $1,660 per person (Stone, 1986). With more rural elders being impoverished, they also rely more on state-funded Medicaid and other public assistance to supplement their Medicare coverage. Since Medicare ceilings or total amount paid for services are lower in rural areas, the costs for health care is shifted to the older adult who has to pay for services from their monthly income. State-funded Medicaid does assist in providing payment for skilled nursing home placement for those rural older adults who meet the federal guidelines for impoverishment and whose cognitive impairment cannot be managed at home.

State-funded Medicaid budgets pay for most mental health services delivered to impoverished older adults; however most of those services are 'carved out' from general health care services to managed care organizations known as managed behavioural health organizations. Therefore, mental health care services are separated from health care services under a different organizational umbrella, creating an extra array of procedures to follow (National Rural Health Association, 1999). For most managed care organizations, their rationale is to provide appropriate services in the most effective way, resulting in a bottom line of eliminating some costly mental health services or reducing the quantity of mental health services. Most of these cost-reduction measures have found their way to reducing the number of outpatient visits and inpatient lengths of stay. In rural areas where community resources and services are more limited than urban areas, earlier discharge from acute care hospitalization is a problem. Support services such as partial hospitalization services, respite services and day hospital treatment facilities are rarely available in rural areas. Therefore, rural residents are more at risk for relapse and readmission for their mental health problems (National Rural Health Association, 1999).

Receiving mental health services in rural areas is more complicated because of differences in insurance coverage. With the advent of managed care in the US, most mental health services are 'carved-out' or not included within general health insurance policies with the result that, for consumers and older adults, many mental health services are not reimbursed through the health insurer. If the mental health services are covered under the health insurance, the costs that the individual pays prior to insurance overage is 50 per cent more than the costs for other health care services. Thus, the individual is paying more 'out of pocket' for mental health services than for general health care services. For some insurance carriers, mental health services are either not covered or the cost of insurance is prohibitive (Center for Mental Health, 1998). Therefore, costs for mental health services for rural elders can be too expensive in the light of poor insurance coverage and poverty of the population.

Access to rural mental health services

Access to health care is defined as the timely use of needed health care in addition to having a usual source of care. Both of these measures, timeliness in receiving care and having a regular source of care, are a de facto measure of appropriateness of health care, the effective use of that health care and the continuity of health care (Aday, 1993; Auchincloss *et al.*, 2001). Most older adults in the US do not have problems accessing the health care services that they need. On the other hand, vulnerable older adults or those who do not have comprehensive health insurance, are poor, have disabilities, are minorities and live in rural areas do have problems in accessing adequate health care services. According to Auchincloss and colleagues (2001), family income and lack of private insurance, living alone, and living in impoverished neighbourhoods decreased access to services. Geographic distance from tertiary care, travel costs and higher poverty rates in rural areas all contribute to this phenomenon.

Although the prevalence rates for some psychiatric disorders (schizophrenia, anxiety disorders and dementias) and chemical dependency are the same for rural and urban residents, use of mental health services differ. Approximately two-thirds of individuals with mental disorders receive less or no care at all for their problems. For those that do receive health care from a provider, more rural residents receive care from a general medical practitioner (45 per cent) than receive care from a mental health specialist (40 per cent) (National Rural Health Association, 1999). Since most rural areas lack mental health providers, specialty mental health services and mental health care professionals are fewer in numbers than in urban areas. Thus, rural residents who have mental health conditions are more likely to rely exclusively on general medical practitioners for treatment (Rost *et al.*, 1998).

Availability of rural mental health services

With the changes in federal reimbursement for Medicare and individual state's deteriorating budgets for Medicaid, most rural communities have experienced a reduction in hospital beds, if not closure and the loss of physician and dental practices. With the closure of hospital beds and, in some instances, the entire hospital, primary care services also have closed leaving the community with fewer physicians as well as public health funding. Several reasons have been attributed for the decline in health services in rural areas:

1. Inadequate Medicare reimbursement;
2. The discrepancy between specialty and family practice reimbursement;
3. Professional isolation; and
4. Heavy workloads (Baldwin *et al.*, 2001).

Not only did primary care practices diminish with the closure of rural hospitals and hospital beds, but mental health services were also forced to close resulting in patients having longer distances to travel to mental health services. Like their primary care counterparts, many mental health providers were affiliated with these hospitals, depending upon them for income. In 1990, only 14 per cent of the total rural hospital beds were designated for psychiatric care (Wagenfeld, 1990). Unfortunately, the decline in acute care mental health services provided by hospitals has not been compensated by an increase in outpatient mental health services. Chemical dependency services, however, are more available in rural areas than general psychiatric services. Usually chemical dependency services for alcohol or drug rehabilitation are located in community health centers (Neese et al., 1999).

Compounding the lack of inpatient psychiatric services and designated community mental health services is the lack of health providers who are specialized in the delivery of psychiatric care such as psychologists, psychiatrists, nurses and other providers of mental health care to rural elderly. Not only is recruitment of mental health providers in rural areas a problem, but also retention of these providers, especially providers specializing in psychogeriatric care. An added insult to the situation is the lower reimbursement rate for mental health services that providers receive from insurance carriers and federally-funded programmes (Neese et al., 1999).

In delivering mental health throughout the world, most studies reveal an uneven distribution and recruitment difficulties of mental health professions in rural versus urban areas (Heriz and Murphy, 1997; Yellowlees and Hemming, 1994). When mental health professionals are recruited to rural areas, they tend to be inexperienced, costing their employer more in training costs, only to leave after a couple of years (Herzig and Murphy, 1997). Problems sustaining health professionals in rural areas are not new. The literature abounds with research and articles citing difficulty gaining trust of the rural residents, professional and social isolation of health professionals, and maintaining clinical competency without educational resources as reasons for lack of retention of health and mental health professionals (Herzig and Murphy, 1997).

While there are fewer and less diverse mental health services provided in rural areas, residents tend to use crisis interventions more than other services (Neese, 1994).

> Major problems that rural mental health services face include the recruitment and morale of staff, difficulties in maintaining clinical standards through education and training, and under-use of services by eligible patients because of perceptions about the remoteness and inconvenience of a centralised service. These are problems frequently complained about in our multicultural inner city areas of Europe, North America and Australasia.
>
> Herzig and Murphy, 1997

Sometimes it is not the availability of services but the variability of services that poses the unique problem in accessing the appropriate and necessary health care (Salmon et al., 1993). For instance, general medical practice may be available in rural areas, however, a trained health professional in gerontology usually is not. Nursing home beds may be available in a rural area, but respite beds to ease the burden for caregivers are unavailable. To counteract this lack of range of services, several different proposals and models of providing care to older adults in rural areas were created to compensate.

Most models link existing community and informal resources to form a matrix of services with corresponding grant funding. Beidler and Bourbonniere (1999) proposed an 'Ageing in Place' model, where older adults remain at home and pre-existing resources and services are connected with state-of-the-art urban health care services. A second model has included rural churches by providing health care services through parish nurses who live in the rural community. Chase-Ziolek and Striepe (1999) found that nurses involved in rural churches tended to deliver health services through home visits and phone calls as well as through the church, whereas parish nurses in urban churches delivered health services primarily through the church. Another model for extending health and mental health services to rural areas is the development of family nurse practitioner practices. Independent nurse-managed, community-based care practices are a viable option. Many of these independent nurse-managed health care offices have been created with Schools of Nursing. In rural northeast Tennessee, an independent nurse-managed health care centre was opened to deliver nurse-managed care during the weekday evening hours (5:00 p.m.–9:00 p.m.) and all day on the weekends, which augmented the services provided by a local health care agency whose hours consisted of only weekdays without evening hours or weekend accessibility. According to Ramsey and colleagues (1993), rural residents were highly satisfied with family nurse practitioners (FNPs) when they used them; however they were less likely to seek the services of FNPs. Of the 22 per cent residents in this rural community who accessed the nurse-managed health care agency, only 3 per cent were older adults compared to 23.1 per cent young adults (Ramsey *et al.*, 1993). Ramsey *et al.* (1993) cited lack of knowledge of the care and services provided by FNPs, being more comfortable with traditional physician care, and lack of morning hours, which may not have been convenient for older adults.

Acceptability of rural mental health services

One of the contributing barriers to utilizing mental health services in rural areas is the stigma attached to having a mental disorder. Psychiatric and mental health disorders and those professionals associated with them have a long history of being stigmatized by society. The stigma is more prominent in rural communities that tend to contain a smaller number of people who tend to know everyone. Therefore, many rural residents seek mental health care under the pretext of a physical complaint. Relying on primary care providers to provide the bulk of psychiatric and mental health care to rural older adults is referred to as a de facto provider system. This de facto provider system of obtaining mental health services not only includes treatment by a non-mental health specialist, but also nursing home care, lay workers, self-help consumer-operated services, the faith community, agricultural extension agents, other health care providers (i.e., pharmacists, chiropractors), and law enforcement (Fox *et al.*, 1995; National Rural Health Association, 1999).

Rural culture, which includes deeply held value systems, ethnicity, religious and patriotic beliefs, may hinder accessing mental health services. Youmans (1977) identified three general value systems that interfere with rural residents utilization of mental health services:

1. Identifying with the surrounding community and a sense of belonging,

2. Work or 'doing' orientation, and

3. A fatalistic attitude.

Rural elders tend to manage their symptoms of mental illness by themselves or with their families. Likewise, discussions of mental health concerns are contained within the nuclear family or a tight network of relatives rather than a health care professional (Stoller and Foster, 1992). While self-sufficiency may be a necessity due to the scarcity of mental health services, more often self-sufficiency among rural elders is from valuing their independence and hard work (National Rural Health Association, 1999). Often mental illness is viewed as a sign of personal weakness, if not defeat (Smith *et al.*, 1997). This fear of being labeled as 'crazy or insane' leads most rural elders to being concerned that they will be 'locked away' in an institution, which may prevent them from seeking mental health care services (Buckwalter *et al.*, 1994).

Although more research has been conducted in the last two decades to examine the differences and methods of best providing culturally sensitive care to minority populations, there remain many gaps in the literature. Understanding the different ethnic community's perspective in service use in rural areas is important to development of services that will be accepted and used. In the rural African American community, the church and kin are primary social and health support resources for older African American adults. In addressing rural service use among minority older adults, social networks and supports need to be examined because it is often those same social supports that can hinder receiving services. Therefore, the social support network influences the utilization of health care and in-home care services (Porter *et al.*, 2000). Within the different rural ethnic cultures, folk healers or indigenous healers, herbalists, root doctors, or shamans are considered initially for various emotional afflications, which vary dramatically from traditional psychiatric practice (Buckwalter *et al.*, 1994).

Conclusion

Although this chapter has focused on the barriers to providing rural mental health services to older adults, there are several advantages to living in rural areas. Scarce health and mental health resources preclude the fragmentation that larger urban settings experience in delivering mental health care to their population. There is less duplication of services and better coordination of both formal and information services within the community because of fewer resources. Likewise, health and mental health providers have learned how to incorporate community resources into effective treatment plans. A good example of this is the use of parish nurses who function through the auspices of the local rural churches. Social institutions including the church, volunteer agencies, clubs and agriculture extension agents are more accessible and often provide informal health care safety nets when older adults are discharged from nursing homes or hospitals. Although stigma will be a barrier to accepting mental health services, rural communities as a whole tend to be more tolerant of peculiar personality traits and abnormal behaviour. Instead of ostracizing an individual with a mental illness, rural residents offer support to family members in time of crisis (Center for Mental Health Services, 1998).

References

Aday, L.A. (1993) *At Risk in America: The Health and Health Care Needs of Vulnerable Populations in the United States.* San Francisco, CA: Jossey-Bass.

American Psychiatric Association (2000) *Diagnostic and Statistical Manual of Mental Disorders Fourth Edition Text Revision (DSM-IV-TR).* Washington, DC: American Psychiatric Association.

Auchincloss, A.H., Van Nostrand, J.F., and Ronsaville, D. (2001) Access to health care for older persons in the United States: personal structural, and neighborhood characteristics. *Journal of Aging and Health,* **13** (3), 329–54.

Baldwin, K.A., Sisk, R.J., Watts, P., McCubbin, J., Brockerschmidt, B., and Marion, L.N. (2001) Acceptance of nurse practitioners and physician assistants in meeting the perceived needs of rural communities. *Public Health Nursing,* **15** (6), 389–97.

Beidler, S.M. and Bourbonniere, M. (1999) Aging in place: a proposal for rural community-based care for frail elders. *Nurse Practitioner Forum,* **10** (1), 33–8.

Blazer, D., Crowell, B.A., and George, L. K. (1987) Alcohol abuse and dependence in the rural South. *Archives of General Psychiatry,* **44**, 736–40.

Blazer, D., George, L., Landerman, R., Pennybacker, M., Melville, M.L., Woodbury, M., Manton, K.G., Jordan, K., and Locke, B. (1985) Psychiatric disorders: a rural/urban comparison. *Archives of General Psychiatric,* **42**, 651–6.

Buckwalter, K.C., Smith, M., and Caston, C. (1994) Mental and social health of rural elderly. In R. Coward, N. Bull, G. Kulkulka, and J. Gallaher (eds.) *Health Services for Rural Elders,* pp. 203–33. New York: Springer.

Bushy, A. (2000) *Orientation to Nursing in the Rural Community.* Thousand Oaks, CA: Sage.

Center for Mental Health Services (1998) *Mental Health, United States, 1998.* R. W. Manderscheid and M. J. Henderson (eds.), DHHS Pub. No. (SMA) 99–3285. Washington, DC: US Government Printing Office.

Chase-Ziolek, M. and Striepe, J. (1999) A comparison of urban versus rural experiences of nurses volunteering to promote health in churches. *Public Health Nursing,* **16** (4), 270–9.

Coburn, A.F. and Bolda, E.J. (1999) The rural elderly and long term care. In T. C. Ricketts (ed.) *Rural Health in the United States,* pp. 179–89. New York, Oxford.

Cohen, R.A., Bloom, B., Simpson, G., and Parsons, P.E. (1997) Access to health care: Part 3. Older Adults. *Vital Stat,* **10** (198). (Available from the National Center for Health Statistics, Hyattsville, MD).

Coward, R.T., Bull, C.N., Kukulka, G., and Galliher, J.M. (1994) *Health Services for Rural Elders.* New York: Springer.

Coward, R.T. and Lee, G.R. (1985) *The Elderly in Rural Society: Every Fourth Elder*. New York: Springer.

Elkind, P., Carlson, J., and Schnable, B. (1998) Agricultural hazards reduction through stress management. *Journal of Agromedicine*, **5** (2), 23–32.

Ermann, D. A. (1990) *Rural Health Care: The Future of the Hospital*. (ANCPR Program Note). Washington, DC: Agency for Health Care Policy and Research.

Fox, J.C., Merwin, E., and Blank, M. (1995) De facto mental health services in the rural south. *Journal of Health Care for the Poor and Underserved*, **6** (4), 434–68.

Harper, M.S., and Alexander, C.D. (1990) Profile of the black elderly. In M.S. Harper (ed.) *Minority aging: Essential curricula content for selected health and allied health professionals*, pp. 193–222. DHHS Publication No. HRS (P-DV-90-4). Washington, DC: US Government Printing Office.

Havens, B. and Kyle, B. (1993) Formal long-term care. In C. Bull (ed.) *Aging in Rural America*, pp. 173–88. Newbury Park, CA: Sage.

Herzig, H. and Murphy, E. (1997) Rural lessons for urban services. *Journal of Mental Health*, **6** (1), 1–11.

Kermis, M.D. (1987) Equity and policy issues in mental health care of the elderly: dilemmas, deinstitutionalization, and DRG's. *Journal of Applied Gerontology*, **6**, 268–83.

Letvak, S. (2002) The importance of social support for rural mental health. *Issues in Mental Health Nursing*, **23**, 249–61.

Magilvy, J.K., Congdon, J.G., and Martinez, R. (1994) Circles of care: home care and community support for rural older adults. *Advanced Nursing Science*, **16** (3), 22–33.

Mulder, P.L., Kenken, M.B., Shellenberger, S., Constantine, M.G., Streigel, R., Sears, S.F., Junper-Thurman, P., Kalodner, M., Danda, C.E., and Hager, A. (2001) The behavioral health care needs of rural women. [On-line]. Available at: http://www.apa.org/rural/ruralwomen.pdf

Murray, C.J.L. and Lopez, A.D. (1996) *The Global Burden of Disease. A Comprehensive Assessment of Mortality and Disability from Diseases, Injuries, and Risk Factors in 1990 and Projected to 2020*. Cambridge, MA: Harvard School of Public Health.

National Rural Health Association (1999) *Mental Health in Rural America*. Online, available at http://www.nrharural.org/dc/issuepapers/ipaper14.html.

Neese, J.B. (1994) Service utilization among rural elders. Doctoral dissertation, University of Virginia, 1994. Dissertation Abstracts International, **55**, 520.

Neese, J.B., Abraham, I.L., and Buckwalter, K.C. (1999) Utilization of mental health services among rural elders. *Archives of Psychiatric Nursing*, **13** (1), 30–40.

Nyman, J.A., Sen, A., Chan, B.Y., and Commins, P.P. (1991) Urban/rural differences in home health patients and services. *The Geronologist*, **31** (4), 457–66.

Office of the Federal Register. (1998) *Code of Federal Regulations*, No. 42, Chapter IV, 10–1–98 edition. College Park, MD: National Archives and Records Administration.

Palmore, E. (1983–1984) Health care needs of the rural elderly. *International Journal of Aging and Human Development*, **18** (1), 39–45.

Porter, E.J., Ganong, L.H., and Armer, J.M. (2000) The church family and kin: An older rural black woman's support network and preferences for care providers. *Qualitative Health Research*, **10** (4), 452–70.

Ramsey, P., Edwards, J., Lenz, C., Odom, J. E., and Brown, B. (1993) Types of health problems and satisfaction with services in a rural nurse-managed clinic. *Journal of Community Health Nursing*, **10** (3), 161–70.

Robbins, L.N. and Regier, D.A. (1994) *Psychiatric Disorders in America: The Epidemiologic Catchment Area Study*. New York: The Free Press.

Roberts, L.W., Battaglia, J., Smithpeter, M., and Epstein, R.S. (1999) An office on main street: Health care dilemmas in small communities. *The Hastings Center Report*, **29** (4), 28–37.

Rosen, C.E., Coppage, S.J., Troglin, S.J., and Rosen, S. (1981) Cost effective mental health services for the rural elderly. In P.K. Kim and S.P. Wilson (ed.) *Toward mental health of rural elderly*. Washington, DC: University Press of America.

Rost, K., Owen, R., Smith, J., and Smith, G.R. (1998) Rural-urban differences in service use and course of illness in bipolar disorder. *The Journal of Rural Health*, **14** (1), 36–43.

Salmon, M., Nelson, G., and Rous, S. (1993) The continuum of care revisited: a rural perspective. *Gerontologist*, **33**, 658–66.

Scheidt, R.J. and Windley, P.G. (1982) Well-being profiles of small town elderly in differing rural contexts. *Community Mental Health Journal*, **18**, 257–67.

Smith, M., Buckwalter, K.C., and DeCroix-Bane, S. (1997) Rural settings. In N. K. Workley (ed.) *Mental Health Nursing in the Community*, pp. 276–89. St. Louis, MO: Mosby.

Stefl, M.E. and Prosperi, D.C. (1985) Barriers to mental health service utilization. *Community Mental Health Journal*, **21** (3), 167–77.

Stoller, E.P. and Foster, L.E. (1992) Patterns of illness behavior among rural elderly: preliminary results of health diary study. *Journal of Rural Health*, **8** (1), 13–26.

Stone, R. (1986) *The Feminization of Poverty and Older Women: An Update*. Report No. NCHSR 86–16. Washington, DC; US Government Printing Office.

US Census Bureau (1992) *CPI-1990 Census population. General Population Characteristics for the United States*. (Table 14). Washington, DC: U. S. Government Printing Office.

US Census Bureau (2000) *Census 2000 urban and rural classification*. Online www.census.gov/geo/www/ua/ua-2k.html.

US Census Bureau (2001) *Census 2000 Summary File 1; 1990 Census of population, General Population Characteristics, United States*. Online www.census.gov/prod/cen2000/doc/sf1.pdf.

US Congress, House of Representatives (1973) *Special Problems of the Rural Aging*. Report No. 93–103. Washington, DC: US Government Printing Office.

US Congress, Office of Technology Assessment (1990) *Health Care in Rural America*. OTA-H-434. Washington, DC: US Government Printing Office.

Wagenfeld, M.O. (1990) Mental health and rural America: a decade review. *The Journal of Rural Health*, **6** (4), 507–22.

Weinert, C. and Burman, M.E. (1996) Nursing of rural elders: myth and reality. In E. A. Swanson and T. Tripp-Reimer (eds.) *Advances in Gertonological Nursing: Issues for the 21st Century*, vol. **1**, pp. 57–79. New York, New York: Springer.

Yellowlees, P.M. and Hemming, M. (1992) Rural mental health. *Medical Journal of Australia*, **157**, 152–4.

Youmans, E.G. (1977) The rural aged. *Annals of the American Academy of Political and Social Science*, **419**, 81–90.

Chapter 19

Involvement of carers, consumers and the broader community

Henry Brodaty and Lee-Fay Low

This chapter will examine the consumer movement as it relates to psychogeriatric services and will include practical suggestions about how to appropriately involve consumers and carers in service planning, management and delivery. Ethical and medico-legal issues will be covered.

Carers

Clinicians working with carers

Who are carers?

A carer, also called a caregiver or caretaker, is defined as a family member (or friend), helping someone on a regular (usually daily) basis with tasks necessary for independent living (Zarit and Edwards, 1996, p. 334). Carers are vital partners in the care of older persons. They have roles in assessment, diagnosis, treatment, and medico-legal functions and are also legitimate targets for interventions in their own right. From a service viewpoint, acknowledgement of the need to provide for carers, even if not of an older age themselves, is crucial in organizing service loads.

A community study of people over 75 years in Australia found that 33 per cent had carers providing at least partial assistance (Broe *et al.*, 1999). A population-based study in England reported that 12 per cent of subjects over 65 years were carers (Livingston *et al.*, 1996). The population study also found that of cohabiting carers, 19 per cent cared for people with dementia, 28 per cent for people with depression and 53 per cent for people with physical disability. Carers of people with psychiatric disorders were more likely to have clinical depression than carers of those with physical disability (Livingston *et al.*, 1996).

The roles of the carer

First is the role of carers in assessment. This extends beyond the obvious provision of history as regards loss of short-term memory in cognitively impaired patients to more subtle changes in the patient such as personality change, apathy, hypomania and executive dysfunction. However, clinicians need to be aware that some carers are unreliable in their reports, especially where they have less contact with the patient (Bassett *et al.*, 1990). In the Honolulu Asia Aging Study, family informants failed to recognize cognitive problems in 21 per cent of community-dwelling persons subsequently diagnosed as having dementia (Ross *et al.*, 1997). Problems were more likely to go undetected by family members if patients were older, were less educated, had intact remote memory or had few behavioural or daily functioning problems. In a study of general practice attenders, Kemp *et al.* (2002) found that 40 per cent of carer accounts were discrepant with subsequent psychometric testing; 24 per cent under-reported and 16 per cent over-reported cognitive deficits. Inaccuracy was associated with patients who had milder impairment, less education and poorer remote memory and perhaps with carers who had less education. Even so, cohabiting family members are most often the person who is likely to become aware of cognitive deficits and be able to report on longitudinal course.

The diagnosis, once made, must be communicated. The carer is pivotal in deciding on the best way to break the news and in supporting the patient afterwards. While 71 per cent of carers say they would want to know the diagnosis if they themselves had Alzheimer's disease, only 17 per cent were wanting to tell their loved one (Maguire *et al.*, 1996).

Treatment

Carers have several roles in treatment of patients, especially for those who lack competence. They are usually the decision-makers as regards whether or not to start a treatment or management programme.

Compliance is a crucial issue, perhaps more so in the older patient. Carers may take on the role of ensuring that treatment regimens are adhered to and will be responsible for monitoring of and reporting about treatment outcomes.

Carers' views can be helpful in evaluation of services, although carers may rate outcome or satisfaction with service quite differently than do the patients (Wattis *et al.*, 1994) or the service providers (Riordan and Mockler, 1996). Wattis *et al.* (1994) used outcome measures that included objective and subjective measures of symptom resolution, carer stress, carer and patient measures of satisfaction and problem resolution. A reasonable level of satisfaction with the outcome was reported, though the correlations between different perceptions for individual patients were not high (Wattis *et al.*, 1994). In an audit of care programmes that involved staff, patients and carers, Riordan and Mockler (1996) found that staff rated their effectiveness significantly more highly than did patients and carers. Particular difficulties were noted in the identification of carers' needs as was also reported a survey of carer satisfaction of quality of care delivered to dementia inpatients (Simpson *et al.*, 1995). In that survey, 59 per cent of carers were dissatisfied about some aspects of the admission and communication was a frequently identified issue.

Clinicians, patients and carers should establish therapeutic alliances based on realistic expectations. Carers may have unrealistic expectations of treatment of which they should be disabused by their treating clinician, e.g. that cholinesterase inhibitors are cures for Alzheimer's disease.

Finally, carers may be the therapists themselves. Teri *et al.* (1997) taught behavioural techniques (with either a problem-solving or pleasant events focus) to carers of patients with Alzheimer's disease. Compared to control patients the carer-treated patients had significantly reduced levels and rates of depression. These improvements were maintained at six months follow-up. Further, the levels of depression in the carers, although not the focus of the intervention, fell too. Similarly but separately, Teri and colleagues (2003) instructed carers on implementation of behavioural management techniques combined with an exercise programme for family members with dementia. Patient depression and physical functioning improved in the group that received caregiver training compared to routine medical care. Improvement in physical functioning and depression (in initially more depressed patients) was maintained at 2 year follow-up.

Medico-legal issues

Informed consent for medical procedures requires the patient to understand what they are being treated for, as well as the risks and the benefits of the treatment, and to be able to communicate these to the treating doctor. Patients who are competent make their own decisions about treatment and other life choices. Where patients are not competent, carers usually provide this consent. For incompetent patients, it is the closest family member who usually becomes the person responsible for making proxy decisions and giving proxy informed consent. In some jurisdictions this role is automatic, in others it must be conferred by a formal process.

Where competence is impaired as in dementia, ethical research procedures require carers to give informed consent and, if possible, for patients to assent to the research. However, carers cannot consent to research over the patient's objections, and where risks are substantial or the research controversial many jurisdictions require that a legal body, such as a Guardianship Tribunal, approve the protocol.

Carers as the second patient

The aphorism holds that when one diagnoses a patient with dementia, there is (almost) always a second patient. Carers of persons with a mental illness such as dementia or depression have high rates of depression themselves, low morale, decreased quality of life, poorer physical health, more psychological morbidity and poorer self care, e.g. visits to the doctor for their own health double after home caring ceases (Grasel, 2002).

Numerous studies have demonstrated increased psychological morbidity in carers of people with dementia and depression levels and rates (e.g. George and Gwyther, 1986; Morris *et al.*, 1988; Brodaty and Hadzi-Pavlovic, 1990; Gallagher *et al.*, 1989; Rosenthal *et al.*, 1993; Schulz and Williamson, 1991; Baumgarten *et al.*, 1992; Mittelman *et al.*, 1995; Haley *et al.*, 1996; Pinquart and Sorensen, 2003). Dementia carers also have poorer physical health than non-carer controls (Schulz *et al.*, 1990; Vitaliano *et al.*, 2003), higher levels of chronic conditions, prescription medications and doctor visits (Haley *et al.*, 1987), and more physical symptoms and poorer self-rated health (Baumgarten *et al.*, 1992).

Significantly higher rates of depression or neurotic disorder have been reported in cohabiting carers of elderly depressed patients (64 per cent) than co-habitants of well elderly (29 per cent) (Denihan *et al.*, 1998). Another study of carers of depressed outpatients reported high levels of distress with 28 per cents creening positive for psychiatric caseness (Scazufca *et al.*, 2002). The level of burden experienced by carers of depressed elderly is similar to that reported for dementia carers (Scazufca *et al.*, 2002). Similarly, carers of stroke survivors report that caregiving results in emotional ill-health (79 per cent), disruption of social activities (79 per cent) and leisure time (55 per cent) (Anderson *et al.*, 1995). This level of burden is similar to that reported by dementia carers (Draper *et al.*, 1992).

Providing care also confers positive benefits on some carers such as feelings of satisfaction, fulfillment, enjoyment having helped the person with dementia, and having meaning in their lives (Sheehan and Nuttall, 1988; Nolan and Lundh, 1999; Cohen *et al.*, 2002).

Interventions for carers

A meta-analysis of 78 interventions with carers of the elderly (including patients with dementia, stroke, mental illness and physical disability) found that mean effects varied depending on the outcome measure, ranging from 0.14 for depression to 0.41 for ability/knowledge (Sorensen *et al.*, 2002). The paper also reports that intervention effects for dementia carers were smaller than the effect size for other groups.

Another meta-analysis including only studies of psychosocial interventions with carers of people with dementia (30 studies included) found that there were significant benefits for caregiver psychological distress, caregiver knowledge, any main caregiver outcome measure and patient mood, but not caregiver burden (Brodaty *et al.*, 2003). They also reported four interventions which demonstrated delays in nursing home admission. Common elements of successful programmes were involvement of patient as well as the carer, involvement of the whole family not just the primary carer, intervention of sufficient duration and intensity and, anecdotally, having consistency and flexibility when helping the carer (Brodaty *et al.*, 2003).

Primary care clinician and carers

The role of the primary care clinician is to provide regular support for the carer, to have a low index of suspicion for diagnosing psychological morbidity in the carer, especially depression, to be vigilant about the physical health of the carer and to liaise with and assist in coordinating support services. Psychogeriatric services generally become involved secondarily such as when the patient is diagnosed or, for carers of patients with dementia, when behavioural or psychological symptoms develop. They may be asked to see the carer as the identified patient.

Researchers working with carers

Psychogeriatric research requires close collaboration with carers to corroborate consent, provide proxy consent if the older research subject is incompetent, and monitor treatment outcome. Secondary outcomes of studies with primary aims of treating dementia increasingly focus on the carer, e.g. measuring carer time, burden and reaction to difficult behaviours in trials of anti-dementia drugs (Shikiar *et al.*, 2000; Tariot and Truyen 2001; Fillit *et al.*, 2002).

Summary

Carers are pivotal partners for psychogeriatric services in routine clinical work. Psychogeriatric services can extend their involvement further to include development of special programmes to train and support carers and in including carers in old age psychiatry research.

Consumer involvement in old age mental health services

The principle of consumer participation in the planning and implementation of health care is increasingly being recognized as critical to the development of health systems which promote the health and well-being of communities (The National Resource Centre for Consumer Participation in Health, 2000, p. iii). Involvement of consumers is now policy in the UK (Department of Health, 2001). Involvement requires more than commenting or completing satisfaction surveys, though these are important, it requires users and carers to be formally integrated within the service, actively planning or delivering mental health services (Simpson and House, 2003).

There is a burgeoning literature on how to involve consumers in mental health. There are several ways that users or carers can become involved in health services: consumerism – users exercising their right of choice can influence service provision, political activism and through self-help groups (see below). Past consumers (patients, carers and family) can also participate as volunteers within services.

Methods, benefits and drawbacks of consumer, carer and representative participation have been published by The National Resource Centre for Consumer Participation in Health (2000):

- Consumer satisfaction surveys provide direct feedback, measurable outcomes and highlight problem areas, but responders are non-representative, usually polarized negatively or positively and may not give their true opinion.

- A complaints mechanism is an essential part of a service, formally ensuring accountability and identification and addressing of special incidents. Drawbacks are that consumers may find the system difficult to navigate on, be reluctant to exacerbate the problem, and that minor complaints may go unnoticed.

- Public meetings are a good forum for raising awareness of and discussing major issues, allowing anyone to present their opinion and providing media coverage.

Drawbacks are that opinions presented will be non-representative and confidentiality may be an issue.

◆ Focus groups are a rich source of direct feedback including feelings and ideas, though poor attendance and confidentiality may be drawbacks

◆ Community representatives on boards, management committees etc. allows a cross section of views leading to healthy debate. Drawbacks are that representatives may have time limitations, may be involved for the 'wrong' reasons and be difficult to keep.

By contrast with the literature on methods of involving consumers, there is little on the effectiveness of consumer involvement in mental health and almost nothing specific to old age psychiatry. Dening and Lawton (1998), in their examination of the role of carers in the evaluation of mental health services for older people, reported there was considerable scope for involving carers in the development and evaluation of services, thought there were also some potential concerns, not least that carers and users may have different perspectives. Several themes emerged in their review:

◆ Health providers need to communicate better (Melzer *et al.*, 1998; Brown *et al.*, 1997).

◆ Carers of people with dementia are less satisfied services than carers of people with non-dementing illnesses and have more unmet needs (Durand *et al.*, 1995; Philp *et al.*, 1995; Bedford *et al.*, 1996).

◆ The need for flexibility of services and concerns about standards of care (Melzer *et al.*, 1998).-0pl. 1

◆ There was little correlation between carers' self- reports and keyworkers' assessments of the level of carer stress.

Dening and Lawton concluded that while carers are a valuable source of feedback regarding services, they are not perfect proxies for the interests of patients and there is a need for a standardized assessment tool for rating carer satisfaction.

Simpson and House (2003), in their excellent review of user and consumer involvement in mental health services in general, point out that user or carer involvement is often seen as intrinsically worthwhile, though not everyone expects useful change as a result. Users or carers can benefit directly through acquiring new skills or social contacts or paid work, or services may improve in many ways.

We could find no empirical data on employment of users or carers as service employees, trainers or research interviewers in old age psychiatry. However, involvement of users with quite severe mental illnesses including bipolar disorders and schizophrenia, in general adult services has been demonstrated to be feasible and to provide benefits, particularly in training health professionals and eliciting more critical (and possibly more valid) responses in satisfaction surveys (Simpson and House, 2002).

Consumers can be encouraged to participate in their individual care. They have the enormous potential to influence their own health outcomes if they are actively involved in shared decision-making and provided with quality information and appropriate self-management tools. Acting on conclusions from a Cochrane systematic review, Lahdensuo (1999) found strong evidence that when adults with asthma are active participants in their care, undergo self-management education, and are supported by written action plans, they have reduced hospital admissions, emergency room visits, unscheduled visits to the doctor, days off work or school and nocturnal asthma with significant cost savings for every dollar spent (The Consumer Focus Collaboration, 2001). Similar evidence is lacking in old age mental health.

Consumer organizations and support groups

In this chapter we use the label 'consumer organization' in reference to not-for-profit, non-government organizations that represent and offer services to members of the community. In contrast, we use 'support group' in reference to groups that meet to offer education, advice, and/or an opportunity to share experiences. Consumer organizations often offer support groups, but not all support groups are necessarily run by consumer organizations.

Consumer organizations

The late twentieth century has witnessed the rise of consumer organizations. Consumer organizations relevant to older people fit into several categories. The first category are those related to specific medical conditions such as the Alzheimer's Association, Parkinson's Disease Society, Stroke Association, Mental Health Association, Manic Depressive Self Help Group, Schizophrenia Fellowship, Royal Blind Society, Aftercare, Arthritis Foundation and Palliative Care Association. Organizations linked to age-associated diseases such as dementia are more likely to cater for older people, whereas organizations serving people in whom the disease presents earlier in life, such as the Schizophrenia Fellowship, appear to have few older members. While most of these organizations are targeted at the persons with the condition, others are more designed to assist the families of patients.

The second category consists of non-medical organizations. Examples of national level non-medical organizations include the Centre for Policy on Ageing in the UK that provides research and policy advice on services, Age Concern (England and New Zealand) that provides information and services for older people, the American Association of Retired Persons that provides information, advocacy and services for older people and the Council on the Ageing that protects and promotes the well-being of older Australians. International non-medical organizations include HelpAge, that provides basic human needs and health care, capacity building, and advocacy for older people and the International Federation on Ageing (IFA), that links associations serving older persons at grassroots levels providing a forum for information exchange and advocacy. The World Health Organization (WHO) and United Nations (UN) both have divisions dedicated to ageing (http://www.un.org/esa/socdev/ageing/index.html, http://www.who.int/hpr/ageing/index.htm).

A third category are lobby groups for particular issues related to the aged. These include the American Seniors Housing Association (ASHA) which is involved in the operation, development and finance of a spectrum of senior housing, the Accommodation Rights Service (for people in supported accommodation), the Grey Panthers, a political lobby group with interests in health care, rights for the disabled, housing, environment and family security, and the Voice of the Elderly (VOTE) who offer instruction and assistance to the elderly (particularly on financial rights). An umbrella organization in the US, the National Quality Forum is working to develop and implement a national strategy for healthcare quality measurement and reporting.

How do support groups help?

Support groups, also known as self-help groups, offer the individual emotional and practical supports and create a feeling of 'universalization', that the person is no longer alone. They also create an identity and sense of purpose. The best-known example of a support group is Alcoholic's Anonymous.

Support groups are distinct from group psychotherapy in that the leader is not necessarily a mental health professional, the group is open to members joining and leaving, there is no set number of groups, fees are usually nominal and clients do not have to participate actively.

Telephone and internet education, and online support networks are becoming more common and utilized by carers (Harvey *et al.*, 1998; White and Dorman, 2000; Pierce *et al.*, 2002; Glueckauf and Loomis, 2003). They may be a more accessible option for carers who have difficulty attending a face-to-face group.

An example of a consumer organization and support groups

Alzheimer's Disease International (ADI) (Graham and Brodaty, 1997) is an umbrella organization that supports and encourages National Alzheimer's Associations. Currently there are 69 countries who are members of ADI. ADI provides information, resources, training, research support and hosts an annual international conference. ADI's major research commitment is the 10/66 Dementia Research group (Prince *et al.*, 2004), a collaboration of researchers from developed and developing countries who share knowledge and skills towards common aims.

National Alzheimer's Associations offer information, support, training and services to dementia carers, promote dementia awareness, lobby the government for funding for dementia care, and may fund research or advocate for research funding.

Alzheimer's Associations run local support groups for carers of people with dementia (not just Alzheimer's disease). These groups meet regularly and frequently, usually monthly and are usually led by a health professional, such as a social worker, often in combination with a carer. Meetings may be structured so that there is a formal speaker, viewing of a video-tape or discussion of a set topic, followed by general discussion; or unstructured in order to allow for more interaction between carers. Some support groups are only for family carers, others include people with dementia.

Evidence for the efficacy of support groups

To the best of our knowledge there has been no literature published on the efficacy of support groups specifically for older people with mental illness. The majority of research on support groups with older members is in the area of caregiver support.

The evidence for the efficacy of support groups for elderly carers is equivocal. Cuijper *et al.* (1996) reviewed eight studies reporting on the outcomes of support groups for carers of dementia and the frail elderly and found that only three demonstrated a beneficial effect on carers' depression, stress and well-being. A study of a dementia caregiver support group published since this review reported that the level of carer distress decreased and quality of life improved (Fung and Chien, 2002).

There have been a few published studies of support groups for carers of people with stroke. Welterman and colleagues (2000) found that stroke carers who attended support groups had good stroke knowledge. In a randomized controlled trial van den Heuvel and colleagues (2000) showed that support group attenders used 'seeking social support' as a coping strategy more than controls.

Support groups may be more beneficial for some carers than for others. Support groups have been found to be more effective for carers isolated from family and friends or other carers, in more stressful situations, more dissatisfied with their role, still in paid employment, having to pay a small cost (between $5–20) for group participation and caring for a person with dementia who was apathetic and/or institutionalized (Cuijpers *et al.*, 1996; Pillemer and Suitor, 1996, 2002).

Summary

Consumer involvement is important and beneficial to psychogeriatric service delivery. Consumer organizations provide education, support and advocacy and support groups improve carer outcomes. Consumer and self-help groups are now available for almost every chronic condition, and should be part of the armamentarium of every clinician.

Broader community

Another approach to improving the mental health of older people is to focus on the broader community rather than on patients presenting for treatment. The percentage of persons with a mental condition in general presenting for treatment is low. In the Australian National Mental Health Survey, only 35 per cent of people with a mental disorder in the previous year had presented for treatment for a mental problem, and most of those who did only saw their general practitioner (Andrews *et al.*, 2001). The elderly are even less likely to access specialist mental health services (Jin *et al.*, 2003).

Psychogeriatric services can address this by seeking to improve access for older people to specialist mental health services or by circumventing specialist services either by working better with primary health care providers or by treating a population.

Improving access

There are several barriers to patients of any age with mental illness or their families seeking help (Goldberg and Huxley, 1992). Patients themselves may be unaware that they have a diagnosable condition. In particular, older people may accept feelings of depression, anergia and poor concentration as normal for their age. If they do seek treatment their primary care physician may not recognize the condition or may glibly attribute symptoms to ageing too. Even if mental disorder is diagnosed, treatment may not be instituted or referral initiated. Australian data indicate that older people attend psychiatrists proportionately less often than the middle aged or younger population and that when they do attend psychiatrists they are likely to have shorter consultations (Draper and Koschera, 2001). Draper and Koschera argued that this was not a result of less psychiatric morbidity, but could not dismiss practical difficulties for many older people in attending for a specialist consultation, such as transport costs. Accessibility is especially relevant in rural and remote communities. In all countries there is a rural-urban maldistribution of psychogeriatric services (see Chapter 18). In developing countries psychogeriatric services are rare or absent. Older people themselves may be reluctant to attend specialist services. Medicine in general and psychiatry no less have been poor communicators of the importance of early diagnosis, of the treatability of many psychiatric conditions and of what the profession has to offer. For example community awareness campaigns can alert family to the risk of suicide in elderly depressives and to information on where to seek help.

Stigma about mental illness is a major barrier to presentation and to diagnosis, in developed (de Mendonca Lima *et al.*, 2003) and more so in developing countries (Patel and Prince, 2001). This is accentuated in psychogeriatrics because of the added stigma of growing old (Freidan, 1993). There is a prevailing attitude that younger people should be prioritized in health care over older people. For example on average, a Swedish person is willing to sacrifice 35 70-year-olds to save one 30-year-old (Johannesson and Johansson, 1996). And public support for care entitlements for the elderly is decreasing. An American study of population-representative cohorts in 1986, 1990 and 1997 reported that over time attitudes became less supportive of expanding social security and Medicare programmes for older people and more supportive of cutting their costs and benefits (Silverstein *et al.*, 2001).

Psychogeriatric services have a role in reducing this dual stigma of mental illness and of old age. If stigma can be reduced, older people may be more likely to present for treatment, family and friends more likely to recognize the seriousness of mental symptoms such as depression and memory loss, and primary care doctors more likely to detect mental illness and to treat patients presenting with them.

A technical consensus statement produced by the Old Age Psychiatry section of the World Psychiatric Association and the World Health Organization describes the causes and consequences of stigma towards older people with mental illness, the ways in which specific disorders are stigmatized, and action that can be taken (Graham *et al.*, 2003). Stigma needs to be approached by whole communities including governments, consumer organizations, professionals, older people with mental disorders, carers and families, the general public, the media, the corporate sector and schools and universities (Graham *et al.*, 2003). The main goals of a strategic plan to reduce stigma towards older people with mental disorders outlined by the World Psychiatric Association (Graham, Lindesay *et al.*, 2003, p. 18) were:

- Ensure that health and social services are adequate to meet needs
- Position mental health of older people on the public agenda
- Promote a greater understanding and acceptance of older people with mental disorder
- Create more supportive environments
- Encourage more research into effective, non-stigmatizing treatments

Population approaches to better mental health

Population health approaches can improve the mental health of the elderly. For example prevention programmes have successfully reduced suicide in the elderly in different East Asian regions (Chiu *et al.*, 2003). The only population-based randomized controlled trial to improve mental health in the elderly of which we are aware is an Australian study of all 1466 self-care unit and hostel residents in a large residential facility (Llewellyn-Jones *et al.*, 2001). A shared care intervention for depression was implemented over 9.5 months, including removing barriers to care through multidisciplinary collaboration, general practitioner and carer education and a health education, promotion and activity programme. This significantly improved level of depressive symptoms in the intervention group compared to controls.

Summary

Population approaches, better access to services, and reduction of stigma may improve the mental health of older people.

Conclusion

Psychogeriatric service delivery occurs within a context of families and carers, consumer organizations and self-help groups and the broader community. Clinicians and researchers should maintain a constant awareness of the limitations bestowed by this context, while utilizing the resources it offers.

References

Anderson, C.S., Linto, J., *et al.* (1995) A population-based assessment of the impact and burden of caregiving for long-term stroke survivors. *Stroke,* **26** (5), 843–9.

Andrews, G., Henderson, S., *et al.* (2001) Prevalence, comorbidity, disability and service utilisation. Overview of the Australian National Mental Health Survey. *British Journal of Psychiatry,* **178**, 145–53.

Bassett, S.S., Magaziner, J., *et al.* (1990) Reliability of proxy response on mental health indices for aged, community-dwelling women. *Psychology and Aging,* **5** (1), 127–32.

Baumgarten, M., Battista, R.N., *et al.* (1992) The psychological and physical health of family members caring for an elderly person with dementia. *Journal of Clinical Epidemiology,* **45** (1), 61–70.

Bedford, S., Melzer, D., Dening, T., Lawton, C., Todd, C., Badger, G., and Brayne, C. (1996) What becomes of people with dementia referred to community psychogeriatric teams? *International Journal of Geriatric Psychiatry,* **11**, 1051–6.

Brodaty, H., Green, A., *et al.* (2003) Meta-analysis of psychosocial interventions for caregivers of people with dementia. *Journal of the American Geriatrics Society,* **51** (5), 657–64.

Brodaty, H. and Hadzi-Pavlovic, D. (1990) Psychosocial effects on carers of living with persons with dementia. *Australian and New Zealand Journal of Psychiatry,* **24** (3), 351–61.

Broe, G.A., Jorm, A.F., *et al.* (1999) Carer distress in the general population: results from the Sydney Older Persons Study. *Age and Ageing,* **28** (3), 307–11.

Brown, J.B., Mc William, C.L., and Mai, V. (1997) Barriers and facilitators to seniors' independence: perceptions of seniors, caregivers, and health care providers. *Canadian Family Physician,* **43**, 469–75.

Chiu, H.F., Takahashi, Y., *et al.* (2003) Elderly suicide prevention in East Asia. *International Journal of Geriatric Psychiatry,* **18** (11), 973–6.

Cohen, C.A., Colantonio, A., *et al.* (2002) Positive aspects of caregiving: rounding out the caregiver experience. *International Journal of Geriatric Psychiatry,* **17**,(2), 184–8.

Cuijpers, P., Hosman, C.M., *et al.* (1996) Change mechanisms of support groups for caregivers of dementia patients. *International Psychogeriatrics,* **8** (4), 575–87.

de Mendonca Lima, C.A., Levav, I., *et al.* (2003) Stigma and discrimination against older people with mental disorders in Europe. *International Journal of Geriatric Psychiatry,* **18** (8), 679–82.

Denihan, A., Bruce, I., *et al.* (1998) Psychiatric morbidity in cohabitants of community-dwelling elderly depressives. *International Journal of Geriatric Psychiatry,* **13** (10), 691–4.

Dening, T. and Lawton, C. (1998) The role of carers in evaluating mental health services for older people. *International Journal of Geriatric Psychiatry,* **13**, 863–70.

Department of Health (2001) *Involving Patients and the Public in Healthcare: A Discussion Document.* Department of Health, London, UK.

Draper, B.M. and Koschera, A. (2001) Do older people receive equitable private psychiatric service provision under Medicare? *Australian and New Zealand Journal of Psychiatry,* **35** (5), 626–30.

Draper, B.M., Poulos, C.J., *et al.* (1992) A comparison of caregivers for elderly stroke and dementia victims. *Journal of the American Geriatrics Society,* **40** (9), 896–901.

Durand, P.J., Krueger, P.D., Chambers, Lo, W., and Grek, A. (1995) Predictors of caregivers' dissatisfaction with community long-term care services for seniors: results from the canadian study of health and aging. *Canadian Journal of Public Health,* **86**, 325–32.

Fillit, H.M., Gutterman, E.M., *et al.* (2002) Impact of donepezil on caregiving burden for patients with Alzheimer's disease. *International Psychogeriatrics,* **12** (3), 389–401.

Freidan, B. (1993) *The Fountain of Age*. New York, Simon and Schulster.

Fung, W.Y. and Chien W.T. (2002) The effectiveness of a mutual support group for family caregivers of a relative with dementia. *Archives of Psychiatric Nursing*, **16** (3), 134–44.

Gallagher, D., Rose, J., *et al.* (1989) Prevalence of depression in family caregivers. *Gerontologist*, **29** (4), 449–56.

George, L.K. and Gwyther L.P. (1986) Caregiver well-being: a multidimensional examination of family caregivers of demented adults. *Gerontologist*, **26** (3), 253–9.

Glueckauf, R.L. and Loomis, J.S. (2003) Alzheimer's caregiver support online: lessons learned, initial findings and future directions. *Neurorehabilitation*, **18** (2), 135–46.

Goldberg, D. and Huxley, P. (1992) *Common Mental Disorders*. Routledge, London.

Graham, N. and Brodaty, H. (1997) Alzheimer's Disease International. *International Journal of Geriatric Psychiatry*, **12** (7), 691–2.

Graham, N., Lindesay, J., *et al.* (2003) Reducing stigma and discrimination against older people with mental disorders: a technical consensus statement. [see comment]. *International Journal of Geriatric Psychiatry*, **18** (8), 670–8.

Grasel, E. (2002) When home care ends–changes in the physical health of informal caregivers caring for dementia patients: a longitudinal study. *Journal of the American Geriatrics Society*, **50** (5), 843–9.

Haley, W.E., Levine, E.G., *et al.* (1987) Stress, appraisal, coping, and social support as predictors of adaptational outcome among dementia caregivers. *Psychology and Aging*, **2** (4), 323–30.

Haley, W.E., Roth, D.L., *et al.* (1996) Appraisal, coping, and social support as mediators of well-being in black and white family caregivers of patients with Alzheimer's disease. *Journal of Consulting and Clinical Psychology*, **64** (1), 121–9.

Harvey, R., Roques, P.K., *et al.* (1998) CANDID–Counselling and Diagnosis in Dementia: a national telemedicine service supporting the care of younger patients with dementia. *International Journal of Geriatric Psychiatry*, **13** (6), 381–8.

Jin, H., Folsom, D.P., *et al.* (2003) Patterns of public mental health service use by age in patients with schizophrenia. *American Journal of Geriatric Psychiatry*, **11** (5), 525–33.

Johannesson, M. and Johansson, P.O. (1996) The economics of ageing: on the attitude of Swedish people to the distribution of health care resources between the young and the old. *Health Policy*, **37** (3), 153–61.

Kemp, N.M., Brodaty, H., *et al.* (2002) Diagnosing dementia in primary care: the accuracy of informant reports. *Alzheimer Disease and Associated Disorders*, **16** (3), 171–6.

Lahdensuo, A. (1999) Guided self management of asthma – how to do it. *BMJ*, **319** (7212), 759–60.

Livingston, G., Manela, M., *et al.* (1996) Depression and other psychiatric morbidity in carers of elderly people living at home. *BMJ*, **312** (7024), 153–6.

Llewellyn-Jones, R.H., Baikie, K.A., *et al.* (2001) How to help depressed older people living in residential care: a multifaceted shared-care intervention for late-life depression. *International Psychogeriatrics*, **13** (4), 477–92.

Maguire, C.P., Kirby, M., *et al.* (1996) Family members' attitudes toward telling the patient with Alzheimer's disease their diagnosis. *BMJ*, **313** (7056), 529–30.

Melzer, D., Pearce, K., Cooper, B., and Brayne, C. (1998) Epidemiologically-based needs assessment: Alzheimer's disease and other dementias (draft) NHS Executive, London (quoted in Dening and Lawton, 1998)

Mittelman, M.S., Ferris, S.H., *et al.* (1995) A comprehensive support program: effect on depression in spouse-caregivers of AD patients. *Gerontologist*, **35** (6), 792–802.

Morris, R.G., Morris, L. W., *et al.* (1988) Factors affecting the emotional wellbeing of the caregivers of dementia sufferers. *British Journal of Psychiatry,* **153**, 147–56.

Nolan, M. and Lundh, U. (1999) Research study. Satisfactions and coping strategies of family carers. *British Journal of Community Nursing,* **4** (9), 470–5.

Patel, V. and Prince, M. (2001) Ageing and mental health in a developing country: who cares? Qualitative studies from Goa, India. *Psychological Medicine,* **31** (1), 29–38.

Pierce, L.L., Steiner, V., *et al.* (2002) In-home online support for caregivers of survivors of stroke: a feasibility study. *CIN: Computers, Informatics, Nursing,* **20** (4), 157–64.

Philp, I., McKee, K.J., Meldrum, P., Ballinger, B.R., Gilhooly, M.L.M., Gordon, D.S., Mutch, W.J., and Whittick, J.E. (1995) Community care for demented and non-demented elderly people: a comparison study of financial burden, service use, and unmet needs in family supporters. *BMJ,* 310, 1503–6.

Pillemer, K. and Suitor, J. (2002) Peer support for Alzheimer's caregivers: is it enough to make a difference? *Research on Aging,* **24** (2), 171–92.

Pillemer, K. and Suitor, J.J. (1996) It takes one to help one: effects of similar others on the well-being of caregivers. *Journals of Gerontology Series B – Psychological Sciences and Social Sciences,* **51** (5), S250–7.

Pinquart, M. and Sorensen, S. (2003) Differences between caregivers and noncaregivers in psychological health and physical health: a meta-analysis. *Psychology and Aging,* **18** (2), 250–67.

Prince, M., Graham, N., *et al.* (2004) Alzheimer Disease International's 10/66 Dementia Research Group-One model for action research in developing countries. *International Journal of Geriatric Psychiatry,* **19** (2), 178–81.

Riordan, J. and Mockler, D. (1996) Audit of care programming in an acute psychiatric admission ward for the elderly. *International Journal of Geriatric Psychiatry,* **11**, 109–18.

Rosenthal, C.J., Sulman, J., *et al.* (1993) Depressive symptoms in family caregivers of long-stay patients. *Gerontologist,* **33** (2), 249–57.

Ross, G.W., Abbott, R.D., *et al.* (1997) Frequency and characteristics of silent dementia among elderly Japanese-American men. The Honolulu-Asia Aging Study. *JAMA,* **277** (10), 800–5.

Scazufca, M., Menezes, P.R., *et al.* (2002) Caregiver burden in an elderly population with depression in Sao Paulo, Brazil. *Social Psychiatry and Psychiatric Epidemiology,* **37** (9), 416–22.

Schulz, R., Visintainer, P., *et al.* (1990) Psychiatric and physical morbidity effects of caregiving. *Journal of Gerontology,* **45** (5), P181–91.

Schulz, R. and Williamson, G.M. (1991) A 2-year longitudinal study of depression among Alzheimer's caregivers. *Psychology and Aging,* **6** (4), 569–78.

Sheehan, N.W. and Nuttall, P. (1988) Conflict, emotion, and personal strain among family caregivers. *Family Relations: Journal of Applied Family and Child Studies,* **37** (1), 92–8.

Shikiar, R., Shakespeare, A., *et al.* (2000) The impact of metrifonate therapy on caregivers of patients with Alzheimer's disease: results from the MALT clinical trial. *Journal of the American Geriatrics Society,* **48** (3), 268–74.

Silverstein, M., Angelelli, J.J., *et al.* (2001) Changing attitudes toward aging policy in the United States during the 1980s and 1990s: a cohort analysis. *Journals of Gerontology Series B –Psychological Sciences and Social Sciences,* **56** (1), S36–43.

Simpson, E.L. and House, A.O. (2002) Involving users in the delivery and evaluation of mental health services: systematic review. *BMJ,* **325** (7375), 1265.

Simpson, E.L. and House, A.O. (2003) User and carer involvement in mental health services: from rhetoric to science. *British Journal of Psychiatry,* **183**, 89–91.

Simpson, R.G., Scothern, G., and Vincent, M. (1995) Survey of carer satisfaction with the quality of care delivered to in-patients suffering from dementia. *J Adv Nurs*, **22**, 517–27.

Sorensen, S., Pinquart, M., *et al.* (2002) How effective are interventions with caregivers? An Updated meta-analysis. *Gerontologist*, **42** (3), 356–72.

Tariot, P.N. and Truyen, L. (2001) *Reminyl (galantamine) Reduces Caregiver Distress (poster)*. Tenth Congress of the International Psychogeriatric Association (IPA), Nice, France.

Teri, L., Gibbons, L.E., *et al.* (2003) Exercise plus behavioral management in patients with Alzheimer disease: a randomized controlled trial. *JAMA*, **290** (15), 2015–22.

Teri, L., Logsdon, R.G., *et al.* (1997) Behavioral treatment of depression in dementia patients: a controlled clinical trial. *Journals of Gerontology Series B – Psychological Sciences and Social Sciences*, **52** (4), P159–66.

The Consumer Focus Collaboration (2001) *The Evidence Supporting Consumer Participation in Health*. Department of Health and Ageing, Canberra.

The National Resource Centre for Consumer Participation in Health (2000) *Feedback, Participation and Consumer Diversity. A Literature Review*. Commonwealth Department of Health and Aged Care, Canberra.

van den Heuvel, E.T., de Witte, L.P., *et al.* (2000) Short-term effects of a group support program and an individual support program for caregivers of stroke patients. *Patient Education and Counseling*, **40** (2), 109–20.

Vitaliano, P.P., Zhang, J., *et al.* (2003) Is caregiving hazardous to one's physical health? A meta-analysis. *Psychological Bulletin*, **129** (6), 946–72.

Wattis, J.P., Butler, A., Martin, C., and Sumner, T. (1994) Outcome of admission to an acute psychiatric facility for older people: a pluralistic evaluation. *International Journal of Geriatrics*.

Weltermann, B.M., Homann, J., *et al.* (2000) Stroke knowledge among stroke support group members. *Stroke*, **31** (6), 1230–3.

White, M.H. and Dorman, S.M. (2000) Online support for caregivers. Analysis of an Internet Alzheimer mailgroup. *Computers in Nursing*, **18** (4), 168–76; quiz 177–9.

Zarit, S.H. and Edwards, A.B. (1996) Family caregiving: research and clinical intervention. *Handbook of the Clinical Psychology of Aging*. Chichester, UK, John Wiley and Sons.

Chapter 20

Evaluation of service delivery

Alastair Macdonald

In this chapter I will question the nature of service evaluation in general, review two other approaches to evaluation of service delivery – clinical audit and routine clinical outcomes measurement (RCOM) – then describe the latter in detail as it applies to old age psychiatry services. The lessons learnt from the literature and 6 years of RCOM in an old age psychiatry service are described.

Service evaluation – a critique

In every professional group and every specialty there is a minority who do research. Most observers have some idea of what this entails from the bland descriptions in papers. There is a much smaller minority who claim to be able to evaluate services – sometimes from outside the specialty. What do they do? Many professionals and managers have only a foggy notion – partly because the results are not nearly as digestible. A research paper often has a conclusion – ('treatment X appears superior to treatment Y'), whereas we read few such reports of evaluation ('service A appears superior to service B'). Evaluation is difficult to do, takes a long time, is hard to write about, and even more difficult to read. So reports have a much tougher time finding their way into the literature. Many evaluations never get there at all, ending up as laminate-bound A4 paperweights, unread, on a special shelf near the ceiling. Yet the clamour for evaluation remains strong, almost exclusively about new services and service developments. Loudest are the purchasers of new developments. Even though by the time the evaluation is complete they may well have been replaced, reorganized or disbanded they often demand that a proportion of start-up costs are spent on evaluation. These calls are obviously legitimate – quite apart from the ethics of delivering useless services to anybody, large amounts of public money are involved and it is perfectly proper for spending to be justified. Yet, so often, the results of these evaluations support no clear decision, are simply ignored, or never appear.

Here is a paradox – in a logical and ordered world, taxpayers should clearly only fund services that are evaluated before becoming 'mainstream', yet the results of such evaluations don't seem to have much to do with whether these services develop or die, and most services have never been evaluated at all. What are the reasons for this?

I believe that the way we think about these issues is, in Bleuler's (1919) original use of the term, autistic. It is a natural human tendency to think on the basis of how we would like things to be rather than how they are. It seems that some groups are more prone to this than others, and top of the tree are the health service evaluators themselves.

The most prevalent desire amongst orthodox health service evaluators is that health service evaluation can and should attain the highest ranks of the hierarchy of evidence used in evidence-based clinical practice (e.g. Dunn, 1994; St. Leger *et al.*, 1992); homogenous systematic reviews of randomised controlled trials (RCTs). This can be achieved by (a) concentrating on the outcome of health services rather than structure and process (Donabedian, 2001), (b) clarification of measurable goals, aims and objectives, and (c) subjecting the latter to empirical testing of effectiveness, preferably by RCT. There are now many critiques of RCTs of complex interventions like health services (for instance Pawson and Tulley, 1997; Wolff, 2000). Service evaluation RCTs violate assumptions about protocol fidelity, blindness, study sample equivalence (unless huge numbers are recruited), and contamination. Standard textbooks of evaluation ignore or minimize these problems (e.g. St. Leger *et al.*, 1992).

Another prominent desire is that clear guidance from economic approaches to evaluation can be expected. Economic evaluation concerns the quantification of value (Bannock *et al.*, 1998) to individuals and groups of services and their alternatives, but cannot itself reconcile conflicts in value between these groups (Richardson, 1999). Furthermore, economic evaluation is entirely dependent on the validity (from the Latin *validus*, meaning strong) of the study. If only it were the case that because economists were involved, certainty would emerge! Economic aspects of evaluation will not be dealt with further here.

There is little agreement as to what health service evaluation is. Evaluators do not all subscribe to the dominant, nomothetically-orientated paradigm described above (Marsden and Oakley, 1991). An ideographic, interpretive approach by social scientists is also available, in which evaluation is seen more as part of the process of change within a service or organization; a means of reflection (formative) rather than a judgement (summative) of effectiveness. It therefore lends itself much more to process rather than outcomes. Evaluators of this sort are more likely to use qualitative than quantitative methods, and the results of their work may be therefore appreciated much more by the particular service studied than services in general, as distinct from the aspirations of dominant paradigm evaluators. However, this activity is predicated upon two questionable assumptions: first, that, however well communicated, narrative material from within a service will influence those outside it, and second, that it will influence those within it. There is very little evidence of the former (Bie Nio Ong, 1993, p. 2), and the latter is probably unknowable. The rest of this chapter will be predicated upon a quantitative rather than qualitative paradigm.

Service policy-makers and purchasers are not much further down the autistic tree. They desire 'scientific' qualities in evaluation most. However, the talk is of 'evidence-based' policy or purchasing, but the walk is of political expediency. There is nothing wrong with political expediency – it is how democracies work. The wistful title of a review of this area – 'Can research influence mental health policy?' (Whiteford, 2001) – itself speaks volumes, decades after the development of purchasing and commissioning. Although many purchasers cling to the desire that evidence from evaluation remains central to policy and purchasing decisions, a disinterested observer must conclude that such evidence has marginal impact. In the case of anti-dementia drug treatment in the UK, despite the limited initial evaluation of this expensive intervention having shown few compelling health gains, this treatment was originally sanctioned because of political pressure.

Clinicians are at the same time the generators of many service developments and not much interested in formal evaluation. This is as true of surgery (Meakins, 2002) as of old age psychiatry. Several factors may constrain their enthusiasm for evaluation. They are, correctly in my view, likely to be suspicious of evidence-based decisions about simple interventions, let alone complex ones. They will 'know' that service A is better than service B (even if service B is theirs) and for whom and in what way it is better (not excluding staff), and strive to change things accordingly, yet at the same time be acutely aware of how difficult it will be to prove it. The more evangelical will try to provide proof, as we did with some aspects of a novel open-access multidisciplinary teams (Collighan et al., 1993, Lindesay et al., 1996) with no discernible impact at all on other local provision. Most services remain a mosaic of inherited development and new enthusiasms, some local and unique, others imposed by fiat, or adopted uncritically from guidelines, themselves barely evidenced. Finally, the demand for evaluation can sometimes be effectively used by those keen to see a development stillborn or die in infancy.

Service providers and managers are less troubled with hierarchies of evidence than even clinicians and, in my experience, sleep well at night without having to justify many decisions on the basis of evidence from service evaluations. They respond to the pressure from their political masters, who in turn respond from the pressure they perceive – in democracies, from voters, mediated by the Press. One reason for this sanguine approach is that the pace of change of top-down priorities is so rapid that no thoughtful evaluation is possible before the service is started, changed or abandoned anyway.

Patients and carers are increasingly expected to become central in the development and evaluation of services – general psychiatry services are ahead of old age psychiatry. More than clinicians, they have almost no scope for self-delusion about services – they see them better than anyone, and the irrelevance of evaluation without their input.

So it would be perhaps fair to say that the nature of health service evaluation is obscure, but that the dominant paradigm of effectiveness evaluation – aspiring as it does to RCTs – is unsatisfactory. St. Leger et al. (1992) helpfully list other approaches (headed 'spurious alternatives to the RCT') and include clinical audit and clinical outcomes databases.

Clinical audit

In the UK, clinical audit emerged in the early 1980s as a vehicle for improved service delivery, and was enshrined in a 1990 White Paper – *Working for Patients*. What was supposed to happen was that standards for clinical procedures would be agreed by the clinicians involved, either by local consensus or national guidelines – as much as possible based on evidence. These standards were to be either themselves measurable or open to surrogate measurement. Then a period of implementation would follow, after which data would be gathered so that performance against standards would be measured. The clinicians would review the results and either adjust the standards to be more realistic or make changes in practice that would bring their attainment closer. After a further period of implementation, a further data collection and review would take place. An upward spiral of quality improvement was to be the result. A significant resource was allocated to this activity – £220m (Sellu, 1996) but despite these rational principles it has proved very difficult to establish its value (Lord and Littlejohns, 1997). It is of note that a major UK scandal took place in a paediatric cardiac surgery unit in a UK hospital trust receiving £250,000 per annum for audit (Bristol Royal Infirmiary Inquiry, 2001). Again, the term audit was not clearly defined – simple descriptive surveys still appear under this title (e.g. Hickie *et al.*, 2000), and routine surgical and perinatal mortality conferences, which preceded the 1990s, are also called 'audit'.

In UK old age psychiatry practice, enthusiasm for clinical audit has waned irrespective of attempts to evaluate it. Reasons for this include repeated failure to attain worthy but unattainable goals, irrelevance of standards that could be easily measured, time pressures (Benbow and Jolley, 2002), diversion of resources – particularly data collection and analysis in the setting of inadequate information systems – to general adult psychiatry, subordination of locally relevant audit themes to regional and national imperatives, and the tendency to slide away from the boring and irksome necessity of revisiting the same topic again and again. Finally, the inability of clinicians to criticize each other's practice without causing offence rendered the whole system unworkable. This difficulty was reasonably excused by the lack of evidence for many of the standards being pursued.

The coup de grace for clinical audit in the UK has been the development of a scandal involving paediatric cardiac surgical mortality under the nose of a standard audit system. (Bristol Royal Infirmary Inquiry, 2001). It is no longer accepted that peer pressure can sustain high standards of care, and external review has now been institutionalized. However, this takes the form of an inspectorate, similar to a system that was in place during the mental hospital scandals of the 1960s.

Routine Clinical Outcomes Measurement (RCOM) in health services

RCOM attempts to transcend some of the problems of service evaluation and audit by directly measuring the changes in patients coming through the service, and relating change to service processes, structures and interventions. This is not an easy system to implement, and a brief history of RCOM in psychiatry in the UK is instructive. First, central government decreed that it must start, despite objections from the experimentalist research community about its philosophical basis (Dunn, 1994), which were ignored. Then it commissioned the rapid development and hasty publication of a rough and ready clinical outcomes measure whose performance in the field failed to satisfy many in the experimentalist research community (e.g. Adams *et al.*, 2000), whose scorn was ignored. Then it demanded that this measure be implemented routinely, with minimal training resources, in the face of non-existent or inadequate IT systems and alongside a host of other costly imperatives which it heaps, as ever, upon clinical services. It ignored objections that it cannot be done, forcing the issue by making funding for services contingent upon completion of this measure at determined intervals, without any plan to collate, analyse and feedback the results to the clinicians who have to do the ratings. Does this sound a recipe for success? It is crucial to appreciate that the use of RCOM represents a sea change in culture which demands first a plausible philosophical basis, and then practical support to ensure maximal benefit. Both are necessary and neither sufficient, so I make no apology for starting with philosophical fundamentals, if merely to satisfy St. Leger *et al.*'s admirable call for clarity of thought (St. Leger *et al.*, 1992) in all matters concerned with evaluation. This is a long game, and there are no quick fixes.

Theoretical basis for outcomes measurement

Donabedian's distinction between structure, process and outcomes (Donabedian, 2001) is helpful, despite inspiring repeated and accelerating structural changes by governments in the mistaken belief that this is a causal chain, and that better outcomes will result. A health service is judged by its outcomes, rather than by its neat organizational structures and watertight processes, in the same way that the impact of anarchical structures and processes on an industrial conglomerate are judged not by their appeal to humanistic principles but by the conglomerate's financial success (Semler, 2003). The outcomes of a health service are less easy to determine – they are often categorized as cure (for example making patients better than they would otherwise be), care (for example helping them maintain the highest quality of life, irrespective of cure), and prevention (primary, secondary or tertiary). It is axiomatic that achievement of these functions must be measured – they cannot be assumed. It is also worth noting at this stage that these outcomes are not just for patients – distinct outcomes for carers, referrers, purchasers, governments and society at large need consideration.

When one reviews the methods by which purchasers and commissioners measure the degree with which desirable structures, processes and outcomes (care, cure and prevention) are achieved, it becomes clear that prevention drops out of contention very early, especially in mental health services. For instance, the NHS performance indicator list for mental health services for 2002 contains 30 indicators, only one of

Table 20.1 NHS performance indicators for Mental Health Trusts 2002

Key targets

Assertive outreach team implementation***

CMHT integration***

Mental health minimum dataset implementation***

Number of outpatients waiting longer than the standard**

Improving working lives***

Hospital cleanliness**

Financial management***

Clinical focus

Clinical negligence***

CPA systems implementation***

Psychiatric readmissions (Adult) **

Psychiatric readmissions (Older people) **

Suicide rate*

Patient focus

Transition of care between adult services and OPMH***

Transition of care between CAMHS and adult services***

Patients with copies of their own care plan**

Patient complaints procedure***

Better hospital food**

Privacy and dignity**

Capacity and capability

Missed outpatient appointments**

Crisis Resolution Team implementation**

Out of catchment area treatments (Adults)***

Out of catchment area treatments (Older people)***

CAMHS service mapping***

Data quality***

Staff opinion survey***

Junior doctors' hours***

Consultant appraisal***

Sickness absence rate***

Information governance***

Fire, Health and Safety***

* Prevention (1)
** Outcome: care: patient (9)
*** Structure or process (20)
NHS Executive 2003 http://www.doh.gov.uk/performanceratings/2003/mh_list.html

which is related to prevention (see Table 20.1). Twenty are related to process or structure and nine are related to outcomes. Of these nine, none could be regarded as a 'cure' outcome – they are all related to care. (Although the UK Mental Health Minimum Data Set has obligatory outcomes measurement in it, the indicator is the degree with which this is implemented rather than what the outcomes are). Similar proportions are seen in other countries, including Australia, whose mental health services have embarked on a massive outcomes project in mental health service which has yet to bear fruit.

From this point this chapter will consider only the development of systems for implementing routine 'cure' outcomes measurement, and no more will be said about care or prevention. At present, in most health services the main guarantor of good 'cure' outcomes is evidence-based practice (Sackett *et al.*, 1996). We assume that if clinicians follow the best evidence in their clinical practice, the 'cure' outcomes for their patients will be optimal. The measurement of process (for instance, uptake of continuing professional development or the degree with which clinicians conform to evidence-based guidelines) becomes a proxy for the measurement of how much better their patients are. Put like that, the flaws are obvious. The evidence base for even quite simple interventions is lacking or contentious. Furthermore, such evidence is difficult to generalize to clinical populations – interventions that work in clinical trials may not work in everyday practice, and vice versa, for a host of reasons (Marks, 2002). In practice almost no intervention is simple – they are all necessarily complex, and thus evidence about them from simplistic trials may be misleading.

In the process of introducing patients and carers to RCOM in an old age psychiatry service in London I have been struck by their incredulity that we don't really have a clue whether patients get better during contact with our services at all. They are not astonished, of course, that we do not trouble to check their own assessment of their outcomes, but are very surprised that we appear to lack sufficient systematic curiosity about their improvement or otherwise during our ministrations to even measure it ourselves. Why is this?

One reason may be lack of confidence – we don't measure outcomes in case they show that we have no impact. Self-doubt may be pervasive in all medical and surgical specialties. Of all health services, old age psychiatry has a pretty good case for this excuse; our patients have a high prevalence of degenerative disorders, and epidemiological evidence for poor long-term outcomes in older functionally ill patients is well-known. We have a reputation for being stronger on care than cure, a reputation we may have considerably absorbed ourselves. Another candidate is more fundamental – the problem of attribution implicit in the definition of outcomes themselves. However, with the possible exception of mortality, the development of RCOM is very patchy in almost all medical and surgical specialties, including cardiology (Spertus *et al.*, 2003). Surprisingly, RCOM is only a few years old even in oncology (Clancy and Lawrence, 2002).

What are outcomes? Most definitions involve three components: change (we hope, improvement) in health status, intervention and attribution of one to the other.

That of the New South Wales Health Department is typical ' a change in the health of an individual, group of people or population which is attributable to an intervention or series of interventions' (NSW Health Department, 1992). It is relatively easy to measure health change, slightly more difficult to document interventions, but attribution is very problematic. For, as experimentalist researchers constantly say, it is simply impossible to prove that health change can be attributed to the intervention. This philosophical challenge lies at the heart of much resistance to the idea of RCOM, and we cannot legitimately avoid a response.

It can be answered thus.

1. Causality represents what Hume (1739) called a custom. 'All our reasonings concerning matters of fact are deriv'd from nothing but custom: and that belief is more properly an act of the sensitive, than of the cogitative part of our natures', and he and most subsequent philosophers have accepted that the search for empirical proof is illusory. This applies equally to complex social theory, the results of homogenous systematic reviews of RCTs, or the most prosaic assumptions about billiard balls.

2. The difference between attributions made on the basis of observational (for example, routine clinical outcomes) as opposed to experimental (i.e. RCT) data is thus not categorical – it is dimensional. St. Leger *et al.* accept that 'small changes to practice without recourse to formal trials' may be justified on the basis of 'insights' gathered from routine outcomes data (St. Leger *et al.*, 1992, p. 107), a position untenable if there was a categorical difference between the two sorts of data.

3. The most likely candidate for the dimension along which assumptions based on these sorts of data can be arranged is plausibility. To a community steeped in the scientific method the plausibility of RCT evidence is automatically greater than that of evidence from observational studies. However, as neither is amenable to empirical proof (after Hume and most philosophers who followed him) this is a judgement made on the basis of 'custom' – in the sense of experience. We do not so much think we acquire more reliable knowledge through the medium of controlled experiment than observation, as feel it.

4. The plausibility of results from a RCT of a simple intervention like a medication will depend on its rigour – but particularly in its generalizability, the Achilles heel of trials. The plausibility of results from a routine outcomes study of a simple intervention like this may never match that of an RCT, even less a homogenous systematic review. However, as soon as one considers a mildly complex intervention and especially complexity implicit in service evaluations, the position is reversed, because of the arguments already aired (Pawson and Tulley, 1997; Wolff, 2000). The RCT becomes unworkably complex, its results open to easy challenge, and the alternative provided by RCOM becomes correspondingly attractive. Datasets sufficiently large to allow control for a wide range of factors are only feasible with routine data.

The plausibility of RCT evidence appears inversely related to the complexity of the intervention being evaluated.

5. Where, on the dimension of this complexity, may equipoise between the advantages and disadvantages of the two methods be found? It is certainly tenable that many psychological treatments, heavily manualized and delivered with maximal model fidelity are still unamenable to RCT (Ablon and Jones, 2002), so that equipoise may well lie on the medication side of this divide. It seems highly unlikely that RCTs will ever be useful in service evaluation, whereas the use of large databases of RCOM is overdue.

A model of routine outcomes

The simple definition above (health change attributable to intervention) has its appeal, but misses an important component – context (Pawson and Tulley, 1997). It is natural to expect different outcomes for similar interventions in different conditions, so three dimension are all necessary for any understanding to emerge from outcomes data – change in health status, intervention, and context, often translated into casemix (Broadbent, 2002). It follows that the practical steps necessary to implement RCOM must yield data on each of these. However, there is another important question to consider – who decides on the content of these dimensions? Whose outcomes are they? Two considerations apply: first, health services owe cure outcomes to others as well as the patient – particularly carers. Second, different interests (patient, relative, clinician, general practitioner, purchaser, policy-maker) may have different views as to what aspects of health state should be measured, how they should be measured, what aspects of context or case mix are relevant, which interventions are documented. Table 20.2 illustrates this. In addition, it is likely that opinions as to what constitutes plausibility in attribution will differ between these groups.

Seen like this, (and this only represents the picture for cure outcomes, and then only for patients) implementation seems daunting in the extreme; a ready excuse for going no further. The two left-hand columns of the matrix are the most important, however, and in mental health services the tendency is to start with the second. You have to start somewhere. In mental health services for working-age adults there is as much interest in an approach based on the patients' perspective on outcomes (Slade, 2002), but for practical reasons alone, starting with the clinician perspective is the least complicated of a very complicated set of options. Although in south London we have begun the development of outcomes measurement based on change in patient's assessments, it is the clinician's perspective upon which the rest of the chapter will focus. (*Lesson No 1: start somewhere.*)

Choice of measure of change in health status for routine use

Objectors to RCOM frequently raise doubts about whether rating scales that are sufficiently easy and quick to be feasible in everyday practice have sufficient validity and

Table 20.2 An outcomes matrix

	Interest group					
	Patient	**Staff**	**Carer**	**GP**	**Purchaser**	**Other**
Most desirable health change in patient	e.g. change in quality of life or function	e.g. change in symptoms	e.g. change in behaviour			
How health change is measured	e.g. change in QOL or ADL scale	e.g. change in clinician-rated scale	e.g. change in informant behavioural rating			
Intervention thought relevant	e.g. social, housing, aids	e.g. medication, admission	e.g. medication, advice			
Context thought relevant	e.g. relationships with family	e.g. condition	e.g. attitude of staff			
How context is measured	e.g. social network measure	e.g. diagnosis	e.g. attitudinal ratings			

reliability to yield meaningful results (Adams *et al.*, 2000). Behind this lies the questionable assumption that the reliability and validity of any measure can be divorced from its use and users; that somehow the utility of a measure is a property of the piece of paper with writing on it, rather than the way in which it is used. It is not, therefore sensible to ask 'is the scale reliable and valid' but, rather, how great or small is its reliability and validity when used by X in Y setting? There is no doubt that the way a scale is constructed and presented will have an impact on these values, as will training manuals and glossaries. But it is self-evident that the same piece of paper will have quite different results in the hands of a carefully trained, experienced researcher with adequate time compared with harassed, busy, poorly-trained members of staff who don't know why they are doing the rating, will never see the results, and don't want to do it anyway. These contextual issues are minimized or ignored in the fruitless discussion of the reliability and validity of rating scales. Once again, the missing factor is context – it is only possible to assess the validity and reliability of scales in the context in which they are used, and the results from one context will be as applicable to another only to the degree with which contexts are similar. Important aspects of context include the training and supporting material available (Rock and Preston, 2001), the knowledge of the patient, the ease of procedures for capturing the ratings in an information system and above all the meaningfulness of the rating to the rater. The latter will depend significantly on feedback of results (Silk, 1991) – either for individual patents (together with intervention data) – or caseload (together with intervention and casemix data).

The idea that scales are valid or invalid, reliable or unreliable, is another weird idea that is rarely mentioned in critiques. Clearly, the reliability and validity of a scale, determined by context, are dimensions, and their importance is quantitative; you need to be able to answer the question – in my service, how far can differences in outcome between patients with a particular diagnosis exposed to different interventions be accounted for by unreliability or invalidity of the scales we are using? This implies that measurement of these, or at least estimation based on data from similar contexts, is an important part of implementing routine outcomes. (*Lesson No 2: Assess or estimate the reliability and validity of your chosen measure in the context in which it is used.*)

It follows, then, that the choice of scale itself is not necessarily crucial, and should be determined by practical issues rather than high psychometrics. These issues include brevity, coverage of relevant domains, and the ease and expense of training. It is obvious, however, that if all teams and services use different scales, then the building of databases large enough to be useful for evaluation of interventions and service effectiveness will be impossible, quite apart from the training implications when staff move. A key practical issue is that everyone in services with similar patients and aims should use the same scale. (*Lesson No 3: It matters less what measure you use than that everyone uses it.*)

Health of the Nation Outcome Scales for Older People (HoNOS65+) (Burns *et al.*, 1999)

This was the group of measures chosen by our service in 1997. It consists of 12 clinician-rated scales scored from 0 to 4, covering symptoms, disabilities and other social decrements. For each scale the scoring is 0 if there is no difficulty whatsoever in the domain, 1 if there is a minor or trivial difficulty, and 2, 3 and 4 represent mild, moderate and severe problems in the domain. The scales are shown in Table 20.3. They are identical in name to those of its parent measure, HoNOS for working age adults (Wing *et al.*, 1998), but the glossaries differ in two main respects. First, detail within each scale represent differences between the age groups covered in the sorts of items included – work, for instance, is more important in HoNOS that HoNOS65+. Second, our experience with an early version of the HoNOS65+ glossary (in fact, the one published in error: Macdonald, 1999) was that it was extremely difficult to train staff using a prose glossary written by a committee. There was far too much ambiguity about crucial matters such as the timescale covered, or whether the rating should represent the clinician's or the patient's judgement. Working in partnership with the original authors of HoNOS and HoNOS65+, a UK national implementation group transmuted the early prose glossary into a tabulated one, with clearer rules, based entirely on training experiences (accessible via www.honosorg.uk). This is the UK standard glossary version, translated into Spanish; translations are being carried out into Danish and Dutch.

We chose HoNOS65+ because they satisfied three key criteria at the time.

◆ Feasibility (Slade *et al.*, 1999): once trained, staff can rate a patient quickly (average now 3 minutes)

Table 20.3 The HoNOS65+ scales

Behavioural disturbance
Non-accidental self-injury
Problem drinking or drug use
Cognitive problems
Problems related to physical illness or disability
Problems associated with hallucinations and delusions
Problems associated with depressive symptoms
Other mental and behavioural problems:

- Phobias
- Anxiety and panic
- Obsessive–compulsive
- Mental strain and tension
- Dissociative or conversion problems
- Somatoform – persisting physical complaints of mainly psychological origin (with little evidence of physical disease) e.g. hypochondriasis
- Eating – over/under
- Sleep – hypersomnia/insomnia
- Sexual
- Other: such as elation, expansive mood, problems not specified elsewhere

Problems with social or supportive relationships
Problems with activities of daily living
Overall problems with living conditions
Problems with work and leisure activities and the quality of the daytime environment

- Face validity: they covered most of the domains important to old age psychiatric services in a rough and ready sort of way (with the possible exception of elated mood), and

- Compatibility: HoNOS65+ and its parent HoNOS represented the first systematic attempt in the UK to initiate an outcomes culture in mental health, and at the time were the only measures of their type, and likely to become the standard measures.

Following the discussion above, it should be clear that we did not choose the HoNOS65+ because it was 'valid' or 'reliable'; we started our outcomes project before many data on HoNOS or any data on HoNOS65+ were published (Allen *et al.*, 1999). We have not been particularly surprised at the way in which enthusiasts' claims of adequacy or objectors' claims of inadequacy appear to be based on similar results and similar misconceptions about the use of measures in general – misconceptions that I hope I have already aired.

It is important to assert that HoNOS65+ are scales completed after a full clinical assessment and are not a substitute for the assessment. Clinicians rate patients based on all that they know about the patient and the circumstances at the time.

Choice of period covered by measurement of health status, frequency of ratings and interval between ratings

These related decisions depend on estimates of how quickly one expects interventions to have an impact, and the frequency of important difficulties in the domains of interest. In old age psychiatry services, we suggest that HoNOS65+ ratings are made covering the preceding two weeks – on each scale, on every occasion, the worst they have been in that period is what is rated. For acute inpatient treatment and assessment we ask for the HoNOS65+ to be completed covering the first and last two weeks of admission. If inpatient stays are short this could be reduced by local agreement, as long as the two ratings cover the same number of days. For community team and outpatient work we similarly ask HoNOS65+ to be completed covering two weeks prior to assessment and the two weeks preceding discharge (this would apply to a day hospital if we used one). For patients in contact for long periods we suggest six-monthly scoring.

Choice of measure of context (case mix)

In order to understand the impact of interventions on outcomes in a mental health service for older people you need to trap minimum data on diagnosis, age and sex. Information on living arrangements (e.g. whether or not in a care home), length of illness, physical health status and medication (as a risk factor rather than an intervention) would also be very useful. Most UK NHS mental health services for older people can collect age and sex data, but many only collect a diagnosis based on one of the international classifications if the patient is assessed by a doctor, and sometimes then only a consultant psychiatrist. Non-medical staff are either shy of the process of 'diagnosis' or considered incapable, despite the evidence from our own specialty that in broad terms non-doctors can make accurate diagnoses (Collighan *et al.*, 1993). Unless some simple systems of categorization according to condition are available, outcomes measurement becomes sterile. (*Lesson No 4: Before starting on outcomes, first start diagnosing.*)

Choice of measure of intervention

In our experience two main factors bedevil this aspect of outcomes measurement. The first is that although there are well-developed international consensus-based classification systems for disorders, the development of similar systems for interventions is in its infancy. Only in the area of physical treatments is it possible to be reasonably certain that two interventions with the same name are the same. For this reason we have latterly spent as much time on developing a taxonomy and glossary for the intervention codes to be used by staff as formerly we spent on the HoNOS65+ glossary. The second factor is the absolute necessity for electronic patient records systems to reduce the burden on staff of collecting intervention data. It is not feasible to collect actual interventions in a meaningful way otherwise. At present, lacking this, we base our crude analysis of interventions on those planned at first assessment, coded according to a glossary and entered into our information system. This list currently used is shown in Table 20.4; clearly, not all interventions are coded. However, even without this detail, it is reasonable to embark on RCOM treating various service components as 'black box' interventions – so comparing change between wards or teams is possible, and, in our experience fruitful, provided the minimum data on case mix is also incorporated into the analysis. (*Lesson No 5: Move up to electronic patient records as soon as possible.*)

Table 20.4 Draft intervention categories for old age psychiatry services

A. Contacts with client

i. Support
  ◆ Practical support
  ◆ Social support
  ◆ Emotional support

ii. Monitoring
  ◆ Mental state and risk
  ◆ Compliance with or side-effects of medication

iii. Psychotherapeutic intervention
  ◆ Client-specific psychological intervention informed by a range of models
  ◆ Psychotherapeutic intervention informed by a single model

B. Contacts with carer(s)

i. Indirectly aimed at client's needs
  ◆ Practical support
  ◆ Social support
  ◆ Emotional support

ii. Aimed primarily at carer's needs only
  ◆ Practical support
  ◆ Social support
  ◆ Emotional support

C. Specialist assessment

i. Psychometric and/or neuropsychological
ii. Social Services core assessment
ii. AMPS1/OT Assessment
iii. Neuroimaging

D. Medical interventions

i. Physical medication prescribed
ii. Psychotropic medication prescribed
  ◆ Anti-psychotic
  ◆ Anti-depressant
  ◆ Sedative/hypnotic
  ◆ Drugs for dementia
  ◆ Lithium
  ◆ Other mood stabilizers
iii. Assess requirement for depot neuroleptic
iv. Administer depot neuroleptic medication
v. ECT

E. Liaising with other agencies

i. Social care services
ii. GP
iii. Other

F. Referral (client not discharged)

i. Inpatient admission
ii. NHS Continuing Care
iii. Specialist service
  (e.g. Psychological Treatment Service)
iv. Outreach service
v. Private/voluntary service

G. Other

[1]Goldman and Fisher, 1997

Implementation

The local aims of implementing of RCOM can include fear of someone else doing it (Johanson, 1999), obedience to central dictat (James and Kehoe, 1999), a call to arms against intransigent purchasers (Rozzini *et al.*, 2002), or a desire to improve patient care (Allen *et al.*, 1999). This motivation will infect the staff implementing it. We know of no old age psychiatry service that has got as far as ours in the UK, motivated as we are mainly by the last, and the UK HoNOS65+ Implementation Group's experience suggest that this is the most enduring motivation. (*Lesson No 6: Whatever the initial impulse for embarking on RCOM, its success will depend on whether it can be seen as possibly improving patient care.*)

A full understanding of the theoretical, and even philosophical, basis described above may not be necessary, although services need to be confident that this is in place. The stages of implementation we followed, and would still suggest following, were as shown in Table 20.5. It can be seen that this is a costly and arduous process, with little in the way of fruit, apart from the novelty of joint training, before two years. It is crucial to retain management support, or at least reluctance to interfere, and also

Table 20.5 Stages of implementation of RCOM in an old age psychiatry service (Allen *et al.*, 1999)

Stage 1: 3 months	Local consultation. Agreement at management level to implement RCOM. This was predicated on the existence of an information system that could support it, and on a culture of multidisciplinary assessment and diagnosis (Macdonald *et al.*, 1994). It was not possible to rely on the organisation's information system at that time.
Stage 2: 6 months	Formation of a steering group who underwent training in HoNOS65+. (Nowadays they would also be required to train as trainers, both of HoNOS65+ and the intervention codes). Completion of local training materials (videos rather than written vignettes)
Stage 3: 6 months	Setting up information systems and training of all current staff.
Stage 4: 6 months	New staff trained as part of induction from now on. A softly, softly rollout. Ratings made compulsory on new cases at assessment/admission and at discharge on old cases only. Culminates in feedback to all teams and wards of crude, mean differences between the two groups.
Stage 5: 6 months	Ratings made compulsory on all new referrals at assessment and discharge. Culminates in feedback to all teams and wards of first paired data on outcomes
Stage 6: Continuous	Ratings made compulsory at 6-month intervals for all long-term patients, and at Care Programme Approach[2] reviews. Regular re-training of all staff (every 2 years). Regular feedback of results to steering group (every 2 months) and all staff (every year). Inter-rater reliability studies using video vignettes. Validation study against published criterion scales, independently rated.

[2] Kingdon, 1994

crucial that the administrators who enter data and chivvy clinicians for ratings are deeply implicated and involved. *(Lesson No 7: Form a team and be prepared for a long haul.)*

Data analysis and presentation

Feedback to the clinicians is crucial. This is described elsewhere (Macdonald, 2002). As the dataset grows, it is possible to refine the information more and more, and we are now in a position to examine categorical change (by consensus over what we mean by 'better') in the most afflicted patients, rather than mean scale score changes in all patients. We have already intervened to stop an intervention that appeared to be associated with an untoward deterioration in depression scale ratings in patients with dementia in an acute assessment ward. This aspect of RCOM requires a well-motivated senior figure with access to analysis and presentation skills. If outcomes data is available to clinicians and can be anticipated to act as a brake on managerial enthusiasm or over-compliance with central directives, RCOM can be slightly subversive, which definitely appeals to clinical staff. *(Lesson No 8: Look for a local Champion who can both retain management support and feedback information in a way that motivates clinicians.)*

Conclusion

A chapter like this is unlikely to stimulate Pauline conversion to RCOM, but if it irritates or stimulates those who believe in the current orthodoxy about service evaluation then it will have served its purpose, and if it helps those services trying to develop a more rational, outcomes-based framework for decisions about structures and processes that allows resistance to the current unbridled pace of reorganization then it will also have done its job. But the real test of an outcomes-based service is whether or not the degree of improvement in patients already occurring and the proportions in which it occurs can rise from whatever baseline we find, and keep on rising. Routine clinical outcomes measurement is more interesting than audit and a lot more fun than being inspected.

For further reading I recommend Lyons *et al.* (1997).

References

Ablon, J.S. and Jones, E.E. (2002) Validity of controlled clinical trials of psychotherapy: findings from the NIMH Treatment of Depression Collaborative Research Program. *Am J Psychiatry*, **159**, 775–83.

Adams, M., Palmer, A., O'Brien, J.T. *et al.* (2000) Health of the nation outcome scales for psychiatry: are they valid? *Journal of Mental Health*, **9**, 193–8.

Allen, L., Bala, S., Carthew, R., *et al.* (1999) Experience and application of HoNOS65+. *Psychiatric Bulletin*, **23**, 203–6.

Bannock, G., Baxter, R., and Davis, E. (1998) *The Penguin Dictionary of Economics*. Penguin, London.

Benbow, S.M. and Jolley, D.J. (2002) Burnout and stress amongst old age psychiatrists. *International Journal of Geriatric Psychiatry*, **17**, 710–14.

Bie Nio Ong (1993) *The Practice of Health Services Research*. Chapman and Hall, London.

Bleuler, E. (1919) Autistic undisciplined thinking in medicine, and how to overcome it. Hafner, Darien, Conn.

Broadbent, M. (2002) Reconciling the information needs of clinicians, managers and commissioners – a pilot project. *Psychiatric Bulletin*, **25**, 423–4.

Bristol Royal Infirmary Inquiry HMSO (2001) http://www.bristol-inquiry.org.uk/index.htm

Burns, A., Beevor, A., Lelliott, P., et al. (1999) Health of the Nation Outcome Scales for elderly people (HoNOS 65+). *British Journal of Psychiatry*, **174**, 424–7.

Clancy, C.M. and Lawrence, W. (2002) Is outcomes research on cancer ready for prime time? *Med Care*, **40**, III92–100.

Collighan, G., MacDonald, A., Herzberg, J., *et al.* (1993) An evaluation of the multidisciplinary approach to psychiatric diagnosis in elderly people. *BMJ* **306**, 821–4.

Donabedian, A. (2001) The quality of care – can it be assessed? *JAMA*, **260**, 1743–8.

Dunn, G. (1994) Statistical methods for measuring outcomes. *Social Psychiatry and Psychiatric Epidemiology*, **29**, 198–204.

Goldman, S.L. and Fisher, A.G. (1997) Cross-cultural validation of the Assessment of Motor and Process Skills (AMPS). *British Journal of Occupational Therapy*, **60**, 77–85.

Hickie, I., Burke, D., Tobin, M., *et al.* (2000) The impact of the organisation of mental health services on the quality of assessment provided to older patients with depression. *Australia and New Zealand Journal of Psychiatry*, **34**, 748–54.

Hume, D. (1978) *A Treatise of Human Nature*. A. Selby-Bigge (ed.) 2nd edn, revised by P. Nidditch. Oxford University Press, Oxford.

James, M. and Kehoe, R. (1999) Using the Health of the Nation Outcome Scales in clinical practice. *Psychiatric Bulletin*, **23**, 536–8.

Johanson, J.F. (1999) Importance of outcomes research in endoscopic practice. *Gastrointestinal Endoscopy Clinics of North America*, **9**, 559–64.

Kingdon, D. (1994) Care programme approach. *Psychiatric Bulletin*, **18**, 68–70.

Lindesay, J., Herzberg, J., Collighan, G., *et al.* (1996) Treatment decisions following assessment by multidisciplinary psychogeriatric teams. *Psychiatric Bulletin*, **20**, 78–81.

Lord, J. and Littlejohns, P. (1997) Evaluating healthcare policies: the case of clinical audit. *BMJ* **315**, 668–71.

Lyons, J.S., Howard, K.I., O'Mahoney, M.T., and Lish, J. (1997) *The Measurement and Management of Clinical Outcomes in Mental Health*. John Wiley, New York.

Macdonald, A., Goddard, C., and Poynton, A. (1994) Impact of 'open access' to specialist services – the case of community psychogeriatrics. *International Journal Of Geriatric Psychiatry*, **9**, 709–14.

Macdonald, A.J. (1999) HoNOS 65+ glossary. *British Journal of Psychiatry*, **175**, 192.

Macdonald, A.J. (2002) The usefulness of aggregate routine clinical outcomes data: the example of HoNOS65+. *Journal of Mental Health*, **11**, 645–6.

Marks, D. (2002) *Perspectives on Evidence-based Practice*. Health Development Agency, Department of Health, London.

Marsden, D. and Oakley, P. (1991) Future issues and perspectives in the evaluation of social development. *Community Development Journal*, **26**, 314–28.

Meakins, J.L. (2002) Innovation in surgery: the rules of evidence. *American Journal of Surgery*, **183**, 399–405.

NSW Health Department (1992) The NSW Health Outcomes Program. *New South Wales Public Health Bulletin*, 3 (12), 135.

Pawson, R. and Tulley, N. (1997) *Realistic Evaluation*. Sage Publications, London.

Richardson, J. (1999) *The Economic Framework for Health Service Evaluation and the Role for Discretion*. Centre for Health Program Evaluation, West Heidelberg, Victoria, Australia.

Rock, D. and Preston, N. (2001) HoNOS: is there any point in training clinicians? *Journal of Psychiatric and Mental Health Nursing*, 8, 405–9.

Rozzini, R., Frisoni, G.B., and Trabucci (2002) Outcome measurement in mental health: the Italian experience in psychogeriatrics. *British Journal of Psychiatry*, 181, 442–3.

Sackett, D., Richardson, W., Rosenberg, W., *et al.* (1996) *Evidence-based Medicine - How to Practice and Teach EBM*. Churchill Livingstone, London.

Sellu, D. (1996) Time to audit audit. *BMJ* 312, 128–9.

Semler, R. (2003) *The Seven Day Weekend*. Random House, London.

Silk, D. (1991) *Planning IT – Creating an Information Management Strategy*. Butterworth-Heinemann, London.

Slade, M. (2002) Routine outcome assessment in mental health services. *Psychological Medicine*, 32, 1339–43.

Slade, M., Thornicroft, G., and Glover, G. (1999) The feasibility of routine outcome measures in mental health. *Social Psychiatry and Psychiatric Epidemiology*, 34, 243–9.

Spertus, J.A., Radford, M.J., Every, N.R., *et al.* (2003) Challenges and opportunities in quantifying the quality of care for acute myocardial infarction. Summary from the acute myocardial infarction working group of the American heart association/American college of cardiology first scientific forum on quality of care and outcomes research in cardiovascular disease and stroke. *Journal of the American College of Cardiology*, 41, 1653–63.

St. Leger, A., Schnieden, H., and Walsworth-Bell, J. (1992) *Evaluating Health Services' Effectiveness*. Open University Press, Buckingham.

Whiteford, H. (2001) Can research influence mental health policy? *Australian and New Zealand Journal of Psychiatry*, 35, 428–34.

Wing, J.K., Beevor, A.S., Curtis, R.H., *et al.* (1998) Health of the Nation Outcome Scales (HoNOS). Research and development. *British Journal of Psychiatry*, 172, 11–18.

Wolff, N. (2000) Using randomized controlled trials to evaluate socially complex services: problems, challenges and recommendations. *Journal of Mental Health Policy and Economics*, 3, 97–109.

Chapter 21

Psychogeriatric service delivery with limited resources

Tom Dening and K. S. Shaji

Developing countries

The current scenario

Growing need for services

Numbers of old people in developing countries are set to increase sharply over the next few decades. The most striking effects of population ageing are to be seen in the most rapidly developing regions: China, India and Latin America. The anticipated doubling over the next 30 years of the numbers of older persons living in these regions will change the global distribution of dementia (Prince, 1997). With its devastating negative effects on carers and families, dementia will soon emerge as a major public health problem in most developing countries. The number of elderly people suffering from depression and other mental health problems will also increase. Given the unprecedented pace of demographic ageing, these less-developed societies will have comparatively little time to develop social and health care policies to deal with the increasing demand for services.

Public awareness

The lack of priority accorded to the health care needs of the elderly in developing countries seems to perpetuate the low level of public awareness about mental health problems of old age. A problem such as dementia is not usually identified as a health condition. Even when it is identified, it does not lead to caregivers receiving practical advice or support (Patel and Prince, 2001; Shaji *et al.*, 2003). Dementia and other mental disorders of older people, remain hidden problems rarely brought to the attention of health care professionals and policy makers. Voluntary organizations like Alzheimer's Disease International (ADI) have been actively trying to develop dementia care services in the developing world. Their attempts have helped to gain media attention for dementia and other geriatric health care issues. Cholinesterase inhibitors (donepezil and rivastigmine) are now available at relatively low prices in countries like India. This might lead to better identification and management of cases of dementia in clinical practice. Similarly, the availability of newer antidepressants with better side effect profiles will probably improve the identification and management of geriatric depression by physicians and general practitioners. Developing psychogeriatric services will become easier when health professionals and the public are more aware of and sensitive to the mental health needs of the elderly.

Health care services

When we think of the development of psychogeriatric services, we need to take account of the current structure of the health care systems in the developing world, and their limitations. Specialist psychiatrists and geriatricians, the most skilled and knowledgeable practitioners in this area, are a rare commodity, and cannot hope to provide care and support for more than the tiny minority of those in need. There are no specialized services for old people in the government-run public health care services in India and most other developing countries. Outpatient care in the government health services typically involves long waits in crowded clinics for brief consultations. The usual focus in these settings is on 'treatable' acute pathologies and not on long-term care. Old people find it difficult to go to these clinics as this usually involves travel and use of transport. Most elderly people are unwilling to use the public transport system, as it is not user-friendly. At the same time, most of them cannot afford the cost of private transport. These factors are serious limitations of clinic-based services for old people needing long-term support and care. However, such services may be useful to people in urban areas where accessibility may be less of a problem.

In rural areas, even primary care doctors are a rare commodity, so minimally trained multipurpose health workers (MPHWs) have become the mainstay of the service. These generic community-based health workers exist in some form in many developing country health and social welfare systems. After achieving a basic standard of education these workers receive additional training in simple health care programmes. They are generally given a catchment area responsibility. They get to know all of the families in their area, as they have to make home visits as part of the community-based mother and child health programme. In many developing regions, MPHWs are the only generally available outreach arm of health care services. In principle, MPHWs could, following appropriate training, extend their role to include basic level family and community interventions for elderly people with dementia and other mental health problems in their area of work.

Mental health services

Within the developing world, there are wide variations in the availability of mental health care. According to the World Health Organization (WHO, 2001) one-third of countries across the world do not report a specific mental health budget, although they presumably devote some resources to mental health. Half of the rest allocate less than 1 per cent of their public health budget to mental health, even though neuropsychiatric problems represent 12 per cent of the total global burden of disease. Such budgetary inadequacies will inevitably result in inadequate financial resources for mental health care in most developing countries. Besides this, most money that is allocated for mental health is spent on maintaining large tertiary care centres like mental hospitals. Community-based mental health services are not available in 38 per cent of the countries.

There is also a wide disparity in the availability of trained manpower between low-income countries and high-income countries. The median number of psychiatrists in low-income countries is estimated to be 0.06 per 100,000 in contrast to 9 per 100,000 in high-income countries (WHO, 2001). There is shortage of other trained mental health professionals too. Community care is absent in most countries and health workers are not linked to mental health service providers. A shortage of trained manpower and inadequate budgetary allocation for mental health will seriously limit the development of specialized psychogeriatric services in developing countries. Instead, the emphasis should be upon integration of psychogeriatric services into general health care by training primary care doctors to identify and manage common conditions like dementia and depression. Development of specialized psychogeriatric services is possible in big general hospitals and teaching hospitals where trained manpower is available.

Current care arrangements

What are the current care arrangements of old people with mental health problems in developing regions of the world? Unfortunately, such information is limited. Insight into the needs of patients and their families are of paramount importance in planning services. All services should aim to use their assessment of these needs to improve the quality of life of the person affected as well as that of the carer.

Most elderly people, even those with disabling conditions like dementia, are usually looked after by their families in spite of the difficulties faced by them. Their distress and burden is made worse by unhelpful attitudes from the health care services and the non-availability of other sources of help (Shaji *et al.*, 2003). A recent comprehensive assessment of care arrangements for people with dementia in the developing world was made by the 10/66 Dementia Research Group. They studied 706 persons with dementia and their caregivers in India, China and South-East Asia, Latin America and the Caribbean and Africa (10/66 Dementia Research Group, 2004). The majority of caregivers were women, living with the person with dementia, in large extended family households. According to region, between one quarter and one half of households contained several generations with one or more children under the age of sixteen years. Traditional extended family households were associated with lower caregiver strain, where the caregiver was co-resident. However, despite the relatively intact traditional apparatus of family care, levels of caregiver psychological strain in developing countries were at least as high as those observed in the developed world. There was also marked economic disadvantage. Caregivers had often cut back on paid work to care and they faced additional expense in terms of paid formal care and heavy health service costs.

Caregivers from the poorest developing countries were particularly likely to have used expensive private medical services, and to have spent more than 20 per cent of their country's per capita GNP on health care for the person with dementia.

Looking after an elderly relative at home is thus associated with substantial economic disadvantage. Few older people in developing countries receive government or occupational pensions, and disability pensions are not usually provided. Caregivers who are in paid employment do not receive any form of caregiver allowance. The combination of reduced family incomes and increased family expenditure on care is obviously particularly stressful in lower income countries where so many households exist at or near to subsistence level.

Home-based care

All over the world, the family has always been and still is the major provider of long-term care for the elderly. This is especially so in developing countries, where the family is the only source of care for disabled or behaviourally disturbed elderly people. Institutional care is costly as well as culturally unacceptable in many of these communities. Rising health care costs makes it necessary to strengthen home-based care as an alternative to clinic-based approaches and institutional care.

But it would be wrong to presume that home-based care is without economic and other costs. More often than not, such care is associated with considerable emotional as well as financial burden (Patel and Prince, 2001; Shaji *et al.*, 2003; The 10/66 Dementia Research Group, 2004). Most caregivers are women and they tend to have very little access to or control of the resources needed to assume this responsibility. Obviously caregivers need to be identified and supported and this can be best done if services are provided at home. Community outreach programmes to support home-based care can be of great help to the families, particularly to those from poorer sections of the society. Home-based care remains a feasible option for long-term care of many elderly people with mental health problems.

However, due to various social, economic and demographic changes, family resources are dwindling (e.g. small family size, migration, changing rural and urban social environments, poverty, family members themselves being old or impaired, etc.). Care of elderly people at home, especially those with disabling mental health conditions like dementia, will become increasingly difficult in the future, as younger women upon whom the duties of care most frequently fall, are increasingly likely to work outside their homes.

Clinic-based services

A wide variety of services can be provided in the general hospitals. Most geriatric psychiatric conditions can be managed in the outpatient setting if follow up visits to the hospital are possible. Caregiver education and support can be provided in such clinics. Special services like dementia clinics or psychogeriatric clinics can be started in general hospitals and, where they are established, such clinics can make effective use of the clinician. For example, a weekly dementia clinic in the Medical College hospital at Thrissur in the state of Kerala in India is jointly run by the departments of neurology and psychiatry. The clinic provides information and education for families and emotional support to caregivers. Follow-up visits often focus on the management of distressing symptoms at home. Most families find this new service very useful and we believe that the service has provided a better quality of care. Redeployment of existing resources to suit the needs of the elderly can help support such initiatives in general hospital settings.

Development of new psychogeriatric services

Goals of services

Where resources are limited, service goals should be based upon realistic assumptions. Community-based services will have to make active attempts to identify their target populations. Clinic-based services can limit themselves only to those who seek help, though of course this means that they may not cater for those in greatest need. Increasing public awareness through health education should always be an important goal. Educating the public about the need to provide services for the elderly in turn may result in more resources being provided for the development of better services.

Mapping of resources

Once the geographical area is selected, it is desirable to identify all existing health and social care facilities in that area. Organizations who could support or help in providing services for elderly people can then be approached. The potential for working together needs to be explored. This might help to make services more acceptable, as well as keeping the costs low.

Obviously, where resources are limited, it is important to make full use of any existing facilities or potential partners.

Identifying people in need of services

When community-based interventions are planned, it is necessary to consider the target population and how relevant cases can best be identified. This is particularly important for conditions like dementia, which are not frequently encountered by clinicians in primary care settings. The 10/66 Dementia Research Group has shown that health workers can be trained to identify cases of dementia in the community (Shaji et al., 2002). With adequate training these health workers are also able to provide simple home-based interventions.

Ingredients of the intervention

Simple, cost-effective interventions are preferred when resources are limited. For example, several interventions, like providing information and education and giving emotional support to caregivers of patients with dementia, can be done by trained health workers. They can also be trained to make brief assessments and deliver appropriate non-pharmacological interventions at home. It is prudent to choose interventions that can be delivered by personnel who are already part of the health care system. Interventions that need to be provided by qualified mental health professionals will have only limited prospect for wider application in the community.

Financial aspects

Psychogeriatric services need to be integrated to existing health care services so that the costs can be kept low. Most governments in the developing countries will soon initiate health care programmes for older people. It is vital that the mental health component gets due importance when funds are allocated for such programmes.

As pension and other social security schemes for the elderly in the developing world are generally grossly inadequate, the vast majority of old people will not be able to meet the costs of treatment. Families will often not be able to support care expenses out of their own pockets so, consequently, other mechanisms will be needed to provide continued financial support for psychogeriatric services.

A developed country: the United Kingdom

Along with other northern European countries, the UK population has aged over several decades and thus will not see such spectacular demographic changes as many other countries, especially those in the developing world. Old age psychiatry began in the UK about 40 years ago (Roth, 1955; Post, 1965; Arie, 1970) and it has been recognized as a separate speciality within psychiatry by the UK Department of Health for over a decade. There are now around 400 consultants in old age psychiatry in the UK. Several accounts describe the development and the current organization of older people's mental health services in the UK (Royal College of Psychiatrists/Royal College of Physicians, 1998; Audit Commission, 2001; Challis *et al.*, 2002; Fairbairn, 2002; Wattis, this volume). Policy in this area is set out in the National Service Framework for Older People (Department of Health, 2001) (though, in the devolved UK, this just applies to England).

Nonetheless, the UK has challenges and difficulties too. From 2001 to 2026 the proportion of the population over the age of 60 will rise from 20 per cent to nearly 28 per cent. Numbers aged 85+ will go on increasing until well into the century, by over 50 per cent in the next 25 years (National Statistics, 2002). Although the UK economy has performed well in recent years, there are current concerns about its ability to afford current labour patterns and trends towards increasingly early retirement. As a result, there is considerable uncertainty over pensions (Jones, 2003; Scott, 2003). The demographic and economic situation for older people will obviously affect the resources available to support mental health services.

Furthermore, despite growing numbers of old age psychiatrists, their distribution across the country is uneven. For example, their catchment area populations range from around 8000 people over 65 to 25,000 or more. Some services have great difficulty recruiting psychiatrists at all. They may depend on locum (temporary) staff, often of variable quality and sometimes recruited at considerable cost through commercial agencies. So the issue in the UK is less often trying to start up a service but either trying to recruit to all the posts that are established or else trying to consolidate what is already in place and respond to increasing demands.

Current challenges

Workforce issues

Psychiatrists

The UK has a separate speciality of old age psychiatry with specialist training programmes for old age psychiatrists. In most other countries, however, older people are served by neurology or geriatric medicine for dementia and general psychiatry for functional disorders. Older people with mental health problems may be regarded as having lower priority than younger patients or those with other diagnoses. Even if this is not so, it is difficult to develop a rational and comprehensive service for older people's mental health without suitable specialists.

As mentioned above, even if old age psychiatry is established, recruitment may be patchy. Not until a training programme has been running for a few years will accredited specialists appear from it. Well-established services find it easier to attract new doctors than those that are struggling. Within psychiatry as a whole, other specialities may prove more attractive depending on their level of resources and perceived prospects for development.

The growth of the older population and increased expectations for older people provide exciting opportunities to develop new approaches. Notable examples include memory clinics and prescribing of anti-dementia drugs (Lindesay *et al.*, 2002), liaison psychiatry (Melding and Draper, 2001; Holmes *et al.*, 2002), and assessments of mental capacity. The latter has grown especially in Scotland following the Adults with Incapacity Act 2000 (Alzheimer Scotland Action on Dementia, 2002) which requires medical assessments and certificates of incapacity. These pressures to expand work in several directions are likely to cause some degree of subspecialization within old age psychiatry.

Although recruitment of old age psychiatrists remains difficult in some places, there are some reasons for optimism. UK Department of Health projections, based on current trends, do not regard old age psychiatry as a shortage speciality. Some general initiatives are likely to improve the recruitment of psychiatrists, for example, increased medical student numbers, including graduate entry programmes for students without the traditional science background. New medical schools, emphasizing community services, and humanities-oriented students may produce more doctors interested in psychiatry. Also, basic training grades are to be revised by expanding the pre-registration period to two years, which could incorporate experience in psychiatry. The UK is also actively recruiting psychiatrists from overseas, notably through its International Fellowship scheme (www.nhs.uk/fellowships).

Recruitment to old age psychiatry as a speciality depends on its inclusion in broad-based psychiatric training schemes, where trainees are often inspired by the appeal of working with older people or by the energy and enthusiasm of their trainers. Where a service is struggling to attract consultants, it may benefit from links with more established services, for example by means of secondments or academic links. Often this may be brought about through the formation of large mental health trusts, covering extended areas, though equity is not necessarily instantly achieved.

Managing workload within reasonable hours is clearly a challenge for many professionals including old age psychiatrists (Benbow and Jolley, 2002). It is essential to prioritize the tasks confronting the service and then to use scarce consultant resources effectively. For example, referrers value prompt assessments especially of emergencies, so some capacity can be preserved by not spending time on the follow-up of routine cases. This may be possible by delegating to other members of the multidisciplinary team or referring back to primary care. Shared protocols with primary care may make this clearer and more acceptable.

Memory clinics are an important development, usually operating as part of the old age psychiatry service (Lindesay *et al.*, 2002). They effectively identify people with dementia at an earlier stage, thus providing opportunities for early treatment (Luce *et al.*, 2001). Developing a memory clinic should be undertaken with the needs of the whole service in mind, so that the resulting demand does not generate unacceptably long waiting lists or detract from the rest of the service provided.

Other professional groups

Recruitment and retention of nurses is a problem in many developed countries. Nursing has become a less attractive career especially for women, as other opportunities have emerged. It is often perceived as poorly paid, as physically and emotionally demanding and as having inconvenient hours. Career progression tends to divert nurses from clinical work into management roles, thus losing many skilled practitioners from patient contact. All these issues apply to older people's mental health, with the additional problem that trainee mental health nurses spend most of their training working with younger patients, so they are often more attracted to jobs in this area.

Various measures may help. First, recruitment is crucial, at all stages from nurses in training to looking overseas for qualified staff. However, language issues may limit the success of overseas recruitment. Second, vigorous attempts to retain existing staff are equally important. This includes providing incentives and a career structure that enable skilled nurses to develop specialist clinical skills and remain in clinical work. The establishment of consultant nurse posts recognizes the invaluable contribution of such nurses (Packer, 2001).

Other health professionals are also in short supply, including psychologists, occupational therapists, physiotherapists and speech therapists. As a result, older people do not have fair access to psychological treatment services or creative therapies (Zarit and Knight, 1996; Hepple *et al.*, 2002; Innes and Hatfield, 2001), even though there is good evidence that they can benefit.

Primary care

Primary care is often criticized for not diagnosing dementia early enough, not communicating the diagnosis and not referring people on to appropriate services (e.g. Briggs and Askham, 1999; Audit Commission, 2000), but this should be set against the relative rarity of dementia for any individual general practitioner. A GP with a list size of 2000 and an average age distribution will see just one or two new cases per year and will have around 14 established cases at different stages of dementia (Iliffe and Drennan, 2001). Although there is certainly scope to improve GPs' knowledge of dementia and other mental health problems, how this is most effectively done remains unclear. Probably the way forward is multifactorial, including adequate online decision-supporting information for GPs (Iliffe *et al.*, 2002), and better access to assessment through memory clinics and specialist mental health services.

In the UK, health funding is allocated through a network of Primary Care Trusts (PCTs), which commission services for their local population needs. PCTs are themselves providers of primary care services and, in some instances, more often in Scotland than in England, they may provide the specialist mental health services too.

For various reasons therefore, a mental health service needs close working relationships with primary care. This includes broad issues and service agreements, development of agreed protocols for referrals and treatments, and discussions between clinicians about individual cases. There are often tensions over resources, like new drug treatments or new services (e.g. young-onset dementia), but certain tasks may be devolved back to primary care, such as lithium monitoring, administration of depot antipsychotic injections, and routine follow-up of stable cases.

Social care

Most formal care for people with dementia in the UK is provided through the social care system, rather than health. Services are either commissioned by local authority social services departments or purchased directly by clients. Thus, the state of the local social care system has a profound effect on the mental health service in that area.

Several problems are common. First, where there are specialist social workers they are key members of the multidisciplinary community mental health team, but often no social workers are specifically designated for mental health in older people, leading to disadvantage for this client group. Their needs are considered along with people with physical health needs, and consequently they often miss out.

Second, provision of domiciliary and other forms of care (e.g. day care) for older people with mental health needs, may be inadequate, either because of funding constraints or lack of available staff. Social services departments usually operate tight eligibility criteria controlled by a process known as Best Value, which is defined as a duty of continuous improvement for local authorities, set out by the Local Government Act 1999. In theory it is an initiative for quality, though in practice it appears more like a rationing measure (Weaver and Parker, 2002). Again, unless there is specific recognition of mental health problems, this older age group is likely to be denied potentially valuable services.

Third, there may be insufficient residential and nursing home places for the needs of the local population. This can place extreme pressure on inpatient beds, delaying discharges and in effect making hospitals into nursing homes. Furthermore, there has been a recent loss of confidence among care home providers, leading to home closures and loss of beds. Staffing is often a problem for care homes. Many care staff are untrained, the work is physically and emotionally demanding and wages are low, leading to poor recruitment and high turnover. This makes it difficult to offer effective training inputs, as the staff group will often change within a short period. One approach is to focus on care home managers as key figures who reinforce positive attitudes in homes and who can give appropriate value to the work of care staff (Cantley, 2001).

Fourth, organizational differences and poor joint working between health and social care agencies can lead to frustration and poor services for older people. Various policy initiatives address this issue, including 'Better Services for Vulnerable People' and the so-called 'Health Act flexibilities' which allow statutory bodies to share budgets and plan more closely together. Many mental health trusts in England now work in partnership with social services, including managing seconded social work staff, and in the future health and social care may possibly merge into care trusts.

Consumer input

Public services in general have moved strongly towards encouraging a stronger voice from their users. For older people, the role of carers in developing services has been recognized for some time (Dening and Lawton, 1998), but only more recently has the need to engage older service users, including those with dementia, been recognized (e.g. Kitwood, 1997; Barnett, 2000). This process is assisted by a strong voluntary sector, especially the national Alzheimer's organizations for people with dementia, but also Age Concern and the Mental Health Foundation, who take an interest in functional disorders.

Involvement of older service users presents particular challenges. They may be physically frail, lacking in confidence and/or without independent transport. The views of people with dementia can be gathered, even from people with marked disability (Allan, 2001; Barnett, 2000). Genuine user and carer input requires resources, as it takes time to get people together, and it may take time and patience to elicit their thoughts. Nonetheless, their full participation in matters of service development, management and evaluation is likely to be of mutual benefit to service providers and consumers.

Meeting the needs of groups within the population

Several groups of people may be overlooked or ignored, even compared with the generality of older people. These include people from minority ethnic groups (Patel *et al.*, 1998), older prisoners or patients in forensic settings (Fazel *et al.*, 2001), people with learning disabilities (Thompson, 2002) and people with early onset dementia (Royal College of Psychiatrists, 2000). Also, people with long-term severe functional illnesses or with substance misuse problems are often at risk of being neglected by services. Space precludes a full discussion of these issues, but the important point is that such needs must be considered when deciding how to balance limited resources. Initiatives may include, for example, working with community elders or religious leaders to improve access for people from minority ethnic backgrounds, or developing novel ways of supporting older people in secure settings (Yorston, 1999).

Practical steps

Despite the importance of money, additional investment in itself will not solve all the difficulties. The training of qualified professionals involves a lag between making the investment and seeing the results. For unqualified staff, there is simply a shortage of personnel, as many areas of the UK are close to full employment.

There is of course no single answer but how to make progress against financial restraints and workforce constraints require action on several fronts, of which the following seem especially important:

- *Leadership and clear goals.* For the service to argue its case and secure its resources, it must know what it wants to do, what its strengths and weaknesses are, and how it wants to use the available evidence in negotiating with service commissioners.

- *Research and development* activities can directly attract new resources, both for staff and for new treatments in clinical trials, but also the stimulus of research activity benefits recruitment and retention and can improve service quality in more general ways.

- *Delegation* of tasks, both within the service (e.g. initial assessments of new referrals may be performed by different members of the multidisciplinary team, not just the consultant psychiatrist) and outside it (e.g. whether or not the service accepts younger people with dementia or 'graduates' from general adult psychiatric teams).

- *Lobbying*, both locally and nationally in various ways. For example, in partnership with the Alzheimer's Society, or through specific campaigns such as the Coalition for Quality in Care (www.cpa.org.uk/events/qualcare.html). Locally, this will include various ways of raising the profile of the service with PCTs, social services, lay groups and the media. It may extend to encouraging patients and carers to contact their Members of Parliament or the press.

◆ *Opportunism* frequently seems to pay off. Funding initiatives are often announced with absurdly short deadlines, so that it is worthwhile having a few projects in the filing cabinet that can be submitted at short notice. Also, it is possible to anticipate the direction of policies and therefore the areas where funding may become available.

◆ *Partnerships*, both with obvious partners such as statutory bodies, users and carers, but also more widely and imaginatively, for example Dementia Services Development Centres (www.stirling.ac.uk/dsdc), architects (Judd *et al.*, 1997) and poets (Killick, 1997). Working with geriatric physicians also remains essential (Callahan, 2001).

◆ *Energy, enthusiasm and commitment* are desirable personal qualities, to which might be added a positive and optimistic outlook. If these attributes become part of the service culture, then much can be achieved.

Resources and rationing
Funding

In all countries of the world, it would be generally agreed that the resources available for older people's mental health services are limited. Obviously, the precise issues vary from country to country. In a developing country, the access to any form of health care may be a problem, but in a developed country the issues may be around access to anti-dementia drugs or the use of MR scans in diagnosis. Even so, the perception that health care is always underfunded has been criticized (Maynard, 2001) with the argument that demand can always be talked up by the supply side, including providers and pharmaceutical companies. The resources available to a service depend on many factors, including the total health budget for the country in question, the allocation of health spending within the total budget, attitudes to providing services for older people and/or those with mental health problems, and the ways in which decisions about rationing are made (see Chapter 4).

Lack of money is not the only issue, as some problems are about the availability of qualified and unqualified staff. However, economic factors are important in many ways:

◆ Older people lack economic power. They are often poor, subsisting on minimal pensions and benefits, so their choices (e.g. about residential care) are often limited.

◆ New drugs, especially anti-dementia drugs, may not have adequate funding allocated. For example, in the UK, despite national guidance (National Institute for Clinical Excellence 2001), funds are not always available to providers, which leads to uneven availability of these drugs across the country, so-called 'postcode prescribing'.

- Money available to finance long term care is inadequate. In the UK, social services departments are virtually monopoly purchasers and they have used this position to drive down prices, to the point that many homes are no longer viable.

- Care staff are paid at very low rates, so they may be unable to afford the cost of living in affluent areas. Care organizations are competing with other employers, such as supermarkets, where work is perceived as easier.

Because of the economic situation of many older people, mental health services are likely to be funded and provided as public services. This provides opportunities for rational planning, but there is also a public expectation that new investments will result in demonstrable improvements in work practices, efficiency and outcomes. There may be real new investment in older people's services, though often most service development has come from closing long term beds in old hospitals and moving the money into community services. In the UK, funding of long-term care has been shifted from the National Health Service to local authorities and private individuals.

Rationing

Age discrimination

Using age as a criterion on which to base rationing decisions has been both proposed (e.g. Daniels, 1988; Shaw, 1994) and opposed (e.g. Rivlin, 1995; Evans, 1997; Clarke, 2001). Two of the main arguments are, among others, the 'long innings' argument and concerns about the expense of treating old people using resources that could be better used elsewhere. The first argument is fallacious as it is clearly wrong to esteem the lives of all younger people above those of all older people simply on the basis of their chronological age. The second argument overlooks the fact that most health spending on older people is not for high-tech acute treatment but for less intensive support for chronic conditions like dementia or arthritis (Rivlin, 1995).

Beyond this it may be held that society has special duties and obligations towards older people to ensure that their needs for care are met (Jecker and Pearlman, 1989). This would be consistent with the often-heard maxim that the quality of society can be ascertained from how it treats its older people. In addition, age discrimination equates to a form of gender discrimination, given the longer life expectancy of women (Jecker, 1991).

Both government and professional consensus are opposed to using age as a criterion for eligibility (e.g. British Geriatrics Society, 2003). 'Rooting out age discrimination' is the first among eight standards in the English National Service Framework for Older People (Department of Health, 2001). It states that 'National Health services will be provided, regardless of age, on the basis of clinical need alone. Social care services will not use age in their eligibility criteria or policies, to restrict access to available services'. Thus, policies that specifically use age as a criterion are outlawed, though whether age is still used covertly is less easy to detect.

Explicit and implicit rationing

Given that there is always likely to be an excess of need (or, if not need, then demand) for health care services above the resources available, decisions need to be made about how spending is allocated and what care is or is not offered to patients (Aday *et al.*, 1999; Callahan, 1999). Rationing has several definitions, for example, failure to offer care or the denial of care from which patients would benefit (Maynard, 1999). Mechanic (1995) distinguishes between explicit and implicit forms of rationing. Recently, explicit rationing has grown with fixed budgets and the development of eligibility criteria and rating systems based on the values given to certain outcomes. Managed care in the US is probably the most developed such system. Methods of determining 'core services' or including the public voice in places such as Oregon and New Zealand have received attention (e.g. Cumming, 1997; New, 1998).

However, in practice, most rationing follows a more mixed course and at all levels people seem reluctant to take really hard decisions. For example, in the UK budgets are set centrally but then the responsibility for them is devolved to local level, with obvious potential risks for efficiency and equity (Sheldon and Smith, 2000). In part, this may reflect politicians' wishes not to be held directly responsible for unpopular decisions.

It remains undecided who should take decisions for tough choices. Some regard the issue as an empirical one, that better research will eventually guide us to the correct choices (Williams, 2001), while others (e.g. Mechanic, 1995) argue that attempts at explicit rationing are unstable as they simply focus conflict and dissatisfaction. It may be useful to arrive at a consensus of 'medically futile treatment' that prolongs survival at all costs, irrespective of any quality of life (Zucker and Zucker, 1997) or to agree limits on the infinite quest for perfect health (Callahan, 1998), but these issues remain controversial.

If rationing is not explicit, then much of the burden falls upon clinicians, who often have reservations about the task (Weinstein, 2001). Despite this, Mechanic (1995) argues largely for implicit rationing, ultimately depending on the discretion of professionals informed by practice guidelines, outcomes research and other relevant information. Rationing remains a contentious topic, with various stakeholders vying for influence but minimal responsibility. Allocation of health care funding is determined by a mixture of influences, and rationing reflects these, though at a more micro level.

So clinicians will continue to play a vital role in deciding how resources will be used in providing mental health services for older people. We have mentioned above the need for leadership and the setting of clear goals and priorities for the service, along with positive personal qualities and attitudes. Managing demand for services is a major challenge for services everywhere. This may be achieved by having waiting lists or by concentrating on particular aspects of the service, e.g. diagnostic assessments. Efficient use of the multidisciplinary team and sharing work with primary care are also important.

We would also argue that old age psychiatry needs a firm epidemiological base, in order to ensure that the population as a whole is receiving the best and fairest service that can be provided. On its own, managing demand is of limited value unless there is also equity of access for those in greatest need. It is necessary to have a picture of the catchment area, to know how many individuals will have dementia and other mental disorders, and to know about the social mixture in the area, for example, areas of poverty or minority ethnic groups.

Conclusion

Providing mental health services for older people will always be a challenge. Across the world services feel as if they are battling insurmountable odds with wholly inadequate resources. There are of course real differences between developed and developing countries, and these are both quantitative and qualitative in nature.

However, our main conclusion is that many of the underlying issues are rather similar. They relate to lack of money, availability of suitable staff, social attitudes and the national political agendas. Similarly, the remedies required are also mixed: some are practical solutions, others require negotiation with partners, and some are political in nature. Across the world, the same characteristics are needed to provide good services – a clear philosophy (WHO, 1997) and clear thinking. Whatever else, the needs and rights of older people are fundamental.

References

Aday, L.A., Begley, C.E., Lairson, D.R., Slater, C.H., Richard, A.J., and Montoya, I.D. (1999) A framework for assessing the effectiveness, efficiency, and equity of behavioral healthcare. *American Journal of Managed Care*, 5, SP25–44.

Allan, K. (2001) *Communication and Consultation: Exploring Ways for Staff to Involve People with Dementia in Developing Services.* Policy Press, Bristol.

Alzheimer Scotland – Action on Dementia (2002) *Dementia: Money and Legal Matters – A Guide.* Alzheimer Scotland – Action on Dementia, Edinburgh.

Arie, T. (1970) The first year of the Goodmayes Psychiatric Service for Old People. *Lancet,* ii, 1179–82.

Audit Commission (2000) *Forget Me Not: Mental Health Services for Older People.* Audit Commission, London.

Barnett, E. (2000) *Including the Person with Dementia in Designing and Delivering Care: 'I Need to be Me!'.* Jessica Kingsley, London.

Benbow, S.M. and Jolley, D.J. (2002) Burnout and stress amongst old age psychiatrists. *International Journal of Geriatric Psychiatry,* 17, 710–14.

Briggs, K. and Askham, J. (1999) *The Needs of People with Dementia and Those Who Care for Them: A Review of the Literature.* Alzheimer's Society, London.

British Geriatrics Society (2003) *Standards of Care for Specialist Services for Older People.* British Geriatrics Society, London.

Callahan, C.M. (2001) Geriatric psychiatry from a geriatrician's viewpoint. Psychiatric Bulletin, 25, 149–50.

Callahan, D. (1998) *False Hopes: Why America's Quest for Perfect Health is a Recipe for Failure.* Simon and Schuster, New York.

Callahan, D. (1999) Balancing efficiency and need in allocating resources to care of persons with serious mental illness. *Psychiatric Services*, **50**, 664–6.

Cantley, C. (2001) Understanding people in organisations. In C. Cantley (eds.) *A Handbook of Dementia Care*, pp. 220–39. Open University Press, Buckingham.

Challis, D., Reilly, S., Hughes, J., Burns, A., Gilchrist, H., and Wilson, K. (2002) Policy, organisation and practice of specialist old age psychiatry in England. *International Journal of Geriatric Psychiatry*, **17**, 1018–26.

Clarke, C.M. (2001) Rationing scarce life-sustaining resources on the basis of age. *Journal of Advanced Nursing*, **35**, 799–804.

Cumming, J. (1997) Defining core services: New Zealand experience. *Journal of Health Services Research and Policy*, **2**, 31–7.

Daniels, N. (1988) *Am I My Brother's Keeper? An Essay on Justice Between the Young and Old.* Oxford University Press, New York.

Dening, T. and Lawton, C. (1998) The role of carers in evaluating mental health services for older people. *International Journal of Geriatric Psychiatry*, **13**, 863–70.

Department of Health (2001) *National Service Framework for Older People.* Department of Health, London.

Evans, J.G. (1997) The rationing debate: rationing health care by age: the case against. *BMJ* **314**, 822–5.

Fairbairn, A.F. (2002) Principles of service provision in old age psychiatry. In R. Jacoby and C. Oppenheimer (eds.) *Psychiatry in the Elderly*, 3rd edn, pp. 423–40. Oxford University Press, Oxford.

Fazel, S., Hope, T., O'Donnell, I., and Jacoby, R. (2001) Hidden psychiatric morbidity in elderly prisoners. *British Journal of Psychiatry*, **179**, 535–9.

Hepple, J., Pearce, J., and Wilkinson, P. (2002) *Psychological Therapies with Older People: Developing Treatments for Effective Practice.* Brunner-Routledge, Hove.

Holmes, J., Bentley, K., and Cameron, I. (2002) *Between Two Stools: psychiatric services for older people in general hospitals.* University of Leeds, Leeds.

Iliffe, S., Austin, T., Wilcock, J., Bryans, M., Turner, S., and Downs, M. (2002) Design and implementation of a computer decision support system for the diagnosis and management of dementia syndromes in primary care. *Methods Information and Medicine*, **41**, 98–104.

Iliffe, S. and Drennan, V. (2001) *Primary Care and Dementia.* Jessica Kingsley, London.

Innes, A. and Hatfield, K. (2001) *Healing Arts Therapies and Person-Centred Dementia Care.* Jessica Kingsley, London.

Jecker, N.S. (1991) Age-based rationing and women. *Journal of the American Medical Association*, **266**, 3012–15.

Jecker, N.S. and Pearlman, R.A. (1989) Ethical constraints on rationing medical care by age. *Journal of the American Geriatrics Society*, **37**, 1067–75.

Jones, R. (2003) Last rites for final salary pensions. *Guardian*, 16 January.

Judd, S., Marshall, M., and Phippen, P. (ed.) (1997) *Design for Dementia.* Hawker, London.

Killick, J. (1997) *You Are Words: Dementia Poems.* Hawker, London.

Kitwood, T. (1997) *Dementia Reconsidered: The Person Comes First.* Open University Press, Buckingham.

Lindesay, J., Marudkar, M., van Diepen, E., and Wilcock, G. (2002) The second Leicester survey of memory clinics in the British Isles. *International Journal of Geriatric Psychiatry*, **17**, 41–7.

Luce, A., McKeith, I., Swann, A., Daniel, S., and O'Brien, J. (2001) How do memory clinics compare with traditional old age psychiatry services? *International Journal of Geriatric Psychiatry*, **16**, 837–45.

Maynard, A. (1999) Rationing health care: an exploration. *Health Policy*, **49**, 5–11.

Maynard, A. (2001) Ethics and health care 'underfunding'. *Journal of Medical Ethics*, **27**, 223–7.

Mechanic, D. (1995) Dilemmas in rationing health care services: the case for implicit rationing. *BMJ* **310**, 1655–9.

Melding, P. and Draper, B. (2001) *Geriatric Consultation Liaison Psychiatry*. Oxford University Press, Oxford.

National Institute for Clinical Excellence (2001) *Guidance on the Use of Donepezil, Rivastigmine and Galantamine for the Treatment of Alzheimer's Disease*. NICE, London.

National Statistics (2002) *Annual Abstract of Statistics*, p. 28. Stationery Office, London.

New, B. (ed.) (1998) *Rationing: Talk and Action in Health Care*. BMJ Publishing Group, London.

Packer, T. (2001) A nurse consultant in dementia care. *Signpost*, **5** (3), 19–22.

Patel, N., Mirza, N.R., Lindblad, P., Amstrup, K., and Samaoli, O. (1998) *Dementia and Minority Ethnic Older People: Managing Care in the UK, Denmark and France*. Russell House, London.

Patel, V. and Prince, M. (2001) Aging and mental health in a developing country: who cares? Qualitative studies from Goa, India. *Psychological Medicine*, **31**, 29–38.

Post, F. (1965) *The Clinical Psychiatry of Late Life*. Pergamon, Oxford.

Prince, M.J. (1997) The need for research on dementia in developing countries. *Tropical Medicine and Health*, **2**, 993–1000.

Rivlin, M.M. (1995) Protecting elderly people: flaws in ageist arguments. *BMJ* **310**, 1179–82.

Roth, M. (1955) The natural history of mental disorder in old age. *Journal of Mental Science*, **101**, 281–301.

Royal College of Psychiatrists (2000) *Services for Younger People with Alzheimer's Disease and Other Dementias*. Royal College of Psychiatrists, London.

Royal College of Psychiatrists/Royal College of Physicians (1998) *The Care of Older People with Mental Illness: Specialist Services and Medical Training*. Royal College of Psychiatrists/Royal College of Physicians, London.

Scott, M. (2003) Pensions 'to fall by a third'. *Observer*, 5 January.

Shaji, K.S., Smitha, Praveen Lal K., and Prince, M.J. (2003) Caregivers of patients with Alzheimer's disease: a qualitative study from the Indian 10/66 dementia research network. *International Journal of Geriatric Psychiatry*, **18**, 1–6.

Shaji, K.S., Arun Kishore, N.R., Praveen Lal, K., and Prince, M.J. (2002) Revealing a hidden problem. An evaluation of a community dementia case-finding program from the Indian 10/66 Dementia Research Network. *International Journal of Geriatric Psychiatry*, **17**, 222–5.

Shaw, A.B. (1994) In defence of ageism. *Journal of Medical Ethics*, **20**, 188–91.

Sheldon, T.A. and Smith, P.C. (2000) Equity in the allocation of health care resources. *Health Economics*, **9**, 571–4.

The 10/66 Dementia Research Group (2004) Care arrangements for people with dementia in developing countries. *International Journal of Geriatric Psychiatry*, **19**, 170–7.

Thompson, D. (2002) *Growing Older with Learning Disabilities: The GOLD Programme*. Mental Health Foundation.

Weaver, M. and Parker, S. (2002) Best value and inspection: the issue explained. *Guardian*, 29 October.

Weinstein, M.C. (2001) Should physicians be gatekeepers of medical resources? *Journal of Medical Ethics*, **27**, 268–74.

Williams, A. (2001) How economics could extend the scope of ethical discourse. *Journal of Medical Ethics*, **27**, 251–5.

World Health Organization (1997) *Organization of Care in Psychiatry of the Elderly: A Technical Consensus Statement.* WHO, Geneva.

World Health Organization (2001) *World Health Report 2001 – Mental Health: New Understanding, New Hope.* WHO, Geneva.

Yorston, G. (1999) Old age forensic psychiatry. *British Journal of Psychiatry*, **174**, 193–5.

Zarit, S.H. and Knight, B.G. (1996) *A Guide to Psychotherapy and Aging.* American Psychological Association, Washington, DC.

Zucker, M.B. and Zucker, H.D. (eds.) (1997) *Medical Futility and the Evaluation of Life-sustaining Interventions.* Cambridge University Press, Cambridge.

Chapter 22

The future of psychogeriatric services

Brian Draper, Henry Brodaty and Pamela Melding

Introduction

What are going to be the key issues that shape psychogeriatric service delivery over the next few decades? In this chapter we will address this question from different perspectives ranging from developing countries to developed countries, from health policy considerations to specific new treatments and technology, and from ethics to economics. As described by John Snowdon and Tom Arie in Chapter 1, psychogeriatrics is a young discipline with a formal history of only about 50 years. Much, however, can be learnt from this brief history when considering the future.

The impact of an ageing world

The ageing population was probably the major demographic factor that shaped the initial development of psychogeriatric services in the UK and it will continue to be the major factor that influences global developments in service delivery over coming years. While this poses challenges for service delivery in developed countries, it is in the developing countries that the rapid ageing of the population will have the greatest impact. In Table 22.1, we have listed population projections for different regions of the world from the ages of 65 and 75 years. It is the increase in the 'old old' aged over 75 that is likely to have the major impact, as the effects of population ageing are amplified by the even larger increase in older people with dementia (Prince, 2001).

Population ageing will continue over the next 30 years in all countries, but while the proportion of older people in the population will be higher in developed countries, the rate of change and the absolute numbers of older people will be much greater in developing countries. This is demonstrated in Table 22.2. In essence, this will largely lead to two different scenarios for psychogeriatrics – one for developed countries and the other for developing countries – though there will be some countries such as Israel, South Africa and some Eastern European countries that share characteristics of both.

Paradoxically, improvement in prevention, treatment and care of other disorders is increasing the demand for psychogeriatric services. Broe and Creasey (1995) pointed out that we are in the age of neurodegenerative disorders. The fall in rates of death from infectious diseases a century ago is now being mirrored by a decline in cardiac and stroke-related mortality. As our bodies survive longer, our brains become more susceptible to the ravages that can be wreaked by old age.

Table 22.1 Percentage of elderly by age: 2000 to 2030

Region	Year	65 years and over	75 years and over
Europe	2000	15.5	6.6
	2030	24.3	11.8
North America	2000	12.6	6.0
	2030	20.3	9.4
Oceania	2000	10.2	4.4
	2030	16.3	7.5
Asia	2000	6.0	1.9
	2030	12.0	4.6
Latin America/	2000	5.5	1.9
Caribbean	2030	11.6	4.6
North East/	2000	4.3	1.4
North Africa	2030	8.1	2.8
Sub-Saharan Africa	2000	2.9	0.8
	2030	3.7	1.3

Source: *An Aging World*, Kinsella, Velkoff and US Census Bureau 2001, p. 9

Table 22.2 Percentage increase in elderly population in selected developed and developing countries, 2000–2030

Developed countries		Developing countries	
Canada	126	Malaysia	277
Australia	108	Colombia	258
USA	102	Indonesia	240
Israel	102	Philippines	240
New Zealand	92	Mexico	227
Luxembourg	87	Egypt	210
Germany	63	Morocco	193
France	56	Brazil	192
United Kingdom	55	India	174
Japan	54	China	170
Italy	43	Pakistan	153

Source: *An Aging World*, Kinsella, Velkoff and US Census Bureau 2001, p. 11

For developed countries the challenge is to determine how existing specialist or secondary services (whether they be specialist psychogeriatric, mental health or aged care services) will cope with the increased workload. This will be influenced by other factors that include the expectations and demands of consumers, resource availability, the effects of technological advances, and increased knowledge about best practice in service delivery. With improvements in the health of the older population and increasing expectations that older people should work beyond the traditional retirement and pension age of 65, one possibility is that the age 'cut-offs' between adult psychiatry and psychogeriatrics could be increased to 75 years. Already it is notable that the healthy 'young old' in the 65–74 year age range have not acquired many of the age-related problems that make psychogeriatrics a specialist field, and their problems might be just as well managed by adult psychiatry.

There may also be cohort effects with population ageing. For example, the baby-boomer generation is likely to make increased demands upon available mental health resources through its larger size, increased knowledge of mental health issues and greater expectations of treatment. Another cohort effect that might occur is increased habitual use of illicit and recreational drugs amongst older people.

For developing countries the challenge will be to determine how existing primary health services, with limited assistance from whatever secondary or tertiary services that are available, will cope with the rapid population ageing. Dening and Shaji comment in Chapter 21 that it will not be financially viable for psychogeriatric services to operate in a stand-alone model. In Chapter 3, Martin Prince and Peter Trebilco have described a possible road map for developing countries. This involves increased public awareness, appropriate research that quantifies the extent of the problems for patients and carers, the development of specialist centres of excellence at a regional or national level, the development of comprehensive community-based primary care at a local level, and provision of regulated residential care. All of this requires an equitable distribution of resources both between and within countries.

Consumer and carer involvement

It is already notable that baby boomers have higher expectations than earlier generations about the quality of health care to which they feel entitled. Allied with this expectation has been the gradual increase in consumer involvement in health service planning, administration and coalface service delivery as described by Henry Brodaty and Lee-Fay Low in Chapter 19. These trends are likely to be accentuated over the next few decades.

In most countries, there is currently minimal involvement of consumers and carers in planning and administration of services. While consumer consultations are widely embraced in service planning, the extent to which they actually influence the outcome is unclear. It can be expected that consumer participation in service administration will increase, with the main effect being to increase the transparency of decision-making. Patient and consumers' rights are likely to receive greater attention and this will further accentuate the tension between autonomy and paternalism in health care. The experiences in Sweden, as described by Sture Eriksson in Chapter 12, where normalization policies intended to enhance the autonomy of mentally impaired people inadvertently resulted in substandard care of older people with dementia and other mental disorders, are an example of how this balance can be difficult to achieve.

A number of innovative programs involving volunteers and family carers that improve the quality of care of older people have already been described. One delirium prevention programme in medical wards in which volunteers assisted in the orientation, feeding, exercising and supporting of 'at-risk' elders was found to significantly reduce rates of delirium (Inouye et al., 1999). Many studies have demonstrated the benefits of carer support and training programmes in reducing stress upon carers and in providing better outcomes for the patients (Brodaty and Gresham, 1989; Mittelman et al., 1996). But there are also considerable benefits for health and welfare services. The delays in institutionalisation that have been reported translate into more efficient resource utilisation without appearing to increase the burden on carers or psychogeriatric services. In Australia, the Alzheimer's Association with funding from the Australian Government is currently conducting 7-week 'Living with Memory Loss' programmes for carers and persons with early dementia. The programme involves education, skills training and support for the carers. If the benefits demonstrated in research can be translated to routine care and allow informal home-based care to be pursued for longer, this would suggest that in the future such programmes should be central to service delivery. In some places, psychogeriatric services may well be the most appropriate option to run such programmes in association with the Alzheimer's Association or similar consumer groups.

Resource availability

One of the effects of an ageing population is to increase the 'aged dependency ratio' in a country. This is the ratio between the working age population 15–64 and the number of persons aged 65 and over. For example, in Australia the aged dependency ratio will increase from less than 20 to 40 per cent in the next 50 years. This means that in 2050 there may be only 2.5 people of working age for every person aged 65 and over, compared with 5 currently (Access Economics, 2001). More telling is the projected change in the composition of the dependent population, which will change from two children for every older person to two older people for every child. In Australia dementia costs about 1 per cent of GDP and this is projected to rise to 3 per cent by 2040 (Access Economics, 2003). So simply to maintain the status quo, services will have to increase or be delivered more efficiently and/or the demand for services will need to decrease. The Australian Government has recently announced policies to encourage older people to remain in the workforce longer to counteract these trends.

Many funding models for health care are being used worldwide. Some are problematic for mental health services in general and psychogeriatric services in particular.

For example in the US, as described by Soo Borson and colleagues in Chapter 6, both private insurance and Government-funded programmes such as Medicare and Medicaid provide less funding for mental conditions than general medical conditions. Among the limitations in Medicare coverage of mental health services are required limits on inpatient psychiatric days, a lack of outpatient prescription drug coverage, 50 percent co-payment for psychotherapy, and limited coverage of day care, respite care, residential care and community health care (Bartels *et al.*, 1999). One of the difficulties in the US, and some other countries such as Australia, is that there are battles between levels of government over responsibility for funding services resulting in service gaps. As costs of both hospital and long term care are projected to increase dramatically in coming years, these gaps may get larger as governments attempt to cope with the dilemma. If the US as the wealthiest country in the world is predicting that funds for hospital services will be exhausted by 2026 unless a radical solution is found (Center for Medicare and Medicaid Services, 2003), then other countries are likely to be facing similar problems.

Financial models and incentives are what drive much of the health service. Clearly if there are malnourished children or raging infectious diseases such as HIV these will take priority, but in the developed world this is not so. One measure that has gained currency is Disability Adjusted Life Years (DALYs), which can disadvantage the elderly. For example, the decision to subsidize medication in Australia is based to some extent on the dollar cost per DALY saved. Models of health service delivery which ration services based on DALYs also disadvantage older people. Older people, merely through their reduced life expectancy, can hardly be expected to achieve the same DALY savings as a young child. As the 'demographic imperative' takes hold, more equitable models will surely be developed.

There is a lack of hard data about optimal models of care that encompass both clinical and financial outcomes. Bartels *et al.* (1999) have suggested that the following features may be important in an optimal model:

- Integration of mental health and general medical services to enable collaborations between primary care, aged care and psychogeriatrics;
- Integration of hospital and community care to form a comprehensive model of acute and long-term care;
- Capitated care arrangements to contain costs and to encourage use of cost-effective services;
- Reallocation of expenditures to support home and community-based alternatives to long-term care;
- Risk adjustment strategies that account for the huge costs associated with comorbid physical and mental disorders in old age;
- Ensuring accountability, advocacy and outcomes.

One direction that is being taken in a number of countries is outcomes-based funding to ensure quality of care. Historically, measurement of outcomes in psychogeriatrics has been infrequently undertaken, though as pointed out by Alastair Macdonald in Chapter 20, routine measurement of clinical outcomes is both feasible and desirable for a range of reasons. Interestingly, when routine outcome measurement using the HoNOS 65+ is undertaken by psychogeriatric services, significant clinical improvement can be demonstrated in both inpatient and community services (Spear *et al.*, 2002). It is envisaged that the use of routine measurement of clinical outcomes will become widespread in coming years, if only as an accepted form of service accountability. However, the outcomes may not simply relate to symptomatic improvement but may also include other measures of the quality of care.

Developments in other branches of medicine will inevitably become routine psychogeriatric practice, viz: use of nurse practitioners, devolvement of assessment and management roles to less expensive but very competent nursing and allied health staff, a greater liaison role for consultants i.e. consulting with other health professionals more than providing direct patient services. Specialization of primary care practitioners to take on roles now handled by aged care psychiatry services is already happening and is likely to continue. For example, in the Netherlands, doctors can specialize in nursing home care, which straddles but differs from geriatrics and psychogeriatrics. These developments should retain the special skill and knowledge that consultant psychogeriatricians bring to a service. Clinicians will also be expected to be more aware of the economic implications of management decisions on individual cases, for example, the relative costs and benefits of drug options; the use of investigations; hospital versus community based care.

The model of institutional aged care may well be revised. Financial incentives have led to larger nursing homes, which can deliver economies of scale. Research indicates that levels of behavioural disturbance are lower in smaller homes (Brodaty *et al.*, 2002). Other models of care such as smaller group homes or community foster care are possible and may become more popular if viable funding models can be developed. It remains to be seen what the effect of long-term care insurance, as is in train in Germany and Japan, will have on the provision of aged care.

Currently old age psychiatry is largely a public health enterprise with few doctors entering private psychogeriatric practice. The many reasons for this include relatively poor remuneration (because of lack of highly paid procedures, need for home visits, longer duration of consultations needed), the lower financial status of older people and the need to work with a multidisciplinary team. As more psychiatrists complete sub- (or supra-) specialty training, and as the affluent baby boomers reach their 70s and 80s, demand and supply for private psychogeriatricians are likely to increase.

The ideal

When a psychogeriatrician becomes Minister for Health and decides that mental health of older people will be the first priority for the health service, we will see:

♦ Availability and promulgation of population based exercise, social and intellectual stimulating activities

- A general awareness programme:

  to educate older people how to 'maintain the brain' and prevent common mental disorders in old age

  about the warning signs of depression, dementia and other common psychiatric disorders

  to reduce stigma associated with mental illness and with ageing

- Adequate funding to enable preventative, early treatment and rehabilitation services for the elderly

- Mandatory training for general practitioners in the detection of early cognitive impairment and depression

- Seamless integration of geriatric, psychogeriatric, primary care and community services

- Group homes for the elderly unable to be managed at home or those without families

- Properly trained staff to provide residential care

- Avoidance of most behavioural problems of dementia through better and more person-orientated care

- Availability of family-carer training packages and support programmes

- Development of better models of long-term care

- Adequate funding of research of service delivery models as well as clinical and basic science endeavours.

Effects of increased scientific knowledge and technological change

As pointed out by John Snowdon and Tom Arie in Chapter 1, the development of psychogeriatric services in the 1960s was closely linked to research on the classification and treatment of mental disorders in old age. Without the development of cost-effective antidepressant and antipsychotic medication, many of the advances of psychogeriatric service delivery may not have been possible. Future developments in the field are also likely to be tied to advances in scientific knowledge that allow not only the early identification and more effective treatment of mental disorders in old age, but also their prevention.

Probably the most important area of scientific development is in the early diagnosis, prevention and treatment of Alzheimer's disease. Reliable presymptomatic diagnosis with a combination of peripheral biomarkers e.g. blood levels of tau protein, A beta protein and amyloid precursor protein, neuroimaging e.g. functional MRI and PET imaging of plaques and cognitive assessment (Burggren et al., 2002; Ritchie and Lovestone, 2002; Hampel et al., 2003; Klunk et al., 2003) will possibly be available within 15 years. Within 20–30 years, interventions may be available to both prevent and treat

Alzheimer's disease. This is likely to involve a combination of therapies that halt the neuropathology e.g. secretase inhibitors, beta-amyloid vaccination, and replace damaged cells e.g. stem cell grafts, gene therapy (Draper, 2004).

Less spectacular but more achievable is the change in lifestyle that may reduce rates of Alzheimer's disease and vascular dementia. More education, greater levels of physical, mental and social activities, rigorous control of high blood pressure, prevention and perhaps more assiduous treatment of diabetes mellitus, use of antioxidants, avoidance of cardiovascular risk factors such as smoking and hypercholesterolaemia may each contribute a small but significant decrease in risk of Alzheimer's disease though the cumulative benefit may be greater (Jorm, 2001). Attention to these same potentially protective factors may have even more impact on reducing vascular cognitive impairment.

The huge strides in molecular biology have had limited impact to date on the practice of psychogeriatrics. However it may be possible to predict who is at risk for particular disorders or even who with a particular disorder will develop certain manifestations, e.g. psychosis or aggression in Alzheimer's disease associated with specific genetic polymorphisms (Sweet *et al.*, 2001). The emerging science of pharmacogenomics may enable the clinician to pinpoint exactly which drug is likely to have the most effect for the least risk of adverse effects.

The impact of such advances upon psychogeriatric services is potentially enormous. Not all services take a frontline role in the early diagnosis and treatment of dementia, but those that do are likely to have a rapidly increasing demand. One question that may be raised in this context, particularly in presymptomatic cases, is whether psychogeriatric services should be involved in diagnosis and management at all. This will be particularly the case in funding systems where the treating service is responsible for the costs of treatment. Of course, these treatments may only be partially effective and significant residual psychopathology may remain, though possibly not sufficient to require long-term care. In theory, effective treatments should result in a marked reduction in the need for long-term residential care for dementia.

However, even in affluent developed countries, there is likely to be only a partial usage of effective Alzheimer treatments. The reasons for this include high treatment costs, ignorance of doctors, patients and carers about the availability of treatment, a failure to detect dementia until a late stage (when treatments may have only limited benefit), and refusal of some people to be treated. Some of these problems might be reduced with increased awareness about dementia, but it is still likely that there will remain a significant number of patients whose dementia is not diagnosed until it reaches a moderate degree of severity. They will continue to require psychogeriatric services in much the same way as they do now.

Depression is the other domain in which advances in prevention and treatment may have an important impact upon psychogeriatric services. The vascular depression hypothesis provides the basis for the development of prevention strategies targeting lifestyle factors and treatment of hypertension in mid-life that may result in the reduction of cerebrovascular disease and associated depression and cognitive impairment in late life (Kivipelto et al., 2001). The extent to which rates of depression might diminish is unclear.

New pharmacological approaches to the treatment of depression may have greater efficacy than current treatments. Even if this efficacy simply involved a faster onset of action of antidepressants (say from an average 2–4 weeks to an average of 1–2 weeks), reduced suffering, carer burden and costs to services would result. Up until about 15 years ago antidepressant drugs were effectively limited to tricyclics with some more adventurous clinicians or more desperate patients using monoamine oxidase inhibitors. In April 2004, there were 21 different antidepressant drugs from six drug classes listed in MIMS Online, the Australian pharmaceutical database (MIMS Online, 2004). Although many are critical of the medicalization of normal human adversity, there is good evidence that many people with clinical depression benefit enormously. The benefits to older people have been mainly in the more favourable side-effect profile, particularly the avoidance of the anticholinergic side effects. The huge sales of antidepressants in the developed (more affluent) countries mean that pharmaceutical companies continue to invest heavily in research and development for drugs to combat depression in general and depression for older people in particular given the projected growth in this market. Novel approaches involving new potential therapeutic targets include the modulation of neuropeptide (substance P, corticotrophin-releasing factor, neuropeptide Y, vasopressin V1b, melanin-concentrating hormone-1), N-methyl-D-aspartate, nicotinic acetylcholine, dopaminergic, glucocorticoid, delta-opioid, cannabinoid and cytokine receptors, gamma-amino butyric acid (GABA) and intracellular messenger systems, transcription, neuroprotective and neurogenic factors (Pacher and Kecskemeti, 2004).

Magnetic Seizure Therapy (MST) is a novel approach to depression treatment currently being evaluated as an alternative to ECT that may be more acceptable to the consumer, with less expense and adverse effects due to not requiring anaesthesia (Lisanby et al., 2003). Other innovative methods of treatment under trial are Repetitive Transcranial Magnetic Stimulation (Padberg and Müller, 2003) and Vagus Nerve Stimulation (Sackheim et al., 2001).

The rise of cognitive behaviour therapy (CBT) over the last twenty years has been a general advance in the treatment of depression. Improvement in the application of techniques specific to older people (Koder et al., 1996) may improve outcome of psychotherapy in older people with depression and those with cognitive impairment. Finally population-based approaches attempting to reduce a whole community's level of depression (e.g. Llewellyn-Jones et al., 1999) may be extended. By analogy, if average levels of blood pressure in the populations can be reduced by decreasing salt intake, can enhancement of social and physical participation in activities and reduction of the isolation so common among the elderly, lower the average of level of depression in the community?

The impact of information technology over the last decade has been enormous with widespread use of cell phones, e-mail and the Internet in general for communication, dissemination of information and literature searches. It is now standard practice for health services to have networked PCs for internal communication and for accessing policies, protocols, patient records and the results of investigations. In some settings, the electronic medical record (EMR) has already largely replaced hard copy records and they have also been successfully introduced into developing countries such as Kenya (Blair and Schutte, 2003; Rotich *et al.*, 2003). This is likely to become standard practice in most public health services in the foreseeable future and will probably involve the widespread use of hand-held PCs. Nebeker *et al.* (2003) have projected a 'future history' of the EMR in geriatrics and have suggested that it will go beyond being simply a replacement for the paper chart. They believe the EMR will involve the participation of the multidisciplinary team, family, patients and other care providers in coordinating data from a variety of novel sources about diet, medication use, falls, mobility and the use of sensors on older people to monitor physiological parameters. Computerized cognitive testing is already available on the Internet and is likely to be used more widely as it becomes refined.

Rural health care is one area where information technology promises to have a big impact. Telepsychiatry using videoconferencing has already been shown to be feasible and cost-effective in linking rural and regional centres to urban psychogeriatric services in Hong Kong and the US (Tang *et al.*, 2001; Sumner, 2001). With further improvement in videoconferencing facilities and reduced costs, the attraction of telepsychiatry as a cost-effective method of providing ongoing support to rural services that often have difficulties in attracting adequate staffing is likely to increase. The danger, of course, is that telepsychiatry may be viewed by some administrators as an alternative to face-to-face care rather than as a supplement.

Knowledge about best-practice in service delivery

As we saw in Chapter 5, over the last 15 years there has been a significant increase in knowledge about best practice in psychogeriatric service delivery. Yet much more is required. For example, the use of treatment guidelines and protocols based upon contemporary research has been shown to improve the quality of care in various settings including critical care, oncology, and adult mental health (Bauer, 2002; Heyland *et al.*, 2003; Emens and Davidson, 2003; Morris, 2003). Presumably similar findings are possible in psychogeriatrics but this has not been examined for clinical outcomes other than in cost containment (Bultema *et al.*, 1996).

The management of depression is one area that is particularly suited to the use of treatment guidelines and protocols. There is already evidence that inadequate treatment of depression in some settings has contributed to poor outcomes (Heeren *et al.*, 1997; Hickie *et al.*, 2000; Philpot *et al.*, 2000). The use of treatment guidelines may improve the outcome of care but needs to be tested.

Ethical issues

As mentioned previously, rationing of health services is a major ethical issue that is already confronting administrators and clinicians alike. Resource allocation based upon chronological age alone is regarded as a social value judgement – ageism – and has been deemed unacceptable by organizations such as the American Medical Association (AMA, 1988). But the circumstances in psychogeriatrics are usually less straightforward than, for example, deciding whether the choice of an expensive medical intervention should be given to the person aged 20 or the person aged 80. The Oregon Health Plan is a good example that prioritises funding for health care not explicitly by age but through systematic and public ranking of medical services into nine 'essential services', four 'very important services' and four 'services valuable to certain individuals' categories (Oberlander et al., 2001). However, few services provided in psychogeriatrics would currently qualify in the top rank 'essential services' (e.g., treatment of suicidal patients, terminal care of dementia); most would qualify as 'very important services' (e.g. treatment of episodes of depression, treatment of BPSD and cognitive decline). In practice, Federal Medicaid recipients continue to receive services excluded under the Oregon Health Plan partly due to service providers finding loopholes in the system (Oberlander et al., 2001). The concern remains that older people remain at risk of discrimination whenever resource allocation is used.

Will euthanasia and physician assisted suicide receive more widespread support around the world and what impact might this have upon psychogeriatric services? The Netherlands and Belgium have legalized euthanasia and the state of Oregon in the US has legalized physician-assisted suicide, while in Switzerland altruistic assisted suicide is legal even when performed by a non-physician. In Oregon patients who seek a lethal prescription have to be certified by two physicians as free from depressive symptoms or other conditions that might affect their ability to make health care decisions. While there is a legally specified role for mental health professionals in Oregon, this is not the case in the other jurisdictions. So even if euthanasia and physician assisted suicide are legalized elsewhere, there may not be a direct impact upon psychogeriatric services, though indirectly it is possible that incompetent patients might be vulnerable if adequate safeguards are not in place. Reports from the Netherlands already suggest that doctors are not complying with the legislation so this is quite possible (van Kolfschooten, 2003).

Conclusion

Psychogeriatrics, the Cinderella of medical specialties, has emerged from rags and fireplace but is still to transform into a beautiful princess. Developments in pharmacology, molecular biology, neuroimaging, diagnostics and other novel treatment modalities are exciting. But unless there are spectacular discoveries, analogous to polio vaccine wiping out that epidemic, the most important development that will most affect the mental health of older people will be in how services are financed, organized and delivered. The challenge of psychogeriatrics, and its allure to many of us in the field is that it is so broad – encompassing the molecule, the gene, the neuron, the person, the family, the community, the economy and the whole population – the future of psychogeriatrics is at all these levels.

References

Access Economics (2001) *Population Ageing and the Economy*. Commonwealth Department of Health and Aged Care, Canberra.

Access Economics (2003) *The Dementia Epidemic: Economic Impact and Positive Solutions for Australia*. Prepared for Alzheimer's Australia, Canberra, by Access Economics Pty Ltd.

American Medical Association Council on Ethical and Judicial Affairs (1988) *Ethical Implications of Age-based Rationing of Health Care*. www.ama-assn.org/ama/ama1/pub/upload/mm/369/15b.pdf accessed 26 April 2004.

Bartels, S.J., Levine, K.J., and Shea, D. (1999) Community-based long-term care for older persons with severe and persistent mental illness in an era of managed care. *Psychiatric Services* **50**, 1189–97.

Bauer, M.S. (2002) A review of quantitative studies of adherence to mental health clinical practice guidelines. *Harvard Review of Psychiatry*, **10** (3), 138–53.

Blair, D. and Schutte, P.C. (2003) The electronic medical record in multi-site family practice, Part 1: the planning phase. *Journal of Medical Practice Management*, **19** (2), 84–8.

Brodaty, H., Draper, B., and Low, L.-F. (2002) What environmental and staffing characteristics predict behavioural and psychological symptoms of dementia in nursing home residents? *Psychogeriatrics*, **2**, 47–53.

Brodaty, H. and Gresham, M. (1989) Effect of a training programme to reduce stress in carers of patients with dementia. *BMJ* **299** (6712), 1375–9.

Broe, G.A. and Creasey, H. (1995) Brain ageing and neurodegenerative diseases: a major public health issue of the twenty-first century. *Perspectives in Human Biology*, **1**: 53–8.

Bultema, J.K., Mailliard, L., Getzfrid, M.K., Lerner, R.D., and Colone, M. (1996) Geriatric patients with depression. Improving outcomes using a multidisciplinary clinical path model. *JONA*, **26**, 31–8.

Burggren, A.C., Small, G.W., Sabb, F.W., and Bookheimer, S.Y. (2002) Specificity of brain activation in people at genetic risk for Alzheimer disease. *American Journal of Geriatric Psychiatry*, **10** (1), 44–51.

Centers for Medicare and Medicaid Services (2003) http://cms.hhs.gov accessed 15 January 2003.

Draper, B. (2004) *Dealing with Dementia*. Allen and Unwin, Sydney.

Emens, L.A. and Davidson, N.E. (2003) The follow-up of breast cancer. *Seminars in Oncology*, **30** (3), 338–48.

Hampel, H., Goernitz, A., and Buerger, K. (2003) Advances in the development of biomarkers for Alzheimer's disease: from CSF total tau and Abeta (1–42) proteins to phosphorylated tau protein. *Brain Research Bulletin*, **61** (3), 243–53.

Heeren, T.J., Derksen, P., Heycop Ten Ham, B.F.v., and Van Gent, P.P.J. (1997) Treatment, outcome and predictors of response in elderly depressed in-patients. *British Journal of Psychiatry*, **170**, 436–40.

Heyland, D.K., Dhaliwal, R., Drover, J.W., Gramlich, L., and Dodek, P. (2003) Canadian clinical practice guidelines for nutrition support in mechanically ventilated critically ill adult patients. *Jpen: Journal of Parenteral and Enteral Nutrition*, **27** (5), 355–73.

Hickie, I., Burke, D., Tobin, M., and Mutch, C. (2000) The impact of the organisation of mental health services on the quality of assessment provided to older patients with depression. *Australian and New Zealand Journal of Psychiatry*, **34**: 748–54.

Inouye, S.K., Bogardus, S.T., Jr., Charpentier, P.A., Leo-Summers, L., Acampora, D., Holford, T.R., and Cooney, L.M., Jr. (1999) A multicomponent intervention to prevent delirium in hospitalized older patients. *New England Journal of Medicine* **340**, 669–76.

Jorm, A. (2001) Prospects for the prevention of dementia. *Australasian Journal on Ageing* **21**, 9–13.

Kinsella, K., Velkoff, V., and U.S. Census Bureau Series P95/01–1 (2001) *An Aging World: 2001*. U. S. Government Printing Office, Washington, DC.

Kivipelto, M., Helkala, E.L., Laakso, M.P., *et al.* (2001) Midlife vascular risk factors and Alzheimer's disease in later life: longitudinal, population based study. *BMJ* **322**, (7300), 1447–51.

Klunk, W.E., Engler, H., Nordberg, A., Bacskai, B.J., Wang, Y., Price, J.C., Bergstrom, M., Hyman, B.T., Langstrom, B., Mathis, C.A. (2003) Imaging the pathology of Alzheimer's disease: amyloid imaging with positron emission tomography. *Neuroimaging Clinics of North America*, **13** (4), 781–9.

Koder, D., Brodaty, H., and Anstey, K. (1996) Cognitive therapy for depression in the elderly: A review. *International Journal of Geriatric Psychiatry*, **11**, 97–107.

Lisanby, S.H., Luber, B., Schlaepfer, T.E., and Sackheim, H. (2003) Safety and feasibility of Magnetic Seizure Therapy (MST) in major depression: randomized within-subject comparison with electroconvulsive therapy. *Neuropsychopharmacology*, **28** (10), 1852–65.

Llewellyn-Jones, R.H., Baikie, K.A., Smithers, H., Cohen, J., Snowdon, J., and Tennant, C.C. (1999) Multifaceted shared care intervention for late life depression in residential care: randomised controlled trial. *BMJ* **319**, 676–82.

MIMS Online (2004) *Antidepressants*. http://mims.hcn.net.au accessed 20 April, 2004.

Mittelman, M.S., Ferris, S.H., Shulman, E., Steinberg, G., and Levin, B. (1996) A family intervention to delay nursing home placement of patients with Alzheimer's disease. A randomized controlled trial. *JAMA*, **276** (21), 1725–31.

Morris, A.H. (2003) Treatment algorithms and protocolized care. *Current Opinion in Critical Care*, **9** (3), 236–40.

Nebeker, J.R., Hurdle, J.F., and Bair, B.D. (2003) Future history: medical informatics in geriatrics. *Journals of Gerontology Series A – Biological Sciences and Medical Sciences*, **58** (9), M820–5.

Oberlander, J., Marmor, T., and Jacobs, L. (2001) Rationing medical care: rhetoric and reality in the Oregon Health Plan. *Canadian Medical Association Journal*, **164** (11), 1583–7.

Pacher, P. and Kecskemeti, V. (2004) Trends in the development of new antidepressants. Is there a light at the end of the tunnel? *Current Medicinal Chemistry*, **11** (7), 925–43.

Padberg, F. and Müller, H. (2003) Repetitive transcranial magnetic stimulation. *CNS Drugs*, **17** (6), 383–403.

Philpot, M., Drahman, I., Ball, C., and Macdonald, A. (2000) The prognosis of late-life depression in two contiguous old age psychiatry services: an exploratory study. *Aging and Mental Health*, **4**, 72–78.

Prince, M. (2001) Dementia in developing countries. *International Psychogeriatrics*, **13**, 389–3.

Ritchie, K. and Lovestone, S. (2002) The dementias. *Lancet*, **360** (9347), 1759–66.

Rotich, J.K., Hannan, T.J., Smith, F.E., Bii, J., Odero, W.W., Vu, N., Mamlin, B.W., Mamlin, J.J., Einterz, R.M., and Tierney, W.M. (2003) Installing and implementing a computer-based patient record system in sub-Saharan Africa: the Mosoriot Medical Record System. *Journal of the American Medical Informatics Association*, **10** (4), 295–303.

Sackheim, H.A., Rush, A.J., George, M.S., Marangell, M.B., Husain, M.M., Nahas, Z., Johnson, C.R., Seidman, S., Giller, C., Haines, S., Simpson, R.K. Jr., and Goodman, RR. (2001) Vagus nerve stimulation (VNS) for treatment-resistant depression: efficacy, side-effects, and predictors of outcome. *Neuropsychopharmacology*, **25** (5), 713–28.

Spear, J., Chawla, S., O'Reilly, M., and Rock, D. (2002) Does the HoNOS 65+ meet the criteria for a clinical outcome indicator for mental health services for older people? *International Journal of Geriatric Psychiatry*, **17**, 226–30.

Sumner, C.R. (2001) Telepsychiatry: challenges in rural aging. *Journal of Rural Health*, **17** (4), 370–3.

Sweet, R.A., Pollock, B.G., Sukonick, D.L., Mulsant, B.H., Rosen, J., Klunk, W.E., Kastango, K.B., DeKosky, S.T., and Ferrell, R.E. (2001) The 5-HTTPR polymorphism confers liability to a combined phenotype of psychotic and aggressive behavior in Alzheimer disease. *International Psychogeriatrics*, **13**, 401–9.

Tang, W.K., Chiu, H., Woo, J., Hjelm, M., Hui, E. (2001) Telepsychiatry in psychogeriatric service: a pilot study. *International Journal of Geriatric Psychiatry*, **16** (1), 88–93.

Van Kolfschooten, F. (2003) Dutch television report stirs up euthanasia controversy. *The Lancet*, **361** (9366), 1352.

Index